All Things Nursing

All Things Nursing

Wolters Kluwer | Lippincott Williams & Wilkins
Health

Philadelphia • Baltimore • New York • London
Buenos Aires • Hong Kong • Sydney • Tokyo

Contributors and consultants

Marguerite Ambrose, APRN, BC, DNSc
Assistant Professor
Immaculata (Pa.) University

Wendy Bowles, RN, MSN, CPNP
Assistant Professor
Kettering (Ohio) College of Medical Arts

Kim Clevenger, RN, MSN,C
Assistant Professor of Nursing
Morehead (Ky.) State University

Lillian Craig, RN, MSN, FNP-C
Adjunct Faculty
Oklahoma Panhandle State University
Goodwell

Shelba Durston, RN, MSN, CCRN
Nursing Instructor
San Joaquin Delta College
Stockton, Calif.
Staff Nurse
San Joaquin General Hospital
French Camp, Calif.

Vivian C. Gamblian, RN, MSN
Professor of Nursing
Collin County Community College
McKinney, Tex.

Julia A. Isen, RN, MS, FNP-C, CNS
Family Nurse Practitioner
University of California at San Francisco
    Medical Center
Assistant Clinical Professor
University of California at San Francisco
    School of Nursing

J. MariBeth Linder, RN, PhD, BC
Director & Associate Professor of
    Nursing
Missouri Southern State University
Joplin

Robin R. Wilkerson, RN, PhD
Assistant Dean for Undergraduate
    Program, Assistant Professor
University of Mississippi School of
    Nursing
Jackson

PART

I

Nursing practice

1 Assessment 2

2 Electrocardiography 66

3 Laboratory tests 117

4 Medications 140

5 Procedures 213

6 Specialized aspects of care 285

7 Maternal-neonatal care 346

8 Pediatric care 410

1 Assessment

Performing a 10-minute assessment

You should perform a rapid assessment whenever you come in contact with a patient. Although not all of these assessment steps will need to be performed with every patient you encounter, they're vital if a patient appears distressed or experiences a drastic change in appearance or actions since you last saw him.

General guidelines
· Perform simultaneous assessments (for example, note skin color and temperature while obtaining vital signs).
· Be flexible with the assessment; let the patient's chief complaint guide your actions.
· Keep the patient calm while maintaining your own composure.
· Avoid quick conclusions.

Observations
· Note the patient's level of consciousness, mental status, and general appearance.

· If the patient is unconscious, follow the ABC's of assessment—airway, breathing, and circulation.
· Initiate emergency resuscitation measures if appropriate.

Vital signs
· Assess the patient's physiologic condition from values obtained.
· Recheck findings if abnormal or drastically different from the last readings.
· Evaluate cardiac rhythm, if available.

Health history
· Ask focused questions to evaluate the patient's chief complaint or cause of condition change.
· If the patient is unconscious, obtain information from his family or visitors, or utilize his chart.

Physical examination
· Begin the examination focusing on the chief complaint and compare it to the previous assessment, if available.
· Perform a complete head-to-toe assessment if necessary.

Evaluating a symptom

Ask the patient to describe the symptom bothering him.

▼

Form a first impression. Does the patient's condition alert you to an emergency?

YES ◄   **NO** ◄

Take a brief history to gather more clues.	Take a thorough history to get an overview of the patient's condition. Ask him about associated signs or symptoms.

▼   ▼

Perform a focused physical examination to quickly determine the severity of the patient's condition.	Thoroughly examine the patient to evaluate the chief sign or symptom and to detect additional signs and symptoms.

▼

Evaluate your findings. Are emergency signs or symptoms present?

YES ◄   **NO** ◄

Based on your findings, intervene appropriately to stabilize the patient. Notify the physician immediately of the assessment findings and carry out the physician's orders.	Evaluate your findings to consider possible causes.

▼   ▼

After the patient's condition is stabilized, review your findings to consider possible causes.	Devise an appropriate treatment plan.

Performing palpation techniques

Palpation uses pressure to assess structure size, placement, pulsation, and tenderness. Ballottement, a variation, involves bouncing tissues against the hand to assess rebound of floating structures. Ballottement can be used to assess a mass in a patient with ascites.

Light palpation

To perform light palpation, press gently on the skin, indenting it 1½" to 3½" (4 to 9 cm). Use the lightest touch possible; too much pressure blunts your sensitivity. Close your eyes to concentrate on feeling.

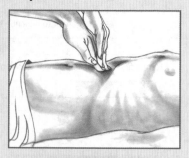

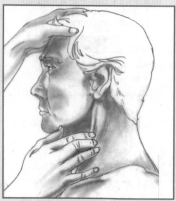

Deep palpation

To perform deep palpation, indent the skin about 1½" (4 cm). Place your other hand on top of the palpating hand to control and guide your movements, as shown top right. To perform a variation of deep palpation that allows you to pinpoint an inflamed area, push down slowly and deeply, then lift your hand away quickly. If the patient complains of increased pain as you release the pressure, you have identified rebound tenderness.

Use both hands (bimanual palpation) to trap a deep, hard-to-palpate organ (such as the kidney or spleen) or to fix or stabilize an organ (such as the uterus) while palpating with the other hand.

Light ballottement

To perform light ballottement, apply light, rapid pressure from quadrant to quadrant of the patient's abdomen. Keep your hand on the surface of the skin to detect tissue rebound.

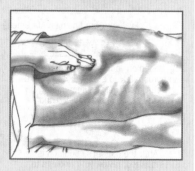

Deep ballottement

To perform deep ballottement, apply abrupt, deep pressure; then release, but maintain contact.

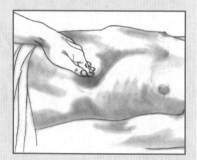

Performing percussion techniques

Percussion has two basic purposes: to produce percussion sounds and to elicit tenderness. It involves three types: indirect, direct, and blunt.

Indirect percussion

The most commonly used method, indirect percussion, produces clear, crisp sounds when performed correctly. To perform indirect percussion, use the second finger of your nondominant hand as the pleximeter (the mediating device used to receive the taps) and the middle finger of your dominant hand as the plexor (the device used to tap the pleximeter). Place the pleximeter finger firmly against a body surface, such as the upper back or abdomen. With your wrist flexed loosely, use the tip of your plexor finger to deliver a crisp blow just beneath the distal joint of the pleximeter. Make sure you hold the plexor perpendicular to the pleximeter. Tap lightly and quickly, removing the plexor as soon as you have delivered each blow.

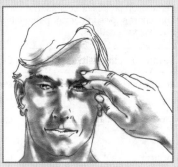

Blunt percussion

To perform blunt percussion, strike the ulnar surface of your fist against the body surface. Alternatively, you may use both hands by placing the palm of one hand over the area to be percussed and then making a fist with the other hand and using it to strike the back of the first hand. Both techniques aim to elicit tenderness—not to create a sound—over organs such as the kidneys. Another blunt percussion method, used in a neurologic examination, involves tapping a rubber-tipped reflex hammer against a tendon to create a reflexive muscle contraction.

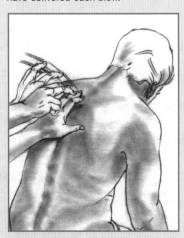

Direct percussion

To perform direct percussion, tap your hand or fingertip directly against the body surface, as shown top right. This method helps assess an adult's sinuses for tenderness.

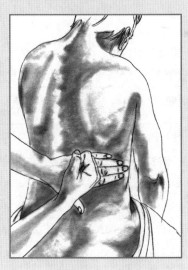

Identifying percussion sounds

Percussion produces sounds that vary according to the tissue being percussed. This chart shows important percussion sounds along with their characteristics and typical locations.

Sound	Intensity	Pitch	Duration	Quality	Source
Resonance	Moderate to loud	Low	Moderate to long	Hollow	Normal lung
Tympany	Loud	High	Moderate	Drumlike	Gastric air bubble or intestinal air
Dullness	Soft to moderate	High	Long	Thudlike	Liver, full bladder, pregnant uterus, or spleen
Hyper-resonance	Very loud	Very low	Long	Booming	Hyperinflated lung (as in emphysema)
Flatness	Soft	High	Short	Flat	Muscle, bone, or tumor

Vital signs

Vital sign ranges vary from neonates to older adults, as shown here.

Age	Temperature		Pulse rate (beats/minute)
	° Fahrenheit	° Celsius	
Neonate	98.6 to 99.8	37 to 37.7	100 to 160
3 years	98.5 to 99.5	36.9 to 37.5	80 to 125
10 years	97.5 to 98.6	36.4 to 37	70 to 110
16 years	97.6 to 98.8	36.4 to 37.1	55 to 100
Adult	96.8 to 99.5	36 to 37.5	60 to 100
Older adult	96.5 to 97.5	35.8 to 36.4	60 to 100

Performing auscultation

Auscultation of body sounds—particularly those produced by the heart, lungs, blood vessels, stomach, and intestines—detects both high-pitched and low-pitched sounds. Although you can perform auscultation directly over a body area using only your ears, you'll typically perform it indirectly, using a stethoscope.

Assessing high-pitched sounds

To properly assess high-pitched sounds, such as breath sounds and first and second heart sounds, use the diaphragm of the stethoscope. Make sure you place the entire surface of the diaphragm firmly on the patient's skin. If the area is excessively hairy, you can improve diaphragm contact and reduce extraneous noise by applying water or water-soluble jelly to the skin before auscultating.

Assessing low-pitched sounds

To assess low-pitched sounds, such as heart murmurs and third and fourth heart sounds, lightly place the bell of the stethoscope on the appropriate area. Don't exert pressure. If you do, the patient's chest will act as a diaphragm and you will miss low-pitched sounds. If the patient is extremely thin or emaciated, use a stethoscope with a pediatric chest piece.

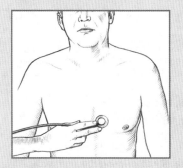

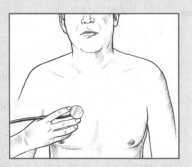

Respiratory rate (breaths/minute)	Blood pressure (mm Hg)
30 to 50	73/45
20 to 30	90/55
16 to 22	96/57
15 to 20	120/80
12 to 20	120/80
15 to 25	120/80

Classifying blood pressure readings

Current blood pressure categories are normal, prehypertension, and stages 1 and 2 hypertension. These are based on the average of two or more readings taken on separate visits after an initial screening. They apply to adults age 18 and older. However, a blood pressure of 130/80 or higher in patients with diabetes or chronic kidney disease is considered high blood pressure.

Category	Systolic		Diastolic
Normal	< 120 mm Hg	and	< 80 mm Hg
Prehypertension	120 to 139 mm Hg	or	80 to 89 mm Hg
Hypertension			
Stage 1	140 to 159 mm Hg	or	90 to 99 mm Hg
Stage 2	≥ 160 mm Hg	or	≥ 100 mm Hg

Pulse oximetry

Performed intermittently or continuously, pulse oximetry is a simple procedure used to monitor arterial oxygen saturation noninvasively. Readings are obtained from the nail bed, earlobe, nose, or forehead. The symbol Spo_2 is used to denote pulse oximetry readings.

Normal Spo_2 levels

Adults and children: 95% to 100%

Neonates (full-term): 93.8% to 100% (by 1 hour after birth)

Note: Lower levels may be acceptable per facility policy or practitioner's order. Pulse oximetry readings may be inaccurate in these situations:

Low readings
· Dark nail polish or artificial nails
· Equipment malfunction
· Excessive light
· Hypotension
· Hypothermia
· Patient movement
· Poor connection
· Vasoconstriction

High readings
· Elevated bilirubin
· Elevated carboxyhemoglobin level

Height and weight conversions

Height conversion
To convert a patient's height from inches to centimeters, multiply the number of inches by 2.54. To convert a patient's height from centimeters to inches, multiply the number of centimeters by 0.394.

Weight conversion
To convert a patient's weight from pounds to kilograms, divide the number of pounds by 2.2 kg; to convert a patient's weight from kilograms to pounds, multiply the number of kilograms by 2.2 lb.

Imperial	Inches	Metric (cm)
4' 8"	56	142.2
4' 9"	57	144.8
4' 10"	58	147.3
4' 11"	59	149.9
5'	60	152.4
5' 1"	61	154.9
5' 2"	62	157.5
5' 3"	63	160
5' 4"	64	162.6
5' 5"	65	165.1
5' 6"	66	167.6
5' 7"	67	170.2
5' 8"	68	172.7
5' 9"	69	175.3
5' 10"	70	177.8
5' 11"	71	180.3
6'	72	182.9
6' 1"	73	185.4
6' 2"	74	188
6' 3"	75	190.5

Pounds	Kilograms
10	4.5
20	9.1
30	13.6
40	18.2
50	22.7
60	27.3
70	31.8
80	36.4
90	40.9
100	45.5
110	50
120	54.5
130	59.1
140	63.6
150	68.2
160	72.7
170	77.3
180	81.8
190	86.4
200	90.9
210	95.5
220	100
230	104.5
240	109.1
250	113.6
260	118.2

Temperature conversion

To convert Fahrenheit to Celsius, subtract 32 from the temperature in Fahrenheit and then divide by 1.8; to convert Celsius to Fahrenheit, multiply the temperature in Celsius by 1.8 and then add 32.

$$(F - 32) \div 1.8 = \text{degrees Celsius}$$

$$(C \times 1.8) + 32 = \text{degrees Fahrenheit}$$

Degrees Fahrenheit (°F)	Degrees Celsius (°C)
89.6	32
91.4	33
93.2	34
94.3	34.6
95.0	35
95.4	35.2
96.2	35.7
96.8	36
97.2	36.2
97.6	36.4
98	36.7
98.6	37
99	37.2
99.3	37.4
99.7	37.6
100	37.8
100.4	38
100.8	38.2
101	38.3
101.2	38.4
101.4	38.6
101.8	38.8
102	38.9
102.2	39
102.6	39.2
102.8	39.3
103	39.4
103.2	39.6
103.4	39.7
103.6	39.8
104	40
104.4	40.2
104.6	40.3
104.8	40.4
105	40.6

Health history review

Obtaining assessment data
· Collect objective data (verifiable data obtained through observation).
· Collect subjective data (data that can be verified only by the patient).

Patient interview
· Select a quiet, private setting.
· Avoid using medical jargon.
· Use appropriate body language.
· Confirm patient statements to avoid misunderstanding.
· Use open-ended questions.

Effective communication
· Use silence effectively.
· Encourage responses.
· Use repetition and reflection to help clarify meaning.
· Use clarification to eliminate misunderstandings.
· Summarize and conclude with, "Is there anything else?"

Components of a health history
· Biographic data, such as the patient's name, address, birth date, and emergency contact information
· Chief complaint
· Past and current health care
· Health of the patient's family
· Psychosocial history (feelings about self, place in society, and relationships with others)
· Activities of daily living

Review of structures and systems
Head
· Headaches
· Past or present head injury

Eyes
· Vision
· Use of glasses or contact lenses
· History of glaucoma, cataracts, color blindness
· Tearing; blurred or double vision; dry, itchy, burning, or inflamed eyes

Ears
· Hearing and balance
· History of ear surgery
· Use of hearing aids
· Ear pain or swelling
· Discharge from ears

Nose
- History of nasal surgery
- Breathing or smelling difficulties
- History of sinusitis or nosebleeds

Mouth and throat
- Dentures
- Mouth sores or dryness
- Loss of taste
- Toothache or bleeding gums
- Sore throat or difficulty swallowing

Neck
- Swelling
- Soreness
- Lack of movement, stiffness, or pain

Respiratory
- Shortness of breath
- Pain or wheezing with breathing
- Cough (productive or nonproductive)
- History of pneumonia, chronic obstructive pulmonary disease, or respiratory tract infections
- Tuberculin skin test and chest X-ray results

Cardiovascular
- Chest pain, palpitations, irregular or fast heartbeat, shortness of breath
- Results of electrocardiogram
- History of high blood pressure, peripheral vascular disease, swelling of the extremities, varicose veins, or intermittent pain in the legs

Breasts
- Women
  - Monthly breast self-examination
  - Lumps, changes in breast contour, pain, discharge from nipples
  - History of breast cancer
  - Results of mammograms
- Men
  - Pain
  - Lumps
  - Change in contour

Gastrointestinal
- Recent weight changes
- Frequency and characteristics of bowel movements
- Laxative use
- Nausea, vomiting, loss of appetite, heartburn, abdominal pain, frequent belching, passing of gas
- Hemorrhoids, rectal bleeding, hernias, gallbladder disease, liver disease

Urinary
- Color of urine
- Nighttime urination
- Burning, incontinence, urgency, retention, reduced urinary flow, or dribbling

Reproductive
- Women
  - Menstruation and menopause
  - Pregnancies
  - Birth control
  - Papanicolaou test results
  - Vaginal infections
  - Sexually transmitted diseases (STDs)
- Men
  - Monthly testicular self-examinations
  - Results of prostate examinations
  - STDs
  - Birth control
  - Penile pain, discharge, or lesions
  - Testicular lumps

Musculoskeletal
- Balance
- Difficulty walking, sitting, or standing
- History of arthritis, gout, back injury, muscle weakness, or paralysis

Neurologic
- Tremors, twitching, numbness, tingling, or loss of sensation
- History of seizures

Endocrine
- Unusual fatigue or tiredness
- Hunger and thirst
- Unexplained weight loss or gain
- Tolerance of heat and cold
- Hair loss or changes
- Hormone medications

Hematologic
- History of anemia, blood abnormalities, or blood transfusions
- Fatigue or bruising

Psychological
- Mood swings or memory loss
- Anxiety, depression, or difficulty concentrating
- Stress and coping mechanisms

Identifying cardiovascular landmarks

These views show where to find critical landmarks used in cardiovascular assessment.

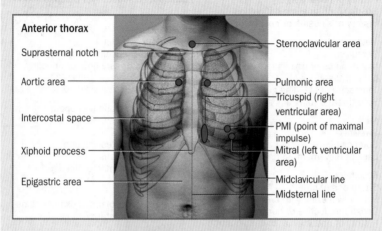

Anterior thorax

Suprasternal notch

Aortic area

Intercostal space

Xiphoid process

Epigastric area

Sternoclavicular area

Pulmonic area

Tricuspid (right ventricular area)

PMI (point of maximal impulse)

Mitral (left ventricular area)

Midclavicular line

Midsternal line

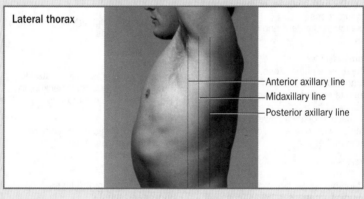

Lateral thorax

Anterior axillary line

Midaxillary line

Posterior axillary line

Positioning the patient for cardiac auscultation

During auscultation, you'll typically stand to the right of the patient, who's in a supine position. The patient may lie flat or at a comfortable elevation.

If heart sounds seem faint or undetectable, try repositioning the patient. Alternate positioning may enhance heart sounds or make them seem louder by bringing the heart closer to the surface of the chest. Common alternate positions include a seated, forward-leaning position and left-lateral decubitus position.

Forward-leaning position
This position is best for hearing high-pitched sounds related to semilunar valve problems such as aortic and pulmonic valve murmurs. To auscultate these sounds, help the patient to the forward-leaning position, and place the diaphragm of the stethoscope over the aortic and pulmonic areas in the right and left second intercostal space.

Left-lateral decubitus position
This position is best for hearing low-pitched sounds related to atrioventricular valve problems, such as mitral valve murmurs and extra heart sounds. To auscultate these sounds, help the patient to the left-lateral decubitus position, and place the bell of the stethoscope over the apical area. If these positions don't enhance heart sounds, try auscultating with the patient standing or squatting.

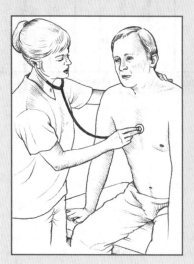

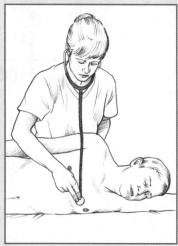

Where extra heart sounds occur in the cardiac cycle

To understand where extra heart sounds fall in relation to systole, diastole, and normal heart sounds, compare the illustrations of normal and extra heart sounds.

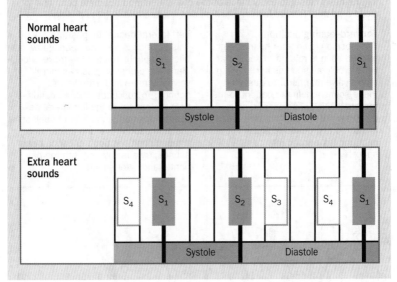

Implications of abnormal heart sounds

Upon detecting an abnormal heart sound, you must accurately identify the sound as well as its location and timing in the cardiac cycle. This information will help you identify the possible cause of the sound. This chart lists abnormal heart sounds with their possible causes.

Abnormal heart sound	Timing	Possible causes
Accentuated S_1	Beginning of systole	Mitral stenosis; fever
Diminished S_1	Beginning of systole	Mitral insufficiency; severe mitral regurgitation with calcified immobile valve; heart block
Accentuated S_2	End of systole	Pulmonary or systemic hypertension
Diminished or inaudible S_2	End of systole	Aortic or pulmonic stenosis
Persistent S_2 split	End of systole	Delayed closure of the pulmonic valve, usually from overfilling of the right ventricle, causing prolonged systolic ejection time
Reversed or paradoxical S_2 split that appears on expiration and disappears on inspiration	End of systole	Delayed ventricular stimulation; left bundle-branch block or prolonged left ventricular ejection time
S_3 (ventricular gallop)	Early diastole	Normal in children and young adults; overdistention of ventricles in rapid-filling segment of diastole; mitral insufficiency or ventricular failure
S_4 (atrial gallop or presystolic extra sound)	Late diastole	Forceful atrial contraction from resistance to ventricular filling late in diastole; left ventricular hypertrophy; pulmonic stenosis; hypertension; coronary artery disease; and aortic stenosis
Pericardial friction rub (grating or leathery sound at left of sternal border; usually muffled, high-pitched, and transient)	Throughout systole and diastole	Pericardial inflammation
Click	Early systole or midsystole	Aortic stenosis; aortic dilation; hypertension; chordae tendineae damage of the mitral valve
Opening snap	Early diastole	Mitral or tricuspid valve abnormalities
Summation gallop	Diastole	Tachycardia

Identifying heart murmurs

Timing	Quality and pitch	Location	Possible causes
Midsystolic (systolic ejection)	Harsh, rough with medium to high pitch	Pulmonic	Pulmonic stenosis
	Harsh, rough with medium to high pitch	Aortic and suprasternal notch	Aortic stenosis
Holosystolic (pansystolic)	Harsh with high pitch	Tricuspid	Ventricular septal defect
	Blowing with high pitch	Mitral, lower left sternal border	Mitral insufficiency
	Blowing with high pitch	Tricuspid	Tricuspid insufficiency
Early diastolic	Blowing with high pitch	Midleft sternal edge (not aortic area)	Aortic insufficiency
	Blowing with high pitch	Pulmonic	Pulmonic insufficiency
Middiastolic to late diastolic	Rumbling with low pitch	Apex	Mitral stenosis
	Rumbling with low pitch	Tricuspid, lower right sternal border	Tricuspid stenosis

Grading murmurs

Murmurs are graded on a scale of 1 to 6. Use the system outlined here to describe the intensity of a murmur:

· Grade I is a barely audible murmur.
· Grade II is audible but quiet and soft.
· Grade III is moderately loud, without a thrust or thrill.
· Grade IV is loud, with a thrill.
· Grade V is very loud, with a palpable thrill.
· Grade VI is loud enough to be heard before the stethoscope comes into contact with the chest.

When recording your findings, use Roman numerals as part of a fraction, always with VI as the denominator. For example, a grade III murmur would be recorded as "grade III/VI."

Palpating arterial pulses

To palpate the arterial pulses, you'll apply pressure with your index and middle fingers positioned as shown here.

Carotid pulse

Lightly place your fingers just medial to the trachea and below the angle of the jaw.

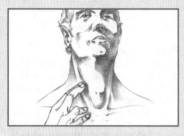

Brachial pulse

Position your fingers medial to the biceps tendon.

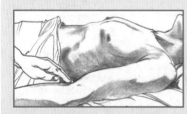

Radial pulse

Apply gentle pressure to the medial and ventral side of the wrist, just below the thumb.

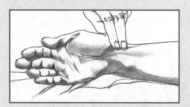

Femoral pulse

Press relatively hard at a point inferior to the inguinal ligament. For an obese patient, palpate in the crease of the groin, halfway between the pubic bone and the hip bone.

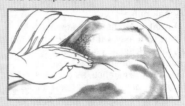

Popliteal pulse

Press firmly against the popliteal fossa at the back of the knee.

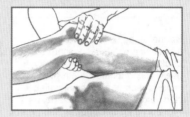

Posterior tibial pulse

Curve your fingers around the medial malleolus, and feel the pulse in the groove between the Achilles' tendon and the malleolus.

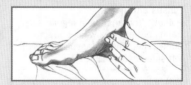

Dorsalis pedis pulse

Lightly touch the medial dorsum of the foot while the patient points the toes down. In this site, the pulse is difficult to palpate and may seem to be absent in some healthy patients.

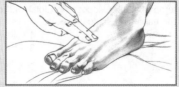

Pulse waveforms

To identify abnormal arterial pulses, check the waveforms below and see which one matches your patient's peripheral pulse.

Weak pulse

A weak pulse has decreased amplitude with a slower upstroke and downstroke. Possible causes of a weak pulse include increased peripheral vascular resistance, as occurs in cold weather or with severe heart failure, and decreased stroke volume, as occurs with hypovolemia or aortic stenosis.

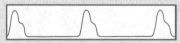

Bounding pulse

A bounding pulse has a sharp upstroke and downstroke with a pointed peak. The amplitude is elevated. Possible causes of a bounding pulse include increased stroke volume, as with aortic insufficiency, or stiffness of arterial walls, as with aging.

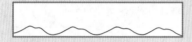

Pulsus alternans

Pulsus alternans has a regular, alternating pattern of a weak and strong pulse. This pulse is associated with left-sided heart failure.

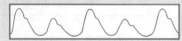

Pulsus bigeminus

Pulsus bigeminus is similar to pulsus alternans but occurs at irregular intervals. This pulse is caused by premature atrial or ventricular beats.

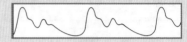

Pulsus paradoxus

Pulsus paradoxus has increases and decreases in amplitude associated with the respiratory cycle. Marked decreases occur when the patient inhales. Pulsus paradoxus is associated with pericardial tamponade, advanced heart failure, and constrictive pericarditis.

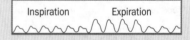

Inspiration   Expiration

Pulsus biferiens

Pulsus biferiens shows an initial upstroke, a subsequent downstroke, and then another upstroke during systole. Pulsus biferiens is caused by aortic stenosis and aortic insufficiency.

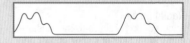

Grading pulses

Pulses should be regular in rhythm and strength. Check carotid, brachial, radial, femoral, popliteal, posterior tibial, and dorsal pedis pulses. Grade them using the numerical scale below.

$$4+ = \text{bounding}$$
$$3+ = \text{increased}$$
$$2+ = \text{normal}$$
$$1+ = \text{weak}$$
$$0 \;\; = \text{absent}$$

Evaluating jugular vein distention

Place the patient in a supine position, with the head of the bed elevated 45 to 90 degrees. (Normally, veins distend only when the patient lies flat.) Locate the angle of Louis (sternal notch). To do so, palpate the clavicles where they join the sternum (suprasternal notch). Place your first two fingers on the suprasternal notch. Then, without lifting them from the skin, slide them down the sternum until you feel a bony protuberance—this is the angle of Louis.

Find the internal jugular vein. Shine a flashlight across the patient's neck to create shadows that highlight his venous pulse. Be sure to distinguish jugular venous pulsations from carotid arterial pulsations; venous pulsations disappear with light finger pressure, whereas arterial pulsations continue.

Locate the highest point along the vein where you can see pulsations. Using a centimeter ruler, measure the distance between that high point and the sternal notch. Record this finding as well as the angle at which the patient was lying. A finding greater than 1⅛" (3 cm) above the sternal notch with the head of the bed at a 45-degree angle indicates jugular vein distention. Additionally, a normal jugular vein is less than 1½" (4 cm) in diameter; a diameter greater than this indicates jugular vein distention.

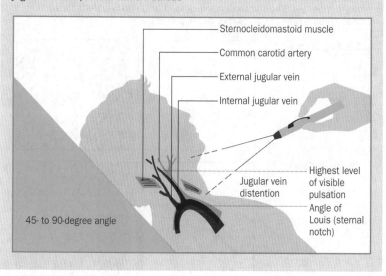

Sternocleidomastoid muscle

Common carotid artery

External jugular vein

Internal jugular vein

Highest level of visible pulsation

Jugular vein distention

Angle of Louis (sternal notch)

45- to 90-degree angle

Capillary refill

Normal: < 3 second
Abnormal: > 3 second

Edema scale

0	None observed
+1	Minimal (< 2 mm)
+2	Depression (2 to 4 mm)
+3	Depression (5 to 8 mm)
+4	Depression (> 8 mm)

Evaluating edema

To assess pitting edema, press firmly for 5 to 10 seconds over a bony surface, such as the tibia, fibula, sacrum, or sternum. Then remove your finger and note how long the depression remains. Document your observation on a scale of +1 (barely detectable depression) to +4 (persistent pit as deep as 1″ [2.5 cm]).

In severe edema, tissue swells so much that fluid can't be displaced, making pitting impossible. The surface feels rock-hard, and subcutaneous tissue becomes fibrotic. Brawny edema may develop eventually.

+1 pitting edema

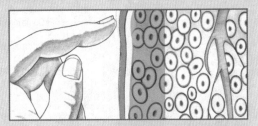

+4 pitting edema

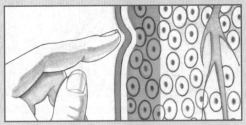

Brawny edema

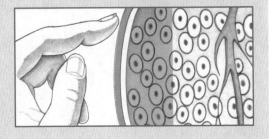

Cardiovascular system: Normal findings

Inspection
• No pulsations are visible, except at the point of maximal impulse (PMI).
• No lifts (heaves) or retractions are detectable in the four valve areas of the chest wall.

Palpation
• No vibrations or thrills are detectable.
• No lifts, or heaves, are detectable.
• No pulsations are detectable, except at the PMI and epigastric area. At the PMI, a localized (less than ½″ [1.3 cm] diameter area) tapping pulse may be felt at the start of systole. In the epigastric area, pulsation from the abdominal aorta may be palpable.

Auscultation
• The first heart sound (S_1), the lub sound, is best heard with the diaphragm of the stethoscope over the mitral area when the patient is in a left lateral position. It sounds longer, lower, and louder there than the second heart sound (S_2). S_1 splitting may be audible in the tricuspid area.

• The S_2 sound, the dub sound, is best heard with the diaphragm of the stethoscope in the aortic area while the patient sits and leans over. It sounds shorter, sharper, higher, and louder there than an S_1. Normal S_2 splitting may be audible in the pulmonic area on inspiration.
• A third heart sound (S_3) in children and slender, young adults with no cardiovascular disease is normal. It usually disappears when adults reach ages 25 to 35. In an older adult, it may signify heart failure. S_3 is best heard with the bell of the stethoscope over the mitral area with the patient in a supine position and exhaling. It sounds short, dull, soft, and low.
• Murmurs may be functional in children and young adults, but are abnormal in older adults. Innocent murmurs are soft, short, and vary with respirations and patient position. They occur in early systole and are best heard in pulmonic or mitral areas with the patient in a supine position.

Respiratory assessment landmarks

Anterior view

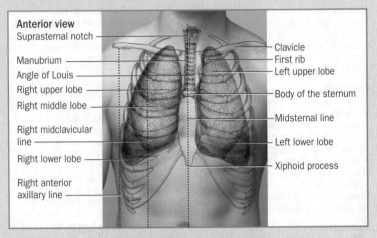

Suprasternal notch

Manubrium

Angle of Louis

Right upper lobe

Right middle lobe

Right midclavicular line

Right lower lobe

Right anterior axillary line

Clavicle

First rib

Left upper lobe

Body of the sternum

Midsternal line

Left lower lobe

Xiphoid process

Posterior view

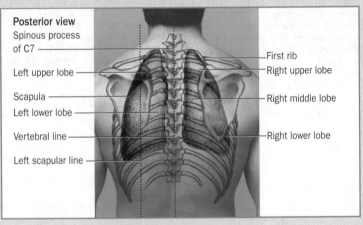

Spinous process of C7

Left upper lobe

Scapula

Left lower lobe

Vertebral line

Left scapular line

First rib

Right upper lobe

Right middle lobe

Right lower lobe

Chest deformities

As you inspect the patient's chest, note deviations in size and shape. The illustrations here show a normal adult chest and four common chest deformities.

Normal adult chest

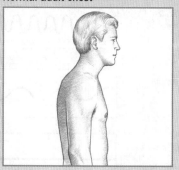

Barrel chest
Increased anteroposterior diameter

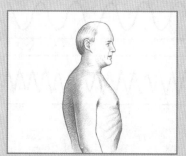

Pigeon chest
Anteriorly displaced sternum

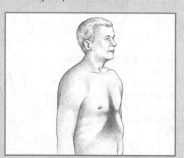

Funnel chest
Depressed lower sternum

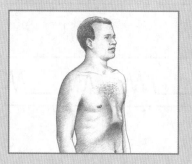

Thoracic kyphoscoliosis
Raised shoulder and scapula, thoracic convexity, and flared interspaces

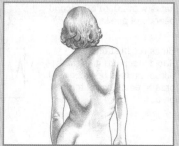

Abnormal respiratory patterns

Here are typical characteristics of the most common abnormal respiratory patterns.

Tachypnea
Shallow breathing with increased respiratory rate

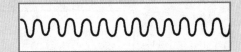

Bradypnea
Decreased rate but regular
breathing

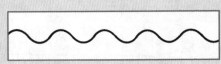

Apnea
Absence of breathing; may be
periodic

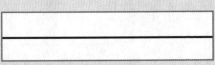

Hyperpnea
Deep, fast breathing

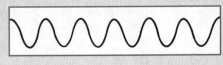

Kussmaul's respirations
Rapid, deep breathing without
pauses; in adults, more than
20 breaths/minute; breathing
usually sounds labored with
deep breaths that resemble
sighs

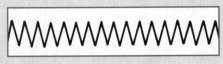

Cheyne-Stokes respirations
Breaths that gradually become
faster and deeper than normal, then slower, during a 30-
to 170-second period; alter-
nates with 20- to 60-second
periods of apnea

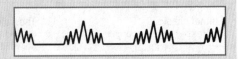

Biot's respirations
Rapid, deep breathing with
abrupt pauses between each
breath; equal depth to each
breath

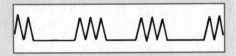

Palpating the chest

To palpate the chest, place the palm of your hand (or hands) lightly over the thorax, as shown. Palpate for tenderness, alignment, bulging, and retractions of the chest and intercostal spaces. Assess the patient for crepitus, especially around drainage sites. Repeat this procedure on the patient's back.

Next, use the pads of your fingers, as shown, to palpate the front and back of the thorax. Pass your fingers over the ribs and any scars, lumps, lesions, or ulcerations. Note the skin temperature, turgor, and moisture. Also note tenderness and bony or subcutaneous crepitus. The muscles should feel firm and smooth.

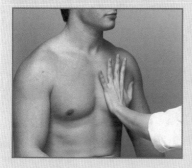
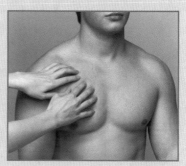

Checking for tactile fremitus

When you check the back of the thorax for tactile fremitus, ask the patient to fold his arms across his chest. This movement shifts the scapulae out of the way.

What to do
Check for tactile fremitus by lightly placing your open palms on both sides of the patient's back, as shown, without touching his back with your fingers. Ask the patient to repeat the phrase "ninety-nine" loud enough to produce palpable vibrations. Then palpate the front of the chest using the same hand positions.

What the results mean
Vibrations that feel more intense on one side than the other indicate tissue consolidation on that side. Less intense vibrations may indicate emphysema, pneumothorax, or pleural effusion. Faint or no vibrations in the upper posterior thorax may indicate bronchial obstruction or a fluid-filled pleural space.

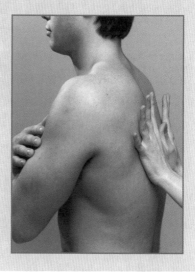

Percussion and auscultation sequences

Follow these sequences to distinguish between normal and abnormal sounds in the patient's lungs. Remember to compare sound variations from one side with the other as you proceed. Carefully describe abnormal sounds you hear and include their locations.

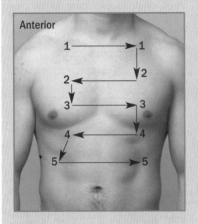

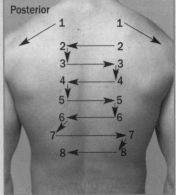

Percussing the chest

To percuss the chest, hyperextend the middle finger of your left hand if you're right-handed or the middle finger of your right hand if you're left-handed. Place your hand firmly on the patient's chest. Use the tip of the middle finger of your dominant hand—your right hand if you're right-handed, left hand if you're left-handed—to tap on the middle finger of your other hand just below the distal joint (as shown).

The movement should come from the wrist of your dominant hand, not your elbow or upper arm. Keep the fingernail you use for tapping short so you won't hurt yourself. Follow the standard percussion sequence over the front and back chest walls.

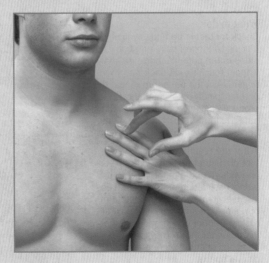

Percussion sounds

Use this chart to help you become more comfortable with percussion and to interpret percussion sounds quickly. Learn the different percussion sounds by practicing on yourself, your patients, and any other person willing to help.

Sound	Description	Clinical significance
Flat	Short, soft, high-pitched, extremely dull, found over the thigh	Consolidation, as in atelectasis and extensive pleural effusion
Dull	Medium in intensity and pitch, moderate length, thudlike, found over the liver	Solid area, as in pleural effusion
Resonant	Long, loud, low-pitched, hollow	Normal lung tissue
Hyperresonant	Very loud, lower-pitched, found over the stomach	Hyperinflated lung, as in emphysema or pneumothorax
Tympanic	Loud, high-pitched, moderate length, musical, drumlike, found over a puffed-out cheek	Air collection, as in a gastric air bubble or air in the intestines

Qualities of normal breath sounds

Breath sound	Quality	Location
Tracheal	Harsh, high-pitched	Over trachea
Bronchial	Loud, high-pitched	Next to trachea
Bronchovesicular	Medium loudness and pitch	Next to sternum
Vesicular	Soft, low-pitched	Remainder of lungs

Abnormal breath sounds

Sound	Description
Crackles	Light crackling, popping, intermittent nonmusical sounds—like hairs being rubbed together—heard on inspiration or expiration
Pleural friction rub	Low-pitched, continual, superficial, squeaking or grating sound—like pieces of sandpaper being rubbed together—heard on inspiration and expiration
Rhonchi	Low-pitched, monophonic snoring sounds heard primarily on expiration but also throughout the respiratory cycle
Stridor	High-pitched, monophonic crowing sound heard on inspiration; louder in the neck than in the chest wall
Wheezes	High-pitched, continual musical or whistling sound heard primarily on expiration but sometimes also on inspiration

Respiratory system: Normal findings

Inspection
• Chest configuration is symmetrical side-to-side.
• Anteroposterior diameter is less than the transverse diameter, with a 1:2 to 5:7 ratio in an adult.
• Chest shape is normal, with no deformities, such as barrel chest, kyphosis, retraction, sternal protrusion, or depressed sternum.
• Costal angle is less than 90 degrees, with the ribs joining the spine at a 45-degree angle.
• Respirations are quiet and unlabored, with no use of accessory neck, shoulder, or abdominal muscles, and no intercostal, substernal, or supraclavicular retractions.
• Chest wall expands symmetrically during respirations.
• Adult respiratory rate is normal, at 16 to 20 breaths/minute. Expect some variation depending on your patient's age.
• Respiratory rhythm is regular, with expiration taking about twice as long as inspiration. Men and children breathe diaphragmatically, whereas women breathe thoracically.
• Skin color matches the rest of the body's complexion.

Palpation
• Skin is warm and dry.
• No tender spots or bulges in the chest are detectable.
• Tactile fremitus is normal bilaterally.

Percussion
• Resonant percussion sounds can be heard over the lungs.

Auscultation
• Loud, high-pitched bronchial breath sounds can be heard over the trachea.
• Intense, medium-pitched bronchovesicular breath sounds can be heard over the mainstem bronchi, between the scapulae, and below the clavicles.
• Soft, breezy, low-pitched vesicular breath sounds can be heard over most of the peripheral lung fields.

Cranial nerves

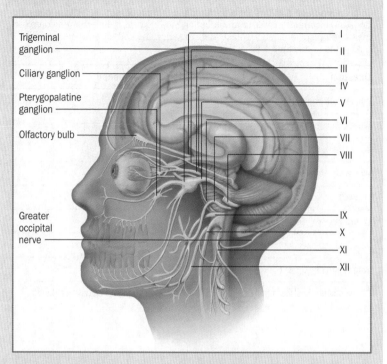

Trigeminal ganglion
Ciliary ganglion
Pterygopalatine ganglion
Olfactory bulb
Greater occipital nerve

I
II
III
IV
V
VI
VII
VIII
IX
X
XI
XII

Cranial nerve function

CN I: **Olfactory**—Smell

CN II: **Optic**—Vision

CN III: **Oculomotor**—Extraocular movement, pupillary constriction, upper eyelid elevation, lens shape change

CN IV: **Trochlear**—Downward and inward eye movement

CN V: **Trigeminal**—Chewing, corneal reflex, face and scalp sensations

CN VI: **Abducens**—Lateral eye movement

CN VII: **Facial**—Expressions in forehead, eye, and mouth; taste

CN VIII: **Acoustic**—Hearing and balance

CN IX: **Glossopharyngeal**—Swallowing, salivating, and taste

CN X: **Vagus**—Swallowing; gag reflex; talking; sensations of throat, larynx, and abdominal viscera

CN XI: **Spinal accessory**—Shoulder movement and head rotation

CN XII: **Hypoglossal**—Tongue movement

Assessing mental status

To quickly screen patients for disordered thought processes, ask these questions. An incorrect answer to any question may indicate the need for a complete mental status examination. Make sure you know the correct answers before asking the questions.

Question	Function screened
What's your name?	Orientation to person
What's your mother's name?	Orientation to other people
What year is it?	Orientation to time
Where are you now?	Orientation to place
How old are you?	Memory
Where were you born?	Remote memory
What did you have for breakfast?	Recent memory
Who's currently the U.S. president?	General knowledge
Can you count backward from 20 to 1?	Attention span and calculation skills

Stages of altered arousal

This chart highlights the six levels or stages of altered arousal and their manifestations.

Stage	Manifestations
Confusion	• Loss of ability to think rapidly and clearly • Impaired judgment and decision making
Disorientation	• Beginning loss of consciousness • Disorientation to time progressing to include disorientation to place • Impaired memory • Lack of recognition of self (last to go)
Lethargy	• Limited spontaneous movement or speech • Easily aroused by normal speech or touch • Possible disorientation to time, place, or person
Obtundation	• Mild to moderate reduction in arousal • Limited responsiveness to environment • Ability to fall asleep easily in absence of verbal or tactile stimulation from others • Minimum response to questions
Stupor	• State of deep sleep or unresponsiveness • Arousable with difficulty (motor or verbal response only to vigorous and repeated stimulation) • Withdrawal or grabbing response to stimulation
Coma	• Lack of motor or verbal response to external environment or any stimuli • No response to noxious stimuli such as deep pain • Can't be aroused by any stimulus

Glasgow Coma Scale

The Glasgow Coma Scale provides an easy way to describe the patient's baseline neurologic status. It can also help detect neurologic changes.

A decreased score in one or more categories may signal an impending neurologic crisis. The best response is scored.

Test	Score	Patient's response
Eye opening		
Spontaneously	4	Opens eyes spontaneously
To speech	3	Opens eyes to verbal command
To pain	2	Opens eyes to painful stimulus
None	1	Doesn't open eyes in response to stimulus
Motor response		
Obeys	6	Reacts to verbal command
Localizes	5	Identifies localized pain
Withdraws	4	Flexes and withdraws from painful stimulus
Abnormal flexion	3	Assumes a decorticate posture
Abnormal extension	2	Assumes a decerebrate posture
None	1	Doesn't respond; just lies flaccid
Verbal response		
Oriented	5	Is oriented and converses
Confused	4	Is disoriented and confused
Inappropriate words	3	Replies randomly with incorrect words
Incomprehensible	2	Moans or screams
None	1	Doesn't respond
Total score		

Identifying abnormal pupil response

Use this chart as a guide to abnormal pupil response.

Pupillary change	Possible causes
Unilateral, dilated (4 mm), fixed, and nonreactive 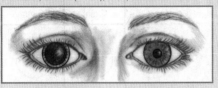	• Uncal herniation with oculomotor nerve damage • Brain stem compression • Increased intracranial pressure • Tentorial herniation • Head trauma with subdural or epidural hematoma • Normal in some people
Bilateral, dilated (4 mm), fixed, and nonreactive 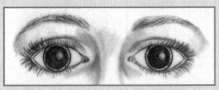	• Severe midbrain damage • Cardiopulmonary arrest (hypoxia) • Anticholinergic poisoning
Bilateral, midsize (2 mm), fixed, and nonreactive 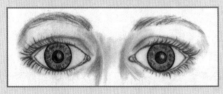	• Midbrain involvement caused by edema, hemorrhage, infarctions, lacerations, contusions
Bilateral, pinpoint (< 1 mm), and usually nonreactive 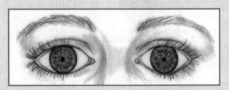	• Lesions of pons, usually after hemorrhage
Unilateral, small (1.5 mm), and nonreactive 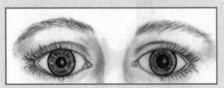	• Disruption of sympathetic nerve supply to the head caused by spinal cord lesion above the first thoracic vertebrae

Grading pupil size

To ensure accurate evaluation of pupillary size, compare the patient's pupils to this scale. Keep in mind that maximum constriction may be less than 1 mm and maximum dilation greater than 9 mm.

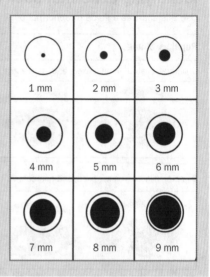

Visual field defects

Here are some examples of visual field defects. The black areas represent vision loss.

	Left	Right
A: Blindness of right eye		
B: Bitemporal hemianopsia, or loss of one-half the visual field		
C: Left homonymous hemianopsia		
D: Left homonymous hemianopsia, superior quadrant		

Assessing deep tendon reflexes

During a neurologic examination, assess the patient's deep tendon reflexes—the biceps, triceps, brachioradialis, patellar or quadriceps, and Achilles reflexes.

Biceps reflex

Position the patient's arm so his elbow is flexed at a 45-degree angle and his arm is relaxed. Place your thumb or index finger over the biceps tendon and your remaining fingers loosely over the triceps muscle. Strike your finger with the pointed end of the reflex hammer, and watch and feel for the contraction of the biceps muscle and flexion of the forearm.

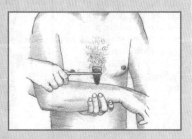

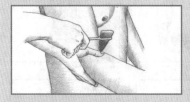

Patellar reflex

Have the patient sit with his legs dangling freely. If he can't sit up, flex his knee at a 45-degree angle, and place your nondominant hand behind it for support. Strike the patellar tendon just below the patella, and look for contraction of the quadriceps muscle in the thigh with extension of the leg.

Triceps reflex

Have the patient adduct his arm and place his forearm across his chest. Strike the triceps tendon about 2″ (5 cm) above the olecranon process on the extensor surface of the upper arm. Watch for contraction of the triceps muscle and extension of the forearm.

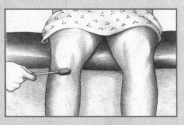

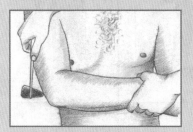

Achilles reflex

Have the patient flex his foot. Then support the plantar surface. Strike the Achilles tendon, and watch for plantar flexion of the foot at the ankle.

Brachioradialis reflex

Ask the patient to rest his elbow. Support the ulnar area with your hand and forearm. Strike the radius (as shown at top of next column). Watch for supination of the hand and flexion of the forearm at the elbow.

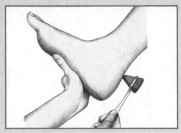

Identifying gait abnormalities

During your assessment, you may identify gait abnormalities. They may result from disorders of the cerebellum, posterior columns, corticospinal tract, basal ganglia, and lower motor neurons. These illustrations identify five gait abnormalities.

Spastic gait

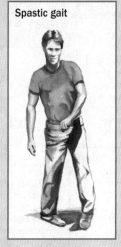

Scissors gait

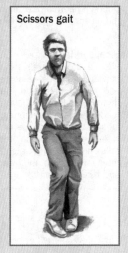

Propulsive gait

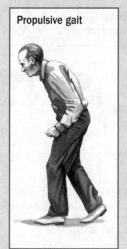

Steppage gait

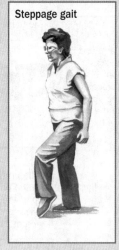

Waddling gait

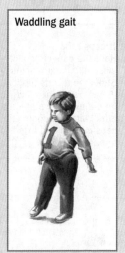

Comparing decerebrate and decorticate postures

Decerebrate posture results from damage to the upper brain stem. In this posture, the arms are adducted and extended, with the wrists pronated and the fingers flexed. The legs are stiffly extended, with plantar flexion of the feet.

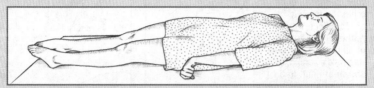

Decorticate posture results from damage to one or both corticospinal tracts. In this posture, the arms are adducted and flexed, with the wrists and fingers flexed on the chest. The legs are stiffly extended and internally rotated, with plantar flexion of the feet.

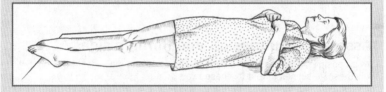

How to elicit Babinski's reflex

To elicit Babinski's reflex, stroke the lateral aspect of the sole of the patient's foot with your thumbnail or another moderately sharp object. Normally, this elicits flexion of all toes (a negative Babinski's reflex), as shown at right. In a positive Babinski's reflex, the great toe dorsiflexes and the other toes fan out, as shown far right.

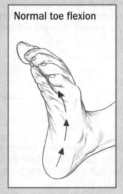
Normal toe flexion

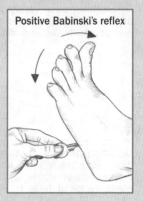
Positive Babinski's reflex

Assessing Brudzinski's and Kernig's signs

When positive, Brudzinski's and Kernig's signs indicate meningeal irritation. Follow these guidelines to test for these two signs.

Brudzinski's sign
With the patient in a supine position, place your hand under his neck and flex it forward, chin to chest. This test is positive if he flexes his ankles, knees, and hips bilaterally. In addition, the patient typically complains of pain when the neck is flexed.

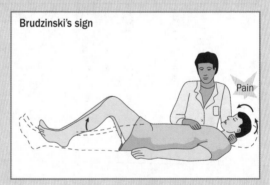
Brudzinski's sign

Kernig's sign
With the patient in the supine position, flex his hip and knee to form a 90-degree angle. Next, attempt to extend this leg. If he exhibits pain, resistance to extension, and spasm, the test is positive.

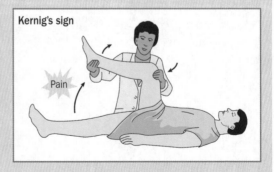
Kernig's sign

Detecting increased ICP

The earlier you can recognize the signs of increased intracranial pressure (ICP), the more quickly you can intervene and better the patient's chance of recovery. By the time late signs appear, interventions may be useless.

	Early signs	Late signs
Level of consciousness	• Requires increased stimulation • Subtle orientation loss • Restlessness and anxiety • Sudden quietness	Unarousable
Pupils	• Pupil changes on side of lesion • One pupil constricts but then dilates (unilateral hippus) • Sluggish reaction of both pupils • Unequal pupils	Pupils fixed and dilated
Motor response	• Sudden weakness • Motor changes on side opposite the lesion • Positive pronator drift; with palms up, one hand pronates	Profound weakness
Vital signs	• Intermittent increases in blood pressure	Increased systolic pressure, profound bradycardia, abnormal respirations (Cushing's syndrome)

Neurologic system: Normal findings

Inspection

• Patient can shrug his shoulders, a sign of an adequately functioning cranial nerve XI (accessory nerve).

• Pupils are equal, round, and reactive to light, a test of cranial nerves II and III.

• Eyes move freely and in a coordinated manner, a sign of adequately functioning cranial nerves III, IV, and VI.

• The lids of both eyes close when you stroke each cornea with a wisp of cotton, a test of cranial nerve V (trigeminal nerve).

• Patient can identify familiar odors, a test of cranial nerve I (olfactory nerve).

• Patient can hear a whispered voice, a test of cranial nerve VIII (acoustic nerve).

• Patient can purse his lips and puff out his cheeks, a sign of an adequately functioning cranial nerve VII (facial nerve).

• Tongue moves easily and without tremor, a sign of a properly functioning cranial nerve XII (hypoglossal nerve).

• Voice is clear and strong; uvula moves upward when the patient says "ah"; gag reflex occurs when the tongue blade touches the posterior pharynx, signs of properly functioning cranial nerves IX and X.

• No involuntary movements are detectable.

• Gait is smooth.

• Patient is oriented to himself, other people, place, and time.

• Memory and attention span are intact.

• Deep tendon reflexes are intact.

Palpation

• Strength in the facial muscles is symmetrical, a sign of adequately functioning cranial nerves V and VII (trigeminal and facial nerves).

• Muscle tone and strength are adequate.

Abdominal quadrants

To perform a systematic GI assessment, visualize the abdominal structures by mentally dividing the abdomen into four quadrants, as shown here.

Right upper quadrant
- Right lobe of liver
- Gallbladder
- Pylorus
- Duodenum
- Head of the pancreas
- Hepatic flexure of the colon
- Portions of the ascending and transverse colon

Left upper quadrant
- Left lobe of the liver
- Stomach
- Body of the pancreas
- Splenic flexure of the colon
- Portions of the transverse and descending colon

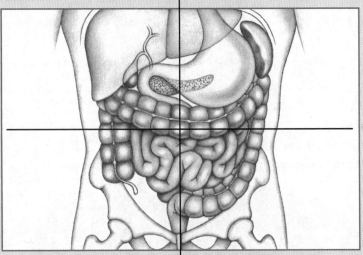

Right lower quadrant
- Cecum and appendix
- Portion of the ascending colon

Left lower quadrant
- Sigmoid colon
- Portion of the descending colon

Vascular sounds

Use the bell of your stethoscope to auscultate for vascular sounds at the sites shown in this illustration.

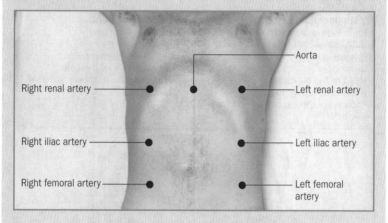

Sites of tympany and dullness

Expect to auscultate tympany and dullness in the areas shown here.

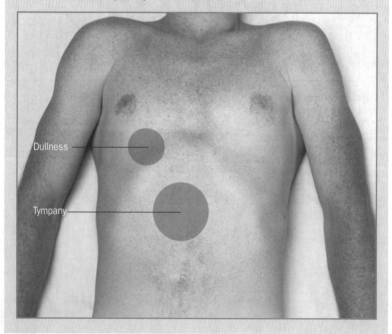

Percussing and measuring the liver

· Identify the upper border of liver dullness. Start in the right midclavicular line in an area of lung resonance, and percuss downward toward the liver. Use a pen to mark the spot where the sound changes to dullness.

· Start in the right midclavicular line at a level below the umbilicus, and lightly percuss upward toward the liver. Mark the spot where the sound changes from tympany to dullness.

· Use a ruler to measure the vertical span between the two marked spots, as shown. In an adult, a normal liver span ranges from 2½″ to 4½″ (6.5 to 11.5 cm).

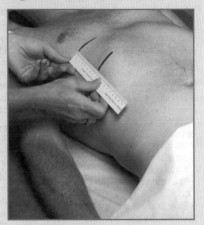

Palpating the liver

These illustrations show the correct hand positions for two ways of palpating the liver.

Method 1: Standard palpation

· Place the patient in the supine position. Standing at his right side, place your left hand under his back at the approximate location of the liver.

· Place your right hand slightly below the mark you made when measuring the liver at its upper border. Point the fingers of your right hand toward the patient's head just under the right costal margin.

· As the patient inhales deeply, gently press in and up on the abdomen until the liver brushes under your right hand. The edge should be smooth, firm, and somewhat round. Note any tenderness.

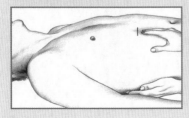

Method 2: Hooking the liver

· Hooking is an alternate way of palpating the liver. To hook the liver, stand next to the patient's right shoulder, facing his feet. Place your hands side by side, and hook your fingertips over the right costal margin, below the lower mark of dullness made when measuring the liver.

· Ask the patient to take a deep breath as you push your fingertips in and up. If the liver is palpable, you may feel its edge as it slides down in the abdomen as he breathes in.

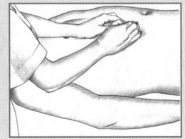

GI system: Normal findings

Inspection
• Skin is free from vascular lesions, jaundice, surgical scars, and rashes.
• Faint venous patterns (except in thin patients) are apparent.
• Abdomen is symmetrical, with a flat, round, or scaphoid contour.
• Umbilicus is positioned midway between the xiphoid process and the symphysis pubis, with a flat or concave hemisphere.
• No variations in the color of the patient's skin are detectable.
• No bulges are apparent.
• The abdomen moves with respiration.
• Pink or silver-white striae from pregnancy or weight loss may be apparent.

Auscultation
• High-pitched, gurgling bowel sounds are heard every 5 to 15 seconds through the diaphragm of the stethoscope in all four quadrants of the abdomen.
• Vascular sounds are heard through the bell of the stethoscope.
• A venous hum is heard over the inferior vena cava.
• No bruits, murmurs, friction rubs, or other venous hums are apparent.

Percussion
• Tympany is the predominant sound over hollow organs, including the stomach, intestines, bladder, abdominal aorta, and gallbladder.
• Dullness can be heard over solid masses, including the liver, spleen, pancreas, kidneys, uterus, and a full bladder.

Palpation
• No tenderness or masses are detectable.
• Abdominal musculature is free from tenderness and rigidity.
• No guarding, rebound tenderness, distention, or ascites are detectable.
• The liver is unpalpable, except in children. (If palpable, the liver edge is regular, sharp, and nontender and felt no more than ¾″ [1.9 cm] below the right costal margin.)
• The spleen is unpalpable.
• The kidneys are unpalpable, except in thin patients or those with a flaccid abdominal wall. (You'll typically feel the right kidney before you feel the left one. When palpable, the kidney is solid and firm.)

External female genitalia

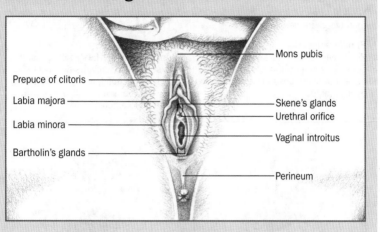

- Mons pubis
- Prepuce of clitoris
- Labia majora
- Labia minora
- Bartholin's glands
- Skene's glands
- Urethral orifice
- Vaginal introitus
- Perineum

Examining the male urethral meatus

To inspect the urethral meatus, compress the tip of the glans, as shown here.

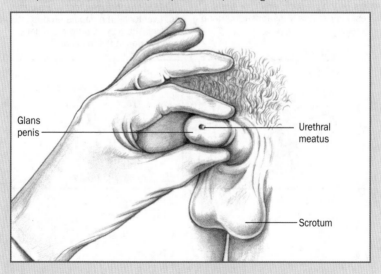

- Glans penis
- Urethral meatus
- Scrotum

Male genital lesions

Several types of lesions may affect the male genitalia. Some of the more common types are described here.

Penile cancer

Penile cancer causes a painless, ulcerative lesion on the glans or prepuce (foreskin), possibly accompanied by discharge.

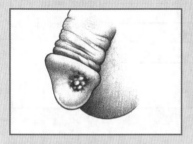

Genital warts

Genital warts are flesh-colored, soft, moist papillary growths that occur singly or in cauliflower-like clusters. They may be barely visible or several inches in diameter.

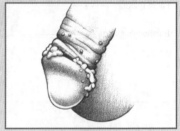

Genital herpes

Genital herpes causes a painful, reddened group of small vesicles or blisters on the prepuce, shaft, or glans. Lesions eventually disappear but tend to recur.

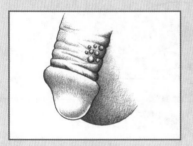

Syphilis

Syphilis causes a hard, round papule on the penis. When palpated, this syphilitic chancre may feel like a button. Eventually, the papule erodes into an ulcer. You may also note swollen lymph nodes in the inguinal area.

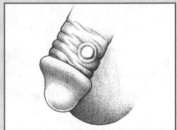

Percussing the urinary organs

Kidney percussion

With the patient sitting upright, percuss each costovertebral angle (the angle over each kidney whose borders are formed by the lateral and downward curve of the lowest rib and the vertebral column). To perform indirect fist percussion, place your left palm over the costovertebral angle and gently strike it with your right fist. Normally, the patient will feel a thudding sensation or pressure during percussion.

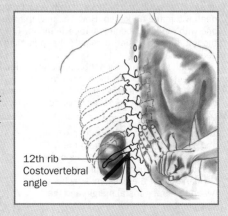
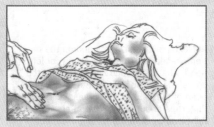

12th rib
Costovertebral angle

Bladder percussion

Using mediate percussion, percuss the area over the bladder, beginning 2″ (5 cm) above the symphysis pubis. To detect differences in sound, percuss toward the bladder's base. Percussion normally produces a tympanic sound. (Over a urine-filled bladder, it produces a dull sound.)

Palpating the urinary organs

In a normal adult, the kidneys usually aren't palpable because they're located deep within the abdomen. However, they may be palpable in a thin patient or in one with reduced abdominal muscle mass. The right kidney, slightly lower than the left, may be easier to palpate. Keep in mind that both kidneys descend with deep inhalation.

An adult's bladder may not be palpable either. However, if it's palpable, it normally feels firm and relatively smooth.

When palpating urinary organs, use bimanual palpation, beginning on the patient's right side and proceeding as follows.

Kidney palpation

1. Help the patient to a supine position, and expose the abdomen from the xiphoid process to the symphysis pubis. Standing at the right side, place your left hand under the back, midway between the lower costal margin and the iliac crest.

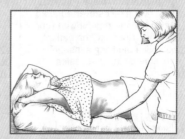

2. Next, place your right hand on the patient's abdomen, directly above your left hand. Angle this hand slightly toward the costal margin. To palpate the right lower edge of the right kidney, press your right fingertips about 1½″ (3.5 cm) above the right iliac crest at the midinguinal line; press your left fingertips upward into the right costovertebral angle.

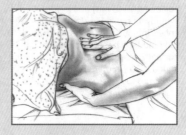

3. Instruct the patient to inhale deeply so that the lower portion of the right kidney can move down between your hands. If it does, note its shape and size. Normally, it feels smooth, solid, and firm, yet elastic. Ask the patient if palpation causes tenderness. (*Note:* Avoid using excessive pressure to palpate the kidney because this may cause intense pain.)

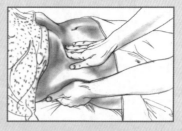

4. To assess the left kidney, move to the patient's left side, and position your hands as described above, but with this change: Place your right hand 2″ (5 cm) above the left iliac crest. Then apply pressure with both hands as the patient inhales. If the left kidney can be palpated, compare it with the right kidney; it should be the same size.

Palpating the urinary organs *(continued)*

Bladder palpation

Before palpating the bladder, make sure the patient has voided. Then locate the edge of the bladder by pressing deeply in the midline 1″ to 2″ (2.5 to 5 cm) above the symphysis pubis. As the bladder is palpated, note its size and location, and check for lumps, masses, and tenderness. The bladder normally feels firm and relatively smooth. During deep palpation, the patient may report the urge to urinate—a normal response.

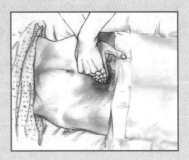

Genitourinary system: Normal findings

Inspection

• No lesions, discoloration, or swelling is apparent on the skin over the kidney and bladder areas.
• No urethral discharge or ulcerations are apparent.
• Pubic area is free from lesions and parasites.

Female
• Labia majora are moist and free from lesions.
• Vaginal discharge is normal. (Discharge varies from clear and stretchy to white and opaque, depending on the menstrual cycle; odorless; and nonirritating to the mucosa).
• Cervix looks smooth and round.

Male
• Penis appears slightly wrinkled, with the color ranging from pink to dark brown, depending on the patient's skin color.
• Smegma is present.
• Urethral meatus is pink and smooth and located in the center of the glans.
• Scrotum is free from swelling and edema but has some sebaceous cysts.

Percussion

• No costovertebral angle tenderness is apparent.
• Tympany is heard over the empty bladder.

Palpation

• Kidneys are unpalpable, except in very thin and elderly patients.
• Bladder is unpalpable.

Female
• Labia feel soft, without swelling, hardness, or tenderness.
• Bartholin's glands are unpalpable.
• Vaginal wall has no nodularity, tenderness, or bulging.
• Cervix is smooth and firm, protrudes ¼″ to 1¼″ (0.5 to 3 cm) into the vagina, and is freely moveable in all directions.

Male
• Penis feels somewhat firm, with the skin smooth and movable.
• Testicles are equally sized, move freely in the scrotal sac, and feel firm, smooth, and rubbery.
• Epididymis is smooth, discrete, nontender, and free from swelling and induration.
• No inguinal or femoral hernias are apparent.
• Prostate gland is smooth and rubbery, is about the size of a walnut, and doesn't protrude into the rectal lumen.

Auscultation

• No bruits can be heard over the renal arteries.

A close look at the skeletal system

Of the 206 bones in the human skeletal system, 80 form the axial skeleton (skull, facial bones, vertebrae, ribs, sternum, and hyoid bone) and 126 form the appendicular skeleton (arms, legs, shoulders, and pelvis). Shown here are the body's major bones.

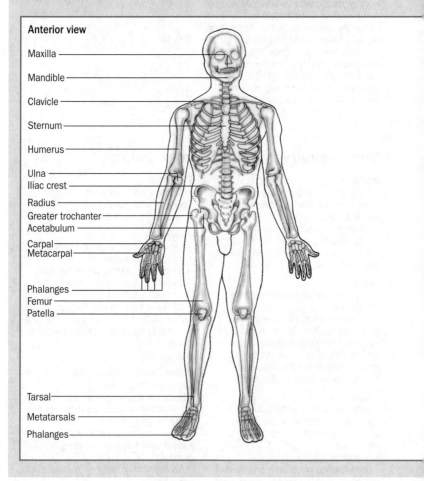

Anterior view

Maxilla

Mandible

Clavicle

Sternum

Humerus

Ulna
Iliac crest

Radius
Greater trochanter
Acetabulum

Carpal
Metacarpal

Phalanges
Femur
Patella

Tarsal

Metatarsals

Phalanges

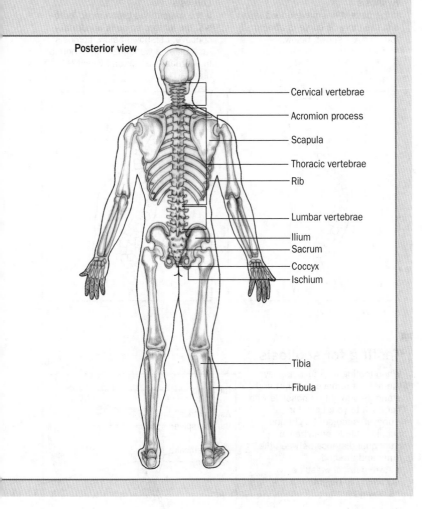

Posterior view

Cervical vertebrae

Acromion process

Scapula

Thoracic vertebrae

Rib

Lumbar vertebrae

Ilium

Sacrum

Coccyx

Ischium

Tibia

Fibula

Kyphosis and lordosis

These illustrations show the difference between kyphosis and lordosis.

Kyphosis
If the patient has pronounced kyphosis, the thoracic curve is abnormally rounded, as shown below.

Lordosis
If the patient has pronounced lordosis, the lumbar spine is abnormally concave, as shown below. Lordosis (as well as a waddling gait) is normal in pregnant women and young children.

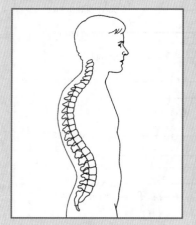

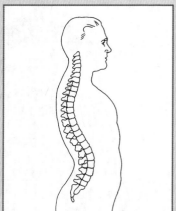

Testing for scoliosis

When testing for scoliosis, have the patient remove her shirt and stand as straight as possible with her back to you. Look for:
· uneven shoulder height and shoulder blade prominence
· unequal distance between the arms and the body
· asymmetrical waistline
· uneven hip height
· sideways lean.

Bent over
Then have the patient bend forward, keeping her head down and palms together. Look for:
· asymmetrical thoracic spine or prominent rib cage (rib hump) on either side
· asymmetrical waistline.

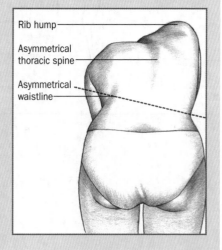

Rib hump

Asymmetrical thoracic spine

Asymmetrical waistline

Testing and grading muscle strength

To test the muscle strength of your patient's arm and ankle muscles, use the techniques shown here.

Biceps strength	Triceps strength
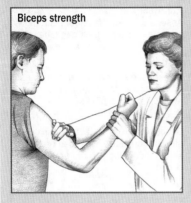	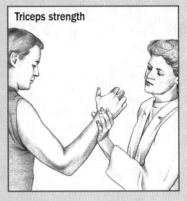

Ankle strength: Plantar flexion	Ankle strength: Dorsiflexion
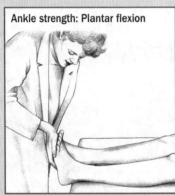	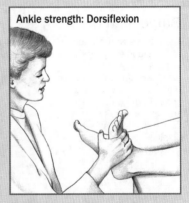

Grading muscle strength

Grade muscle strength on a scale of 0 to 5, as follows:

• 5/5: normal; patient moves joint through full range of motion (ROM) and against gravity with full resistance

• 4/5: good; patient completes ROM against gravity with moderate resistance

• 3/5: fair; patient completes ROM against gravity only

• 2/5: poor; patient completes full ROM with gravity eliminated (passive motion)

• 1/5: trace; patient's attempt at muscle contraction is palpable but without joint movement

• 0/5: zero; no evidence of muscle contraction.

The 5 P's of musculoskeletal injury

To swiftly assess a musculoskeletal injury, remember the 5 P's—pain, paresthesia, paralysis, pallor, and pulse.

Pain
Ask the patient whether he feels pain. If he does, assess the location, severity, and quality of the pain.

Paresthesia
Assess the patient for loss of sensation by touching the injured area with the tip of an open safety pin. Abnormal sensation or loss of sensation indicates neurovascular involvement.

Paralysis
Assess whether the patient can move the affected area. If he can't, he might have nerve or tendon damage.

Pallor
Paleness, discoloration, and coolness on the injured side may indicate neurovascular compromise.

Pulse
Check all pulses distal to the injury site. If a pulse is decreased or absent, blood supply to the area is reduced.

Bulge sign

The bulge sign indicates excess fluid in the joint. To assess the patient for this sign, ask him to lie down so that you can palpate his knee. Then give the medial side of his knee two to four firm strokes, as shown, to displace excess fluid.

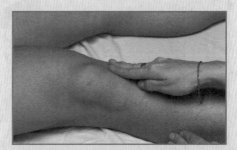

Lateral check
Next, tap the lateral aspect of the knee while checking for a fluid wave on the medial aspect, as shown.

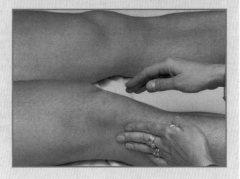

Musculoskeletal system: Normal findings

Inspection
- No gross deformities are apparent.
- Body parts are symmetrical.
- Body alignment is good.
- No involuntary movements are detectable.
- Gait is smooth.
- All muscles and joints have active range of motion with no pain.
- No swelling or inflammation is visible in the joints or muscles.
- Bilateral limb length is equal and muscle mass is symmetrical.

Palpation
- Shape is normal, with no swelling or tenderness.
- Bilateral muscle tone, texture, and strength are equal.
- No involuntary contractions or twitching is detectable.
- Bilateral pulses are equally strong.

A close look at the skin

Skin is made up of separate layers that function as a single unit. Two distinct layers of skin, the epidermis and dermis, lie above a layer of subcutaneous fatty tissue (sometimes called the *hypodermis*).

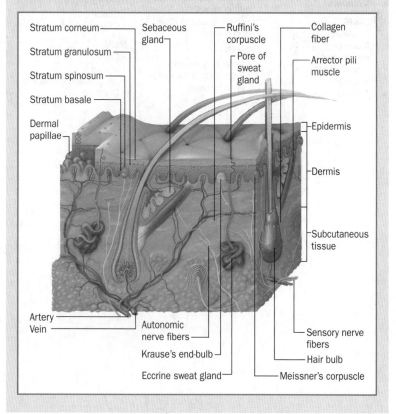

Functions of the skin

- Protects internal structures
- Aids in sensory perception
- Regulates temperature
- Regulates fluid and electrolyte retention and excretion
- Produces vitamin D (crucial to metabolism of calcium and phosphate)
- Absorbs medication
- Communicates through non-verbal cues of facial expression

Comprehensive skin assessment

Examine these factors when assessing a patient's skin.

Color
- Bruising
- Erythema
- Pallor
- Duskiness
- Jaundice
- Cyanosis

Texture
- Thickness
- Mobility
- Roughness
- Smoothness
- Fragility
- Thinness

Moisture
- Excessive dryness
- Excessive moisture
- Edema

Temperature
- Generalized or localized coolness
- Generalized or localized warmth

Smell
- Normal body odor
- Presence of foul odor
- Poor hygiene

Lesions
- Vascular changes
- Hemangiomas
- Telangiectases
- Petechiae
- Purpura
- Ecchymoses
- Scars
- Other lesions

Nails
- Color
- Shape
- Texture and thickness
- Clubbing

Skin color variations

To interpret skin color variation findings faster, refer to this chart.

Color	Distribution	Possible cause
Absent	• Small circumscribed areas • Generalized	• Vitiligo • Albinism
Blue	• Around lips, buccal mucosa, or generalized	• Cyanosis (Note: In blacks, blue gingivae are normal.)
Deep red	• Generalized	• Polycythemia vera (increased red blood cell count)
Pink	• Local or generalized	• Erythema (superficial capillary dilation and congestion)
Tan to brown	• Facial patches	• Chloasma of pregnancy; butterfly rash of lupus erythematosus
Tan to brown-bronze	• Generalized (not related to sun exposure)	• Addison's disease
Yellow to yellowish brown	• Sclera or generalized	• Jaundice from liver dysfunction (Note: In blacks, yellowish brown pigmentation of sclera is normal.)
Yellowish orange	• Palms, soles, and face; not sclera	• Carotenemia (carotene in the blood)

Evaluating skin turgor

To assess skin turgor in an adult, gently squeeze the skin on the forearm or sternal area between your thumb and forefinger, as shown top right. In an infant, roll a fold of loosely adherent abdominal skin between your thumb and forefinger. Then release the skin.

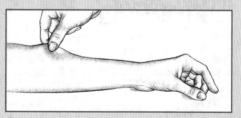

If the skin quickly returns to its original shape, the patient has normal turgor. If it returns to its original shape slowly over 30 seconds or maintains a tented position, as shown bottom right, the skin has poor turgor.

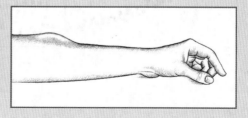

Recognizing common lesion configurations

Identify the configuration of your patient's skin lesion by matching it to one of these diagrams.

Discrete
Individual lesions are separate and distinct.

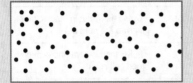

Grouped
Lesions are clustered together.

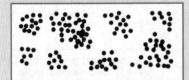

Confluent
Lesions merge so that individual lesions aren't visible or palpable.

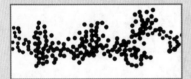

Linear
Lesions form a line.

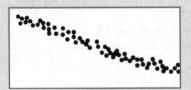

Annular
Lesions are arranged in a single ring or circle.

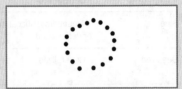

Arciform
Lesions form arcs or curves.

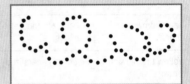

Polycyclic
Lesions are arranged in multiple circles.

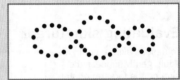

Reticular
Lesions form a meshlike network.

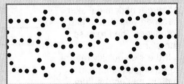

Identifying primary lesions

Are you having trouble identifying your patient's lesion? Here's a quick look at three common lesions. Remember to keep a centimeter ruler handy to accurately measure the size of the lesion.

Macule
Flat, circumscribed area of altered skin color, generally less than 1 cm; examples: freckle, flat nevus

Papule
Raised, circumscribed, solid area; generally less than 1 cm; examples: elevated nevus, wart

Vesicle
Circumscribed, elevated lesion; contains serous fluid; less than 1 cm; example: early chickenpox

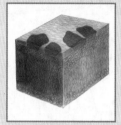 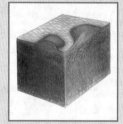 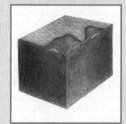

Illuminating lesions

Illuminating a lesion can help you see it better and learn more about its characteristics. Here are two techniques worth perfecting.

Macule or papule?
To determine whether a lesion is a macule or a papule, use this technique: Reduce the direct lighting and shine a penlight or flashlight at a right angle to the lesion. If the light casts a shadow, the lesion is a papule. Macules are flat and don't produce shadows.

Solid or fluid-filled?
To determine whether a lesion is solid or fluid-filled, use this technique: Place the tip of a flashlight or penlight against the side of the lesion. Solid lesions don't transmit light. Fluid-filled lesions transilluminate with a red glow.

Evaluating clubbed fingers

Think hypoxia when you see a patient whose fingers are clubbed. To quickly examine a patient's fingers for early clubbing, gently palpate the bases of his nails. Normally, they'll feel firm, but in early clubbing, they'll feel springy.

To evaluate late clubbing, have the patient place the first phalanges of the forefingers together. Normal nail bases are concave and create a small, diamond-shaped space when the first phalanges are opposed, as shown at top right.

In late clubbing, the now convex nail bases can touch without leaving a space, as shown at bottom right. This condition is associated with pulmonary and cardiovascular disease. When you spot clubbed fingers, think about the possible causes, such as emphysema, chronic bronchitis, lung cancer, and heart failure.

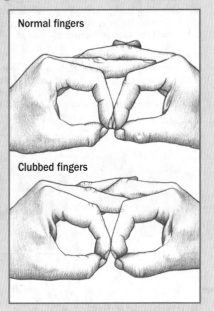

Normal fingers

Clubbed fingers

Integumentary system: Normal findings

Inspection
· Color should be uniform.
· Skin lesions may be present.
· Lesion assessment:
 – Classify the lesion as primary or secondary.
 – Determine if it's solid or fluid-filled.
 – Check the borders to see if they're regular or irregular.
 – Note the lesion's color, pattern, location, and distribution.
 – Skin integrity should be intact.

Palpation
· Texture should be smooth.
· Skin should feel dry and warm to touch.
· Skin should return quickly to its original shape when pinched.
· Nail beds should feel firm.

Psychiatric disorders

Anxiety disorder
Type: Obsessive-compulsive

Symptoms
· Repetitive thoughts causing stress
· Repetitive behaviors (for example, hand washing, counting, checking and rechecking door)
· Social impairment due to compulsive behaviors

Treatments
· Behavioral techniques
· Relaxation techniques
· Medications: Benzodiazepines, monoamine oxidase inhibitors, selective serotonin reuptake inhibitors (SSRIs), tricyclic antidepressants (TCAs)

Mood disorder
Type: Bipolar (manic-depressive)

Symptoms
· Manic: Elation, euphoria, agitation, hyperexcitability, hyperactivity, rapid thought and speech, decreased sleep
· Depressive: Inertia, social withdrawal, apathy, difficulty concentrating, slowed speech, psychomotor retardation, weight loss, slow gait

Treatments
· Manic: Lithium, valproic acid (Depakote)
· Depressive: Antidepressants (use cautiously; can trigger manic episode)

Personality disorder
Type: Borderline personality

Symptoms
· Unstable relationships
· Unstable self-image
· Unstable emotions
· Impulsivity

Treatments
· Psychotherapy
· Group therapy
· Family therapy
· Medications: Antidepressants, anxiolytics, antimanics, antipsychotics

Psychotic disorder
Type: Schizophrenia

Symptoms
· Delusions, hallucinations
· Apathy, blunted affect
· Asociality
· Thought disorder
· Bizarre behavior
· Poverty of speech

Treatments
· Psychosocial treatment and rehabilitation
· Psychotherapy
· Medications: Conventional antipsychotics, atypical antipsychotics (for example, clozapine)

Somatoform disorder
Type: Hypochondriasis

Symptoms
· Preoccupation with normal body functions
· Sensory, motor, or neurologic symptoms that don't follow a recognizable pattern of organic dysfunction and aren't related to abnormal physical findings

Treatments
· Psychotherapy
· Cognitive and behavioral therapy
· Medications: Benzodiazepines, SSRIs, TCAs

PQRST: The alphabet of pain assessment

Use the PQRST mnemonic device to obtain more information about the patient's pain. Asking these questions elicits important details about his pain.

Provocative or palliative
· What provokes or worsens your pain?
· What relieves the pain or causes it to subside?

Quality or quantity
· What does the pain feel like? Is it aching, intense, knifelike, burning, or cramping?
· Are you having pain right now? If so, is it more or less severe than usual?
· To what degree does the pain affect your normal activities?
· Do you have other symptoms along with the pain, such as nausea or vomiting?

Region and radiation
· Where is your pain?

· Does the pain radiate to other parts of your body?

Severity
· How severe is your pain? How would you rate it on a 0-to-10 scale, with 0 being no pain and 10 being the worst pain imaginable?
· How would you describe the intensity of your pain at its best? At its worst? Right now?

Timing
· When did your pain begin?
· At what time of day is your pain best? What time is it worst?
· Is the onset sudden or gradual?
· Is the pain constant or intermittent?

Numerical rating scale

A numerical rating scale can help the patient quantify his pain. Have him choose a number from 0 (indicating no pain) to 10 (indicating the worst pain imaginable) to reflect his current pain level. He can either circle the number on the scale itself or verbally state the number that best describes his pain.

No
pain   0   1   2   3   4   5   6   7   8   9   10   **Pain as
bad as it
can be**

Visual analog scale

To use the visual analog scale, ask the patient to place a mark on the scale to indicate his current level of pain as shown below.

No
pain
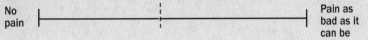
Pain as
bad as it
can be

Wong-Baker faces pain-rating scale

A pediatric patient or an adult patient with language difficulties may not be able to express the pain he's feeling. In such cases, use the pain intensity scale below. Ask the patient to choose the face that best represents the severity of his pain on a scale from 0 to 10.

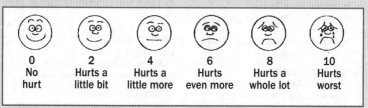

0	2	4	6	8	10
No hurt	Hurts a little bit	Hurts a little more	Hurts even more	Hurts a whole lot	Hurts worst

From Wong, D.L., et al. *Wong's Essentials of Pediatric Nursing*, 6th ed. St. Louis: Mosby–Year Book, Inc., 2001. Reprinted with permission.

Differentiating acute and chronic pain

Acute pain may cause certain physiologic and behavioral changes that you won't observe in a patient with chronic pain.

Type of pain	Physiologic evidence	Behavioral evidence
Acute	• Increased respirations • Increased pulse • Increased blood pressure • Dilated pupils • Diaphoresis	• Restlessness • Distraction • Worry • Distress
Chronic	• Normal respirations, pulse, blood pressure, and pupil size • No diaphoresis	• Reduced or absent physical activity • Despair, depression • Hopelessness

Age-related changes

Musculoskeletal system
- Alterations in joint surfaces, ligaments, tendons, and connective tissues
- Decreased bone density
- Decreased number and size of muscle fibers
- Atrophy of muscle tissue; replaced with fibrous tissue

Respiratory system
- Loss of elastic lung recoil
- Increased airway resistance
- Reduced vital capacity
- Decreased chest wall compliance
- Decreased gas exchange

Cardiovascular system
- Slight decrease in heart size
- Loss of cardiac contractile strength and efficiency
- Decrease in cardiac output of 30% to 35% by age 70
- Thickening of heart valve, causing incomplete valve closure (as well as a systolic murmur)
- Increase in left ventricular wall thickness of 25% between ages 30 and 80
- Fibrous tissue of sinoatrial node and internodal atrial tracts, causing atrial fibrillation and flutter
- Dilation and stretching of veins

- Decline in coronary artery blood flow of 35% between the ages 20 and 60
- Increased aortic rigidity
- Increased amount of time necessary for heart rate to return to normal after exercise
- Decreased strength and elasticity of blood vessels, contributing to arterial and venous insufficiency
- Decreased ability to respond to physical and emotional stress.

Central nervous system
- Reduced nerve conduction speed
- Decreased rate and magnitude of reflex response
- Decreased sensory activity
- Decreased myoneural transmission
- Decreased muscle contraction speed
- Increased postural sway (contributes to balance problems)
- Development of muscle tremors

Integumentary system
- Decreased subcutaneous adipose tissue
- Decreased elasticity of connective tissue
- Loss of sweat and sebaceous glands

How skin ages

This table lists skin changes that normally occur with aging.

Change	Findings in elderly people
Pigmentation	• Pale color
Thickness	• Wrinkling, especially on the face, arms, and legs • Parchmentlike appearance, especially over bony prominences and on the dorsal surfaces of the hands, feet, arms, and legs
Moisture	• Dry, flaky, and rough
Turgor	• "Tents" and stands alone, especially if the patient is dehydrated
Texture	• Numerous creases and lines

Effects of aging on the skin

These illustrations show the physical effects of aging on the skin. Notice how the flattened papillary dermis causes reduced contact between the epidermal and dermal layers of the skin.

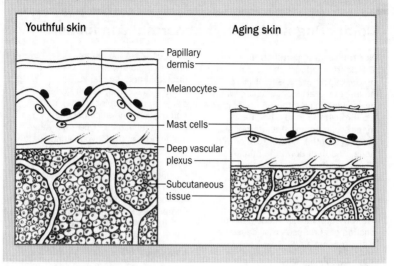

Electrocardiography

Comparing normal and abnormal conduction

Normal cardiac conduction

The heart's conduction system, shown below, begins at the sinoatrial (SA) node—the heart's pacemaker. When an impulse leaves the SA node, it travels through the atria along Bachmann's bundle and the internodal pathways to the atrioventricular (AV) node, and then down the bundle of His, along the bundle branches and, finally, down the Purkinje fibers to the ventricles.

Abnormal cardiac conduction

Altered automaticity, reentry, or conduction disturbances may cause cardiac arrhythmias.

Altered automaticity

Altered automaticity is the result of partial depolarization, which may increase the intrinsic rate of the SA node or lateral pacemakers, or may induce ectopic pacemakers to reach threshold and depolarize.

Automaticity may be altered by drugs, such as epinephrine, atropine, and digoxin, and such conditions as acidosis, alkalosis, hypoxia, myocardial infarction (MI), hypokalemia, and hypocalcemia. Examples of arrhythmias caused by altered automaticity include atrial fibrillation and flutter; supraventricular tachycardia; premature atrial, junctional, and ventricular complexes; ventricular tachycardia and fibrillation; and accelerated idioventricular and junctional rhythms.

Reentry

Ischemia or a deformity causes an abnormal circuit to develop within conductive fibers. Although current flow is blocked in one direction within the cir-

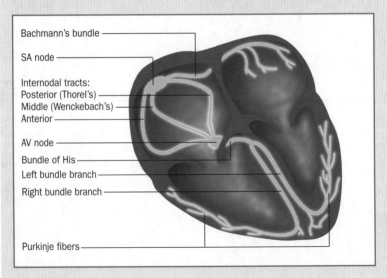

Bachmann's bundle ———

SA node ———

Internodal tracts:
Posterior (Thorel's) ———
Middle (Wenckebach's) ———
Anterior ———

AV node ———

Bundle of His ———
Left bundle branch ———
Right bundle branch ———

Purkinje fibers ———

cuit, the descending impulse can travel in the other direction. By the time the impulse completes the circuit, the previously depolarized tissue within the circuit is no longer refractory to stimulation, allowing reentry of the impulse and repetition of this cycle.

Conditions that increase the likelihood of reentry include hyperkalemia, myocardial ischemia, and the use of certain antiarrhythmic drugs. Reentry may be responsible for such arrhythmias as paroxysmal supraventricular tachycardia; premature atrial, junctional, and ventricular complexes; and ventricular tachycardia.

An alternative reentry mechanism depends on the presence of a congenital accessory pathway linking the atria and the ventricles outside the AV junction; for example, Wolff-Parkinson-White syndrome.

Conduction disturbances

Conduction disturbances occur when impulses are conducted too quickly or too slowly. Possible causes include trauma, drug toxicity, myocardial ischemia, MI, and electrolyte abnormalities. The AV blocks occur as a result of conduction disturbances.

Einthoven's triangle

The axes of the three bipolar limb leads (I, II, and III) form a shape known as *Einthoven's triangle.* Because the electrodes for these leads are about equidistant from the heart, the triangle is equilateral.

The axis of lead I extends from shoulder to shoulder, with the right-arm lead being the negative electrode and the left-arm lead being the positive electrode. The axis of lead II runs from the negative right-arm lead electrode to the positive left-leg lead electrode. The axis of lead III extends from the negative left-arm lead electrode to the positive left-leg lead electrode.

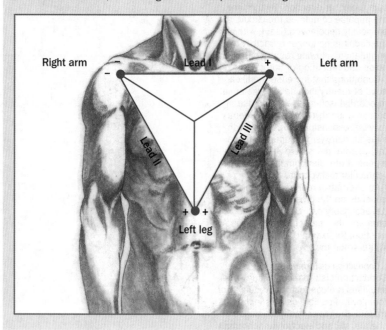

Augmented leads

Leads aV$_R$, aV$_L$, and aV$_F$ are called *augmented leads.* They measure electrical activity between one limb and a single electrode. Lead aV$_R$ provides no specific view of the heart. Lead aV$_L$ shows electrical activity coming from the heart's lateral wall. Lead aV$_F$ shows electrical activity coming from the heart's inferior wall.

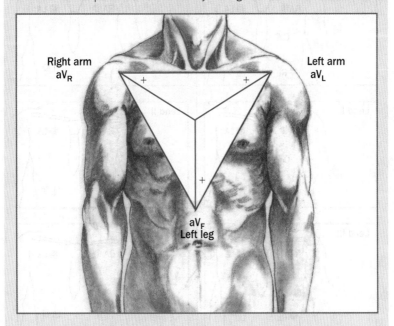

Positioning cardiac monitoring leads

Five-leadwire system	Three-leadwire system
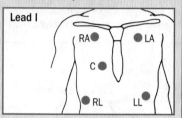 Lead I	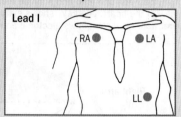 Lead I
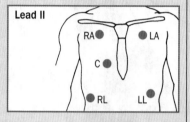 Lead II	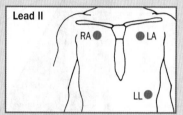 Lead II
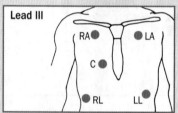 Lead III	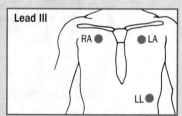 Lead III
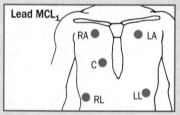 Lead MCL$_1$	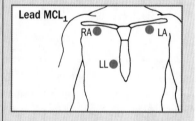 Lead MCL$_1$
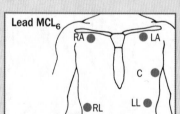 Lead MCL$_6$	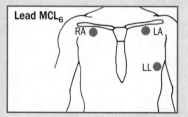 Lead MCL$_6$

Normal ECG

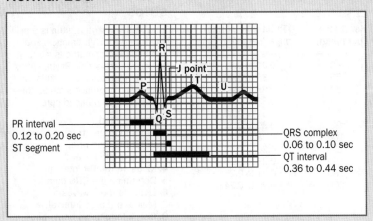

PR interval
0.12 to 0.20 sec
ST segment

QRS complex
0.06 to 0.10 sec
QT interval
0.36 to 0.44 sec

ECG grid

This electrocardiogram (ECG) grid shows the horizontal axis and vertical axis and their respective measurement values.

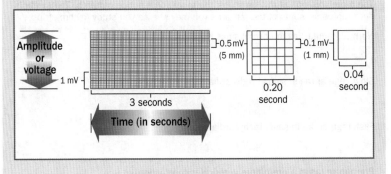

Normal QTc intervals

Heart rate (per minute)	QTc interval normal range (seconds)
40	0.41 to 0.51
50	0.38 to 0.46
60	0.35 to 0.43
70	0.33 to 0.41
80	0.32 to 0.39
90	0.30 to 0.36
100	0.28 to 0.34
120	0.26 to 0.32
150	0.23 to 0.28
180	0.21 to 0.25
200	0.20 to 0.24

Interpreting rhythm strips

Interpreting a rhythm strip is a skill developed through practice. You can use several methods, as long as you're consistent. Rhythm strip analysis requires a sequential and systematic approach such as the 8-step method outlined here.

8-step method

1. Determine the rhythm.
2. Determine the rate.
3. Evaluate the P wave.
4. Measure the PR interval.
5. Determine the QRS duration.
6. Examine the T waves.
7. Measure the QT interval.
8. Check for ectopic beats and other abnormalities.

Rhythm strip patterns

The more you look at rhythm strips, the more you'll notice patterns. The symbols here represent some of the patterns you may see as you study rhythm strips.

Normal, regular (as in normal sinus rhythm)

Slow, regular (as in sinus bradycardia)

Fast, regular (as in sinus tachycardia)

Premature (as in a premature ventricular contraction)

Grouped (as in type I second-degree atrioventricular block)

Irregularly irregular (as in atrial fibrillation)

Paroxysm or burst (as in paroxysmal atrial tachycardia)

Methods of measuring rhythm

Paper-and-pencil method

· Place the electrocardiogram (ECG) strip on a flat surface.
· Position the straight edge of a piece of paper along the strip's baseline.
· Move the paper up slightly so the straight edge is near the peak of the R wave.
· With a pencil, mark the paper at the R waves of two consecutive QRS complexes, as shown below. This is the R-R interval.
· Move the paper across the strip lining up the two marks with succeeding R-R intervals. If the distance for each R-R interval is the same, the ventricular rhythm is regular. If the distance varies, the rhythm is irregular.
· Use the same method to measure the distance between P waves (the P-P interval) and determine whether the atrial rhythm is regular or irregular.

Calipers method

· With the ECG on a flat surface, place one point of the calipers on the peak of the first R wave of two consecutive QRS complexes.
· Adjust the calipers' legs so the other point is on the peak of the next R wave, as shown below. The distance is the R-R interval.
· Pivot the first point of the calipers toward the third R wave and note whether it falls on the peak of that wave.
· Check succeeding R-R intervals in the same way. If they're all the same, the ventricular rhythm is regular. If they vary, the rhythm is irregular.
· Using the same method, measure the P-P intervals to determine whether the atrial rhythm is regular or irregular.

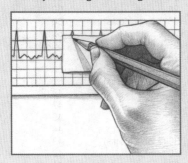

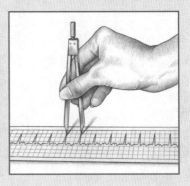

Calculating heart rate

This table can help make the sequencing method of determining heart rate more precise. After counting the number of blocks between R waves, use this table to find the rate. For example, if you count 20 small blocks or 4 large blocks between R waves, the heart rate is 75 beats/minute. To calculate the atrial rate, follow the same method using P waves.

Rapid estimate

This rapid-rate calculation is also called the *countdown method*. Using the number of large blocks between R waves or P waves as a guide, you can rapidly estimate ventricular or atrial rates by memorizing the sequence "300, 150, 100, 75, 60, 50."

Number of small blocks	Heart rate
5 (1 large block)	300
6	250
7	214
8	188
9	167
10 (2 large blocks)	150
11	136
12	125
13	115
14	107
15 (3 large blocks)	100
16	94
17	88
18	83
19	79
20 (4 large blocks)	75
21	71
22	68
23	65
24	63
25 (5 large blocks)	60
26	58
27	56
28	54
29	52
30 (6 large blocks)	50
31	48
32	47
33	45
34	44
35 (7 large blocks)	43
36	42
37	41
38	39
39	38
40 (8 large blocks)	37

Precordial lead placement

To record a 12-lead electrocardiogram, place electrodes on the patient's arms and legs (with the ground lead on the patient's right leg). The three standard limb leads (I, II, and III) and the three augmented leads (aV$_R$, aV$_L$, and aV$_F$) are recorded using these electrodes. Then, to record the precordial chest leads, place electrodes as follows:

V$_1$—Fourth intercostal space (ICS), right sternal border
V$_2$—Fourth ICS, left sternal border
V$_3$—Midway between V$_2$ and V$_4$
V$_4$—Fifth ICS, left midclavicular line
V$_5$—Fifth ICS, left anterior axillary line
V$_6$—Fifth ICS, left midaxillary line

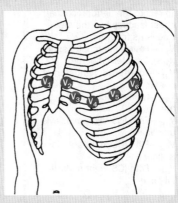

V$_1$

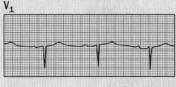

V$_4$

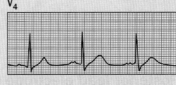

V$_2$

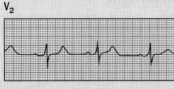

V$_5$

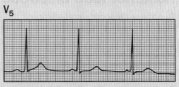

V$_3$

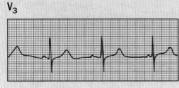

V$_6$

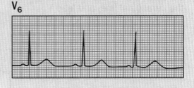

Right precordial lead placement

To record the right precordial chest leads, place the electrodes as follows:

V_{1R}—Fourth intercostal space (ICS), left sternal border

V_{2R}—Fourth ICS, right sternal border

V_{3R}—Halfway between V_{2R} and V_{4R}

V_{4R}—Fifth ICS, right midclavicular line

V_{5R}—Fifth ICS, right anterior axillary line

V_{6R}—Fifth ICS, right midaxillary line

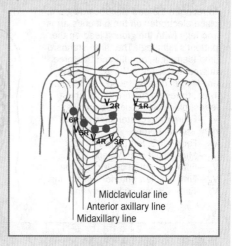

Midclavicular line
Anterior axillary line
Midaxillary line

Posterior lead electrode placement

To ensure an accurate electrocardiogram reading, make sure the posterior electrodes V_7, V_8, and V_9 are placed at the same level horizontally as the V_6 lead at the fifth intercostal space. Place lead V_7 at the posterior axillary line, lead V_9 at the paraspinal line, and lead V_8 halfway between leads V_7 and V_9.

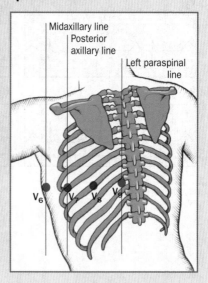

Midaxillary line
Posterior axillary line
Left paraspinal line

Limb lead placement

Proper lead placement is critical for accurate recording of cardiac rhythms. These drawings show correct electrode placement for the six limb leads. RA stands for right arm; LA, left arm; RL, right leg; and LL, left leg. A plus sign (+) indicates a positive pole, a minus sign (–) indicates a negative pole, and G indicates a ground. Below each drawing is a sample electrocardiogram strip for that lead.

Lead I
Connects the right arm (negative pole) with the left arm (positive pole).

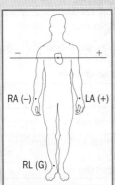

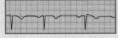

Lead II
Connects the right arm (negative pole) with the left leg (positive pole).

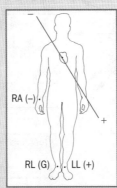

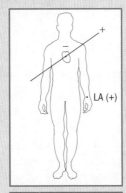

Lead III
Connects the left arm (negative pole) with the left leg (positive pole).

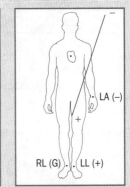

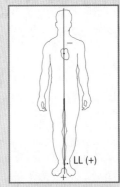

Lead aV$_R$
Connects the right arm (positive pole) with the heart (negative pole).

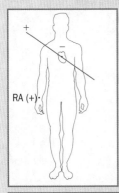

Lead aV$_L$
Connects the left arm (positive pole) with the heart (negative pole).

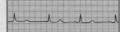

Lead aV$_F$
Connects the left leg (positive pole) with the heart (negative pole).

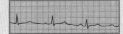

Electrical activity and the 12-lead ECG

Each of the leads on a 12-lead electrocardiogram (ECG) views the heart from a different angle. These illustrations show the direction of electrical activity (depolarization) monitored by each lead and the 12 views of the heart.

Views reflected on a 12-lead ECG

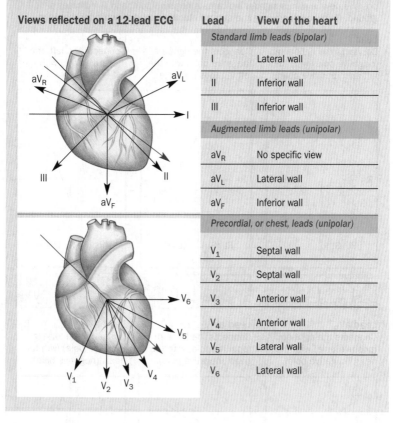

Lead	View of the heart
Standard limb leads (bipolar)	
I	Lateral wall
II	Inferior wall
III	Inferior wall
Augmented limb leads (unipolar)	
aV_R	No specific view
aV_L	Lateral wall
aV_F	Inferior wall
Precordial, or chest, leads (unipolar)	
V_1	Septal wall
V_2	Septal wall
V_3	Anterior wall
V_4	Anterior wall
V_5	Lateral wall
V_6	Lateral wall

Electrical axis determination: Quadrant method

This chart will help you quickly determine the direction of a patient's electrical axis. Observe the deflections of the QRS complexes in leads I and aV$_F$. Lead I indicates whether impulses are moving to the right or left, and lead aV$_F$ indicates whether they're moving up or down. Then check the chart to determine whether the patient's axis is normal or has a left,

right, or extreme right deviation.
• Normal axis: QRS-complex deflection is positive or upright in both leads.
• Left axis deviation: Lead I is upright and lead aV$_F$ points down.
• Right axis deviation: Lead I points down and lead aV$_F$ is upright.
• Extreme right axis deviation: Both waves point down.

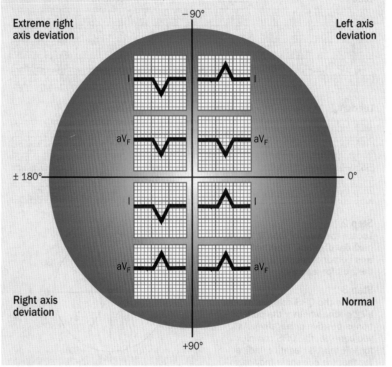

Electrical axis determination: Degree method

The degree method provides a more precise measurement of the electrical axis. It allows you to identify a patient's electrical axis by degrees on the hexaxial system, not just by quadrant. It also allows you to determine the axis even if the QRS complex isn't clearly positive or negative in leads I and aV$_F$. To use this method, take these steps.

Step 1
Identify the limb lead with the smallest QRS complex or the equiphasic QRS complex. In this example, it's lead III.

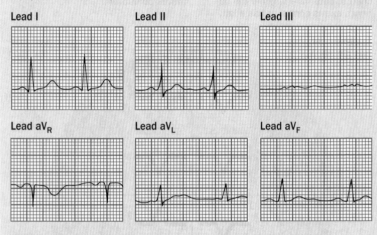

Lead I   Lead II   Lead III

Lead aV$_R$ Lead aV$_L$ Lead aV$_F$

Step 2
Locate the axis for lead III on the hexaxial diagram. Then find the axis perpendicular to it, which is the axis for lead aV$_R$.

Step 3
Examine the QRS complex in lead aV$_R$, noting whether the deflection is positive or negative. As you can see, the QRS complex for this lead is negative, indicating that the current is moving toward the negative pole of aV$_R$, which is in the right lower quadrant at +30 degrees on the hexaxial diagram. So the electrical axis here is normal at +30 degrees.

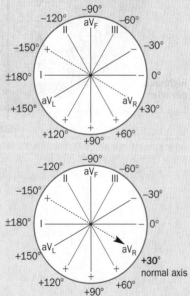

ECG changes in angina

These are some classic electrocardiogram (ECG) changes involving the T wave and ST segment that you may see when monitoring a patient with angina.

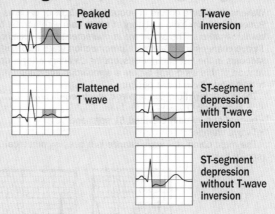

Peaked T wave

T-wave inversion

Flattened T wave

ST-segment depression with T-wave inversion

ST-segment depression without T-wave inversion

ECG changes in Prinzmetal's angina

This illustration shows a 12-lead electrocardiogram (ECG) of a patient with Prinzmetal's angina. Marked ST-segment elevations appear in leads that are monitoring the heart area where the coronary artery spasm occurs. The elevation occurs during chest pain and resolves when pain subsides. T waves are usually of normal size and configuration.

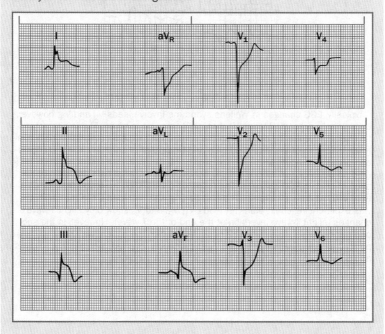

Recognizing Wellens syndrome

Wellens syndrome occurs in about 14% to 18% of patients with unstable angina. Patients typically have a history of chest pain with normal or slightly elevated cardiac markers. The syndrome is characterized by specific ST-segment and T-wave changes that indicate a preinfarction state involving a critical proximal stenosis in the left anterior descending coronary artery. Identification and intervention of this syndrome before a myocardial infarction (MI) can reduce morbidity and mortality in these patients.

The characteristic precordial-lead electrocardiogram (ECG) changes include:
· no pathologic Q waves
· normal or minimally elevated ST segments
· T-wave changes.

The most common T-wave change is a deep symmetrical T-wave inversion (shown here).

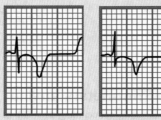

Less common is a biphasic T-wave pattern (shown here).

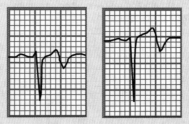

Typically, ECG changes in Wellens syndrome involve leads V_2 and V_3; however, occasionally precordial leads V_1 through V_6 may be involved. These characteristic changes frequently occur when the patient isn't experiencing chest pain. Early identification of Wellens syndrome and treatment of coronary artery stenosis can prevent an acute MI.

Some patients experience a delay between the onset of pain and the appearance of certain ECG changes. The following pages show 12-lead ECGs for a patient with Wellens syndrome. The first tracing was recorded while the patient was experiencing chest pain. Yet leads V_1, V_2, and V_3 show only slight T-wave changes (slight T-wave inversion at the end of the T wave). However, in the second tracing, which was taken 12 hours later when the patient was no longer experiencing pain, leads V_2 through V_6 show deeply inverted, symmetrical T waves and ST-segment abnormalities typical of Wellens syndrome.

ECG changes during anginal pain

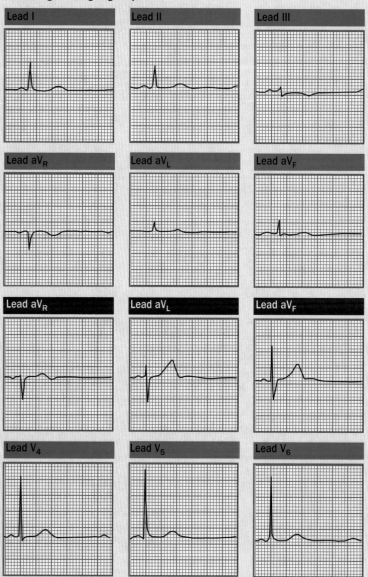

(continued)

Recognizing Wellens syndrome *(continued)*

ECG changes after cessation of anginal pain

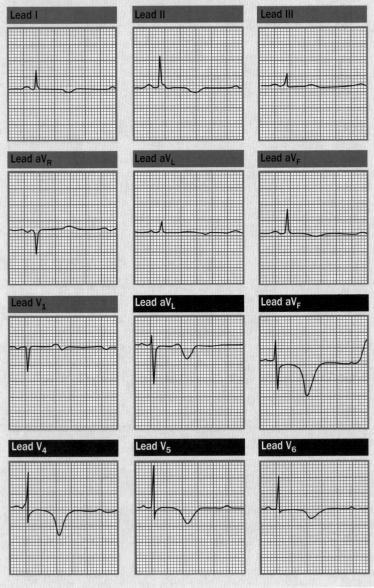

Stages of myocardial ischemia, injury, and infarct

Ischemia

Ischemia is the first stage and indicates that blood flow and oxygen demand are out of balance. It can be resolved by improving flow or reducing oxygen needs. Electrocardiogram (ECG) changes indicate ST-segment depression or T-wave changes.

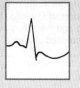

Myocardial ischemia
- T-wave inversion
- ST-depression

Injury

The second stage, injury, occurs when the ischemia is prolonged enough to damage the area of the heart. ECG changes usually reveal ST-segment elevation (usually in two or more contiguous leads).

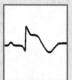

Myocardial injury
- ST-segment elevation
- T-wave inversion

Infarct

Infarct is the third stage and occurs with actual death of myocardial cells. Scar tissue eventually replaces the dead tissue, and the damage caused is irreversible.

In the earliest stage of a myocardial infarction (MI), hyperacute or very tall T waves may be seen on the ECG. Within hours, the T waves become inverted and ST-segment elevation occurs in the leads facing the area of damage. The pathologic Q wave is the last change to occur in the evolution of an MI and is the only permanent ECG evidence of myocardial necrosis.

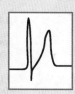

Myocardial infarction
- Hyperacute T waves (earliest stage)

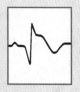

- ST-segment elevation
- T-wave inversion
- Pathologic Q waves
  – in 90% of ST-segment elevation MI
  – in 25% non–ST-segment elevation MI

Locating myocardial damage

After you've noted characteristic lead changes in an acute myocardial infarction, use this table to identify the areas of damage. Match the lead changes (ST-segment elevation, abnormal Q waves) in the second column with the affected wall in the first column and the artery involved in the third column. The fourth column shows reciprocal lead changes.

Wall affected	Leads	Artery involved	Reciprocal changes
Anterior	V_1, V_2, V_3, V_4	Left coronary artery, left anterior descending (LAD)	II, III, aV_F
Anterolateral	I, aV_L, V_3, V_4, V_5, V_6	LAD and diagonal branches, circumflex and marginal branches	II, III, aV_F
Anteroseptal	V_1, V_2	LAD	None
Inferior	II, III, aV_F	Right coronary artery (RCA)	I, aV_L
Lateral	I, aV_L, V_5, V_6	Circumflex branch of left coronary artery	II, III, aV_F
Posterior	V_1, V_2	RCA or circumflex	V_1, V_2, V_3, V_4 (R greater than S in V_1 and V_2, ST-segment depression, elevated T wave)
Right ventricular	V_{4R}, V_{5R}, V_{6R}	RCA	None

Left ventricular hypertrophy

Left ventricular hypertrophy can lead to heart failure or myocardial infarction. The rhythm strips shown here illustrate key electrocardiogram changes of left ventricular hypertrophy as they occur in selected leads: a large S wave (shaded area in left strip) in V_1 and a large R wave (shaded area in right strip) in V_5. If the depth (in mm) of the S wave in V_1 added to the height (in mm) of the R wave in V_5 exceeds 35 mm, then the patient has left ventricular hypertrophy.

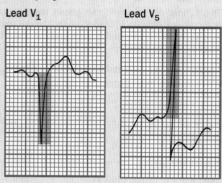

Lead V_1 Lead V_5

Understanding RBBB

In right bundle-branch block (RBBB), the initial impulse activates the interventricular septum from left to right, just as in normal activation (arrow 1). Next, the left bundle branch activates the left ventricle (arrow 2). The impulse then crosses the interventricular septum to activate the right ventricle (arrow 3).

In this disorder, the QRS complex exceeds 0.12 second and has a different configuration, sometimes resembling rabbit ears or the letter "M." Septal depolarization isn't affected in lead V_1, so the initial small R wave remains.

The R wave is followed by an S wave, which represents left ventricular depolarization, and a tall R wave (called *R prime,* or *R'*), which represents late right ventricular depolarization. The T wave is negative in this lead; however, the negative deflection is called a *secondary T-wave change* and isn't clinically significant.

The opposite occurs in lead V_6. A small Q wave is followed by depolarization of the left ventricle, which produces a tall R wave. Depolarization of the right ventricle then causes a broad S wave. In lead V_6, the T wave should be positive.

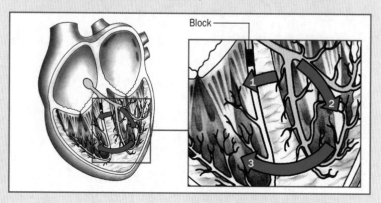

Block

Recognizing RBBB

This 12-lead electrocardiogram shows the characteristic changes of right bundle-branch block (RBBB). In lead V_1, note the rsR′ pattern and T-wave inversion. In lead V_6, note the widened S wave and the upright T wave. Also note the prolonged QRS complexes.

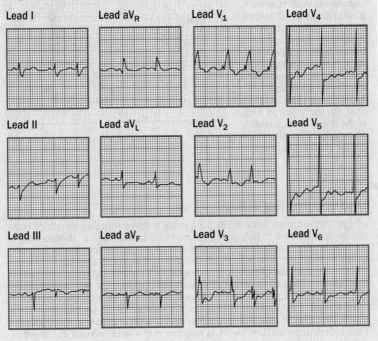

Understanding LBBB

In left bundle-branch block (LBBB), an impulse first travels down the right bundle branch (arrow 1). Then it activates the interventricular septum from right to left (arrow 2) ventricle, the opposite of normal activation. Finally, the impulse activates the left ventricle (arrow 3).

On an electrocardiogram, the QRS complex exceeds 0.12 second because the ventricles are activated sequentially, not simultaneously. As the wave of depolarization spreads from the right ventricle to the left, a wide S wave appears in lead V_1 with a positive T wave. The S wave may be preceded by a Q wave or a small R wave.

In lead V_6, no initial Q wave occurs. A tall, notched R wave, or a slurred one, appears as the impulse spreads from right to left. This initial positive deflection is a sign of LBBB. The T wave is negative.

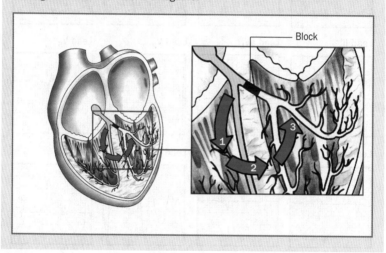

Recognizing LBBB

This 12-lead electrocardiogram shows characteristic changes of left bundle-branch block (LBBB). All leads have prolonged QRS complexes. In lead V_1, note the QS wave pattern. In lead V_6, note the slurred R wave and T-wave inversion. The elevated ST segments and upright T waves in leads V_1 and V_4 are also common in this condition.

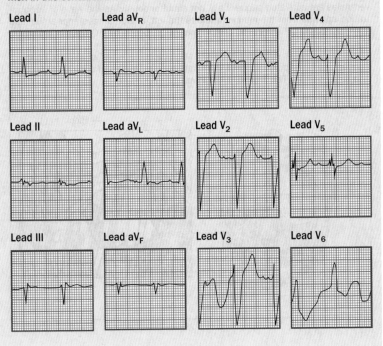

Lead I   Lead aV_R Lead V_1 Lead V_4

Lead II   Lead aV_L Lead V_2 Lead V_5

Lead III   Lead aV_F Lead V_3 Lead V_6

Pericarditis

Electrocardiogram changes in acute pericarditis evolve through two stages:
• Stage 1—Diffuse ST-segment elevations of 1 to 2 mm in most limb leads and most precordial leads reflect the inflammatory process. Upright T waves appear in most leads. The ST-segment and T-wave changes are typically seen in leads I, II, III, aV_R, aV_F, and V_2 through V_6.
• Stage 2—As pericarditis resolves, the ST-segment elevation and accompanying T-wave inversion resolves in most leads.

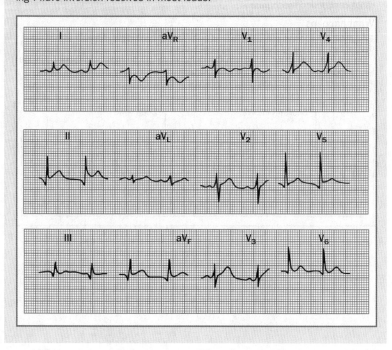

Wolff-Parkinson-White syndrome

Electrical impulses don't always follow normal conduction pathways in the heart. In Wolff-Parkinson-White (WPW) syndrome, electrical impulses enter the ventricles from the atria through an accessory pathway that bypasses the atrioventricular junction.

WPW syndrome is clinically significant because the accessory pathway—in this case, Kent's bundle—may result in paroxysmal tachyarrhythmias by reentry and rapid conduction mechanisms.

What happens
· A delta wave occurs at the beginning of the QRS complex, usually causing a distinctive slurring or hump in its initial slope.
· On a 12-lead electrocardiogram the delta wave will be most pronounced in the leads looking at the part of the heart where the accessory pathway is located.
· The delta wave shortens the PR interval in WPW syndrome.

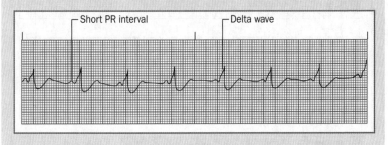

Normal sinus rhythm

To recognize an arrhythmia, you first must recognize normal sinus rhythm. Normal sinus rhythm records an impulse that starts in the sinus node and progresses to the ventricles through the normal conduction pathway. Alterations in this pathway may lead to cardiac arrhythmias. The normal sinus rhythm shown here represents normal impulse conduction through the heart.

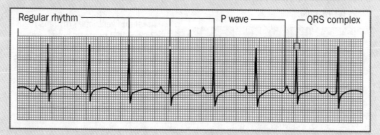

Regular rhythm — — P wave — — QRS complex

Lead II
Atrial rhythm: regular
Ventricular rhythm: regular
Atrial rate: 60 to 100 beats/minute (80 beats/minute shown)
Ventricular rate: 60 to 100 beats/minute (80 beats/minute shown)
P wave: normally shaped (All P waves have a similar size and shape; a P wave precedes each QRS complex.)
PR interval: within normal limits (0.12 to 0.20 second) and constant (0.20-second duration shown)

QRS complex: within normal limits (0.06 to 0.10 second) (All QRS complexes have the same configuration. The duration shown here is 0.12 second.)
T wave: normally shaped; upright and rounded (Each QRS complex is followed by a T wave.)
QT interval: within normal limits (0.36 to 0.44 second) and constant (0.44-second duration shown)

Types of cardiac arrhythmias

This chart reviews many common cardiac arrhythmias and outlines their features, causes, and treatments.

Arrhythmia	Features

Sinus tachycardia

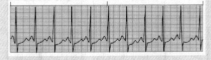

- Atrial and ventricular rhythms regular
- Rate > 100 beats/minute; rarely, > 160 beats/minute
- Normal P wave preceding each QRS complex

Sinus bradycardia

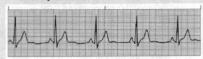

- Atrial and ventricular rhythms regular
- Rate < 60 beats/minute
- Normal P waves preceding each QRS complex

Paroxysmal supraventricular tachycardia

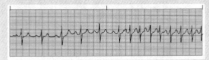

- Atrial and ventricular rhythms regular
- Heart rate > 160 beats/minute; rarely exceeds 250 beats/minute
- P waves regular but aberrant; difficult to differentiate from preceding T wave
- P wave preceding each QRS complex
- Sudden onset and termination of arrhythmia

Causes	Treatment
• Normal physiologic response to fever, exercise, anxiety, pain, and dehydration; may also accompany shock, left ventricular failure, cardiac tamponade, hyperthyroidism, anemia, hypovolemia, pulmonary embolism (PE), and anterior wall myocardial infarction (MI) • May also occur with atropine, epinephrine, isoproterenol, quinidine, caffeine, alcohol, cocaine, amphetamine, and nicotine use	• Correction of underlying cause • Beta-adrenergic blockers or calcium channel blockers
• Normal in a well-conditioned heart, as in an athlete • Increased intracranial pressure; increased vagal tone due to straining during defecation, vomiting, intubation, or mechanical ventilation; sick sinus syndrome; hypothyroidism; and inferior wall MI • May also occur with anticholinesterase, beta-adrenergic blocker, digoxin, and morphine use	• Correction of underlying cause • Advanced cardiac life support (ACLS) protocol for administration of atropine for low cardiac output, dizziness, weakness, altered level of consciousness, or low blood pressure • Temporary or permanent pacemaker • Dopamine or epinephrine infusion
• Intrinsic abnormality of atrioventricular (AV) conduction system • Physical or psychological stress, hypoxia, hypokalemia, cardiomyopathy, congenital heart disease, MI, valvular disease, Wolff-Parkinson-White syndrome, cor pulmonale, hyperthyroidism, and systemic hypertension • Digoxin toxicity; use of caffeine, marijuana, or central nervous system stimulants	• If patient is unstable, immediate cardioversion • If patient is stable, vagal stimulation: Valsalva's maneuver, carotid sinus massage, and adenosine • If cardiac function is preserved, treatment priority: calcium channel blocker, beta-adrenergic blocker, digoxin, and cardioversion; then consider procainamide or amiodarone, if each preceding treatment is ineffective in rhythm conversion • If the ejection fraction is less than 40% or if the patient is in heart failure, treatment order: digoxin, amiodarone, then diltiazem

(continued)

Types of cardiac arrhythmias *(continued)*

Arrhythmia	Features
Atrial flutter 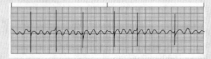	• Atrial rhythm regular; rate 250 to 400 beats/minute • Ventricular rate variable, depending on degree of AV block (usually 60 to 100 beats/minute) • No P wave; atrial activity appears as flutter waves (F waves); sawtooth configuration common in lead II • QRS complexes uniform in shape, but usually irregular in rate
Atrial fibrillation 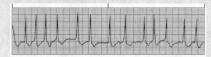	• Atrial rhythm grossly irregular; rate > 400 beats/minute • Ventricular rhythm grossly irregular • QRS complexes of uniform configuration and duration • PR interval indiscernible • No P waves; atrial activity appears as erratic; irregular, baseline fibrillatory waves (f waves)
Junctional rhythm 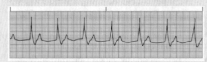	• Atrial and ventricular rhythms regular; atrial rate 40 to 60 beats/minute; ventricular rate usually 40 to 60 beats/minute (60 to 100 beats/minute is accelerated junctional rhythm) • P waves preceding, hidden within (absent), or after QRS complex; usually inverted if visible • PR interval (when present) < 0.12 second • QRS complex configuration and duration normal, except in aberrant conduction
First-degree AV block 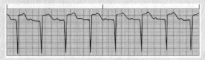	• Atrial and ventricular rhythms regular • PR interval > 0.20 second • P wave precedes QRS complex • QRS complex normal

Causes	Treatment
• Heart failure, tricuspid or mitral valve disease, PE, cor pulmonale, inferior wall MI, and pericarditis • Digoxin toxicity	• If patient is unstable with a ventricular rate > 150 beats/minute, immediate cardioversion • If patient is stable, follow ACLS protocol for cardioversion and drug therapy, which may include calcium channel blockers, beta-adrenergic blockers, amiodarone, or digoxin • Anticoagulation therapy may also be necessary • Radio-frequency ablation to control rhythm
• Heart failure, chronic obstructive pulmonary disease, thyrotoxicosis, constrictive pericarditis, ischemic heart disease, sepsis, PE, rheumatic heart disease, hypertension, mitral stenosis, atrial irritation, or complication of coronary bypass or valve replacement surgery • Nifedipine and digoxin use	• If patient is unstable with a ventricular rate > 150 beats/minute, immediate cardioversion • If patient is stable, follow ACLS protocol and drug therapy, which may include calcium channel blockers, beta-adrenergic blockers, amiodarone, or digoxin • Anticoagulation therapy may also be necessary • In a patient with refractory atrial fibrillation uncontrolled by drugs, radio-frequency catheter ablation
• Inferior wall MI or ischemia, hypoxia, vagal stimulation, and sick sinus syndrome • Acute rheumatic fever • Valve surgery • Digoxin toxicity	• Correction of underlying cause • Atropine for slow rate that produces symptoms • Pacemaker insertion if patient doesn't respond to drugs • Discontinuation of digoxin if appropriate
• May be seen in healthy persons • Inferior wall MI or ischemia, hypothyroidism, hypokalemia, and hyperkalemia • Digoxin toxicity; use of quinidine, procainamide, beta-adrenergic blockers, calcium channel blockers, or amiodarone	• Correction of underlying cause • Possibly atropine if severe bradycardia develops and produces symptoms • Cautious use of digoxin, calcium channel blockers, and beta-adrenergic blockers

(continued)

Types of cardiac arrhythmias *(continued)*

Arrhythmia	Features

Second-degree AV block Mobitz I (Wenckebach)

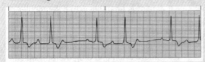

- Atrial rhythm regular
- Ventricular rhythm irregular
- Atrial rate exceeds ventricular rate
- PR interval progressively longer with each cycle until QRS complex disappears (dropped beat); PR interval shorter after dropped beat

Second-degree AV block Mobitz II

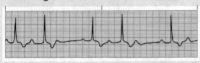

- Atrial rhythm regular
- Ventricular rhythm regular or irregular, with varying degree of block
- P-R interval constant for conducted beats
- P waves normal size and configuration, but some P waves not followed by a QRS complex

Third-degree AV block (complete heart block)

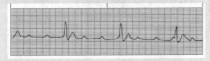

- Atrial rhythm regular
- Ventricular rhythm regular and rate slower than atrial rate
- No relation between P waves and QRS complexes
- No constant PR interval
- QRS duration normal (junctional pacemaker) or wide and bizarre (ventricular pacemaker)

Premature ventricular contraction (PVC)

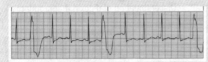

- Atrial rhythm regular
- Ventricular rhythm irregular
- QRS complex premature, usually followed by a complete compensatory pause
- QRS complex wide and distorted, usually > 0.12 second
- Premature QRS complexes occurring alone, in pairs, or in threes, alternating with normal beats; focus from one or more sites
- Ominous when clustered, multifocal, or with R wave on T pattern

Causes	Treatment
• Inferior wall MI, cardiac surgery, acute rheumatic fever, and vagal stimulation • Digoxin toxicity; use of propranolol, quinidine, or procainamide	• Treatment of underlying cause • Atropine or temporary pacemaker for bradycardia that produces symptoms • Discontinuation of digoxin if appropriate
• Severe coronary artery disease (CAD), anterior wall MI, and acute myocarditis • Digoxin toxicity	• Temporary or permanent pacemaker • Atropine, dopamine, or epinephrine for bradycardia that produces symptoms • Discontinuation of digoxin, if appropriate
• Inferior or anterior wall MI, congenital abnormality, rheumatic fever, hypoxia, postoperative complication of mitral valve replacement, postprocedure complication of radio-frequency ablation in or near AV nodal tissue, Lev's disease (fibrosis and calcification that spreads from cardiac structures to the conductive tissue), and Lenègre's disease (conductive tissue fibrosis) • Digoxin toxicity	• Temporary or permanent pacemaker • Atropine, dopamine, or epinephrine for bradycardia that produces symptoms
• Heart failure; old or acute MI, ischemia, or contusion; myocardial irritation by ventricular catheter or a pacemaker; hypercapnia; hypokalemia; hypocalcemia and hypomagnesemia • Drug toxicity (digoxin, aminophylline, tricyclic antidepressants, beta-adrenergic blockers, isoproterenol, or dopamine) • Caffeine, tobacco, or alcohol use • Psychological stress, anxiety, pain, or exercise	• If warranted, amiodarone, procainamide, or lidocaine I.V. • Treatment of underlying cause • Discontinuation of drug causing toxicity • Potassium chloride I.V. if PVCs are induced by hypokalemia • Magnesium sulfate I.V. if PVCs are induced by hypomagnesemia

(continued)

Types of cardiac arrhythmias *(continued)*

Arrhythmia	Features
Ventricular tachycardia 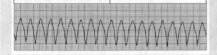	• Ventricular rate 100 to 220 beats/minute, rhythm usually regular • QRS complexes wide, bizarre, and independent of P waves • P waves not discernible • May start and stop suddenly
Ventricular fibrillation 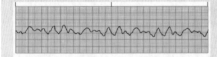	• Ventricular rhythm and rate chaotic and rapid • QRS complexes wide and irregular; no visible P waves
Asystole 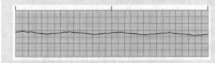	• No atrial or ventricular rate or rhythm • No discernible P waves, QRS complexes, or T waves

Causes	Treatment
• Myocardial ischemia, MI, or aneurysm; CAD; rheumatic heart disease; mitral valve prolapse; heart failure; cardiomyopathy; ventricular catheters; hypokalemia; hypercalcemia; hypomagnesemia; and PE • Digoxin, procainamide, epinephrine, or quinidine toxicity • Anxiety	• With pulse: If hemodynamically stable with monomorphic QRS complexes, administration of amiodarone, procainamide, sotalol, or lidocaine (follow ACLS protocol); if drug is unsuccessful, cardioversion • If polymorphic QRS complexes and normal QT interval, administer amiodarone, beta-adrenergic blockers, lidocaine, procainamide, or sotalol (follow ACLS protocol); if drug is unsuccessful, cardioversion • If polymorphic QRS and QT interval is prolonged, magnesium I.V., then overdrive pacing if rhythm persists; may also administer isoproterenol, phenytoin, or lidocaine • If pulseless, initiate cardiopulmonary resuscitation (CPR); follow ACLS protocol for defibrillation and administration of epinephrine or vasopressin, followed by amiodarone or lidocaine and, if ineffective, magnesium sulfate or procainamide • Implanted cardioverter-defibrillator if recurrent ventricular tachycardia
• Myocardial ischemia, MI, untreated ventricular tachycardia, R-on-T phenomenon, hypokalemia, hyperkalemia, hypercalcemia, hypoxemia, alkalosis, electric shock, and hypothermia • Digoxin, epinephrine, or quinidine toxicity	• CPR; follow ACLS protocol for defibrillation and administration of epinephrine or vasopressin, amiodarone, or lidocaine and, if ineffective, magnesium sulfate or procainamide • Implanted cardioverter-defibrillator if at risk for recurrent ventricular fibrillation
• Myocardial ischemia, MI, aortic valve disease, heart failure, hypoxia, hypokalemia, severe acidosis, electric shock, ventricular arrhythmia, AV block, PE, heart rupture, cardiac tamponade, hyperkalemia, and electromechanical dissociation • Cocaine overdose	• CPR; follow ACLS protocol for transcutaneous pacing and administration of epinephrine and atropine

Safety issues with defibrillation

Precautions must be taken when defibrillating a patient. A defibrillator delivers electrical current that could cause harm to bystanders. Note the following precautions and special situations when using a defibrillator.

Defibrillating a patient

Make sure that no one is in contact with the patient before discharging the defibrillator to avoid the electrical charge transferring from the patient to a bystander or rescuer.

Defibrillating a patient with an implantable cardioverter-defibrillator or pacemaker

Avoid placing the defibrillator paddles or pads directly over the implanted device. Place them at least 1″ (2.5 cm) away from the device.

Defibrillating a patient with a transdermal medication patch

Avoid placing the defibrillator paddles or pads directly on top of a transdermal medication patch, such as a nitroglycerin, nicotine, analgesic, or hormone replacement patch. The patch can block delivery of energy and cause a small burn to the skin. Remove the medication patch and wipe the area clean before defibrillation.

Defibrillating a patient near water

Water is a conductor of electricity and may provide a pathway for energy from the defibrillator to the rescuers treating the victim. Remove the patient from freestanding water and dry his chest before defibrillation.

Using an automated external defibrillator

It's estimated that 70% of sudden cardiac arrests are due to ventricular fibrillation (VF). An automated external defibrillator, or AED, is a defibrillator that can interpret the cardiac rhythm to detect VF and ventricular tachycardia (VT). After these rhythms are detected, the fully automated device charges itself and delivers a shock. This reduces the time required for defibrillation.

Speedy defibrillation is the most important determinant of survival in a patient with VF. The longer it takes for defibrillation to occur, the less likely it becomes for defibrillation to be able to convert VF to a rhythm with a pulse. Defibrillation should occur before CPR is started in an unresponsive and pulseless patient unless a defibrillator isn't immediately available or if the AED indicates that the heart rhythm detected, such as asystole, shouldn't be shocked.

Types of AEDs

There are two basic types of AEDs: semiautomated (or shock-advisory) and fully automated. A semiautomated AED signals that the patient has a shockable arrhythmia (VF or pulseless VT with a rate greater than a preset rate set by the manufacturer), but the nurse must push the button for defibrillation to occur. The fully automated AED assesses the heart rhythm and automatically defibrillates if it detects VF or rapid VT—it requires only that the operator attach the defibrillator pads and turn on the device.

Using a semiautomated AED

Until the advanced cardiac life support (ACLS) team arrives, follow this procedure if your patient is unresponsive.

• First, assess the patient. If he's unresponsive, not breathing, and pulseless, call for help as you get an AED and attach it to the patient. Start CPR if there's a delay in obtaining or attaching the AED.

• Turn on the power to the AED. Place one electrode pad on the chest, just below the right clavicle. Place the other pad at the cardiac apex to the left of the nipple line with the center of the electrode in the midaxillary line. The standard anterior-posterior positions may also be used as an acceptable alternative approach.

• Press the button to analyze the patient's heart rhythm. If the AED indicates that the patient has a shockable rhythm, make sure everyone is clear of the bed, and push the shock button.

• Defibrillate if indicated. If the AED indicates that no further shocks are required, check for spontaneous pulse and respirations. Otherwise, check for pulse and breathing after the third defibrillation.

• If there's no pulse, perform CPR for 1 minute, then check the pulse. If it's still absent, press the AED button to analyze the rhythm. If the AED indicates that the patient has a shockable rhythm, defibrillate as indicated.

• Continue this sequence until either shock is no longer advised (in which case, continue CPR), the pulse returns (in which case, assess vital signs, support airway and breathing, and provide appropriate medications for blood pressure and heart rate and rhythm), or until the ACLS team arrives.

Monophasic and biphasic defibrillators

Monophasic defibrillators

Monophasic defibrillators deliver a single current of electricity that travels in one direction between the two pads or paddles on the patient's chest. To be effective, a large amount of electrical current is required for monophasic defibrillation.

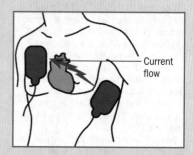

Current flow

Biphasic defibrillators

Biphasic defibrillators have the same pad or paddle placement as with the monophasic defibrillator. The difference is that during biphasic defibrillation, the electrical current discharged from the pads or paddles travels in a positive direction for a specified duration and then reverses and flows in a negative direction for the remaining time of the electrical discharge.

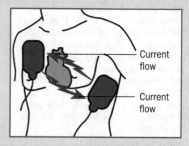

Current flow

Current flow

Energy efficient

The biphasic defibrillator delivers two currents of electricity and lowers the defibrillation threshold of the heart muscle, making it possible to successfully defibrillate ventricular fibrillation (VF) with smaller amounts of energy.

Adjustable

The biphasic defibrillator can adjust for differences in impedance or resistance of the current through the chest. This reduces the number of shocks needed to terminate VF.

Less myocardial damage

Because the biphasic defibrillator requires lower energy levels and fewer shocks, damage to the myocardial muscle is reduced. Biphasic defibrillators used at the clinically appropriate energy level may be used for defibrillation and, in the synchronized mode, for synchronized cardioversion.

Defibrillator paddle placement

Anterolateral placement

Place one paddle to the right of the upper sternum, just below the right clavicle, and the other over the fifth or sixth intercostal space at the left anterior axillary line.

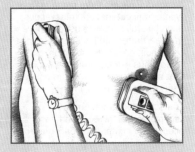

Anteroposterior placement

Place the anterior paddle directly over the heart at the precordium, to the left of the lower sternal border. Place the flat posterior paddle under the patient's body beneath the heart and just below the left scapula (but not under the vertebral column).

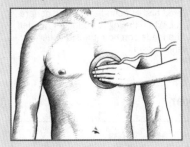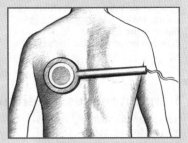

Synchronized cardioversion

How it works

In synchronized cardioversion, an electric current is delivered to the heart to correct an arrhythmia. This procedure may be elective in a stable patient with recurrent atrial fibrillation or urgent in an unstable patient with such arrhythmias as paroxysmal supraventricular tachycardia, atrial flutter, atrial fibrillation, and ventricular tachycardia with a pulse.

Compared with defibrillation, synchronized cardioversion uses much lower energy levels and is synchronized to deliver an electric charge to the myocardium on the peak R wave.

What it does

The procedure causes immediate depolarization, interrupting reentry circuits (abnormal impulse conduction that occurs when cardiac tissue is activated two or more times, causing reentry arrhythmias) and allowing the sinoatrial node to resume control.

Synchronizing the electric charge with the R wave ensures that the current won't be delivered on the vulnerable T wave and disrupts repolarization. This reduces the risk that the current will strike during the relative refractory period of a cardiac cycle and induce ventricular fibrillation.

Types of temporary pacemakers

Temporary pacemakers come in three types: transcutaneous, transvenous, and epicardial. They're used to pace the heart after cardiac surgery, during cardiopulmonary resuscitation, and when sinus arrest, sinus bradycardia that produces symptoms, or complete heart block occurs.

Transcutaneous pacemaker

Completely noninvasive and easily applied, a transcutaneous pacemaker proves especially useful in an emergency. To begin pacing with the device, the electrodes are placed on the skin directly over the heart and connected to a pulse generator.

Transvenous pacemaker

This balloon-tipped pacing catheter is inserted via the subclavian or jugular vein into the right ventricle. The procedure can be done at the bedside or in the cardiac catheterization laboratory. A transvenous pacemaker offers better control of the heartbeat than a transcutaneous pacemaker does. However, electrode insertion takes longer, limiting its usefulness in emergencies.

Epicardial pacemaker

Implanted during open-heart surgery, an epicardial pacemaker permits rapid treatment of postoperative complications. During surgery, the surgeon attaches the leads to the heart and runs them out through the chest incision. Afterward, the leads are coiled on the patient's chest, insulated, and covered with a dressing. If pacing is needed, the leads are simply uncovered and attached to a pulse generator. When pacing is no longer needed, the leads can be removed under local anesthesia.

Transcutaneous pacemaker

Transcutaneous pacing, also referred to as *external* or *noninvasive pacing,* involves the delivery of electrical impulses through externally applied cutaneous electrodes. The electrical impulses are conducted through an intact chest wall using skin electrodes placed in either anterior-posterior or sternal-apex positions. (An anterior-posterior placement is shown here.)

When to use it

Transcutaneous pacing is the pacing method of choice in emergency situations because it's the least invasive technique and it can be instituted quickly.

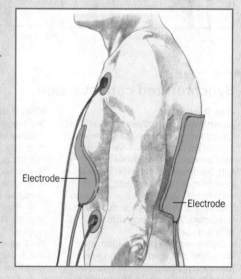

Electrode

Electrode

Temporary pulse generator

The settings on a temporary pulse generator may be changed in various ways to meet the patient's specific needs. This illustration shows a single-chamber temporary pulse generator and gives brief descriptions of its various parts.

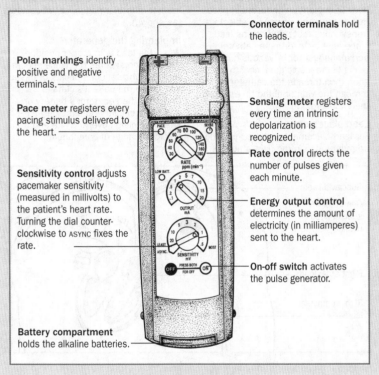

Connector terminals hold the leads.

Polar markings identify positive and negative terminals.

Pace meter registers every pacing stimulus delivered to the heart.

Sensing meter registers every time an intrinsic depolarization is recognized.

Rate control directs the number of pulses given each minute.

Sensitivity control adjusts pacemaker sensitivity (measured in millivolts) to the patient's heart rate. Turning the dial counterclockwise to ASYNC fixes the rate.

Energy output control determines the amount of electricity (in milliamperes) sent to the heart.

On-off switch activates the pulse generator.

Battery compartment holds the alkaline batteries.

Placing a permanent pacemaker

Implanting a pacemaker is a simple surgical procedure performed with local anesthesia and moderate sedation. To implant an endocardial pacemaker, the surgeon usually selects a transvenous route and begins lead placement by inserting a catheter percutaneously or by venous cutdown. Using fluoroscopic guidance, the surgeon then threads the catheter through the vein until the tip reaches the endocardium.

Lead placement

For lead placement in the atrium, the tip must lodge in the right atrium or coronary sinus, as shown. For placement in the ventricle, it must lodge in the right ventricular apex in one of the interior muscular ridges, or trabeculae (as shown).

Implanting the generator

When the lead is in proper position, the surgeon secures the pulse generator in a subcutaneous pocket of tissue just below the patient's clavicle. Changing the generator's battery or microchip circuitry requires only a shallow incision over the site and a quick exchange of components.

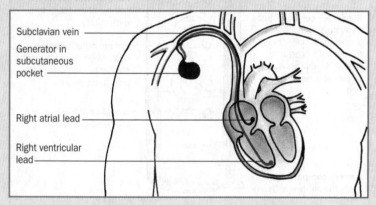

Subclavian vein

Generator in subcutaneous pocket

Right atrial lead

Right ventricular lead

Understanding pacing leads

Unipolar lead

In a unipolar (one lead) system, electrical current moves from the pulse generator through the leadwire to the negative pole. From there, it stimulates the heart and returns to the pulse generator's metal surface (the positive pole) to complete the circuit.

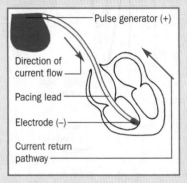

Bipolar lead

In a bipolar (two lead) system, current flows from the pulse generator through the leadwire to the negative pole at the tip. At that point, it stimulates the heart and then flows back to the positive pole to complete the circuit.

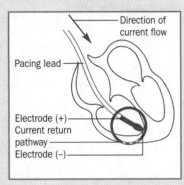

Biventricular lead placement

A biventricular pacemaker, also called *cardiac resynchronization therapy*, uses three leads: one to pace the right atrium, one to pace the right ventricle, and one to pace the left ventricle. The left ventricular lead is placed in the coronary sinus. Both ventricles are paced at the same time, causing them to contract simultaneously, which improves cardiac output.

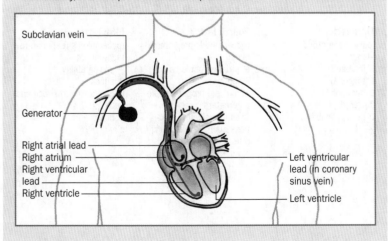

Pacemaker spikes

Pacemaker impulses—the stimuli that travel from the pacemaker to the heart—appear as spikes on an electrocardiogram tracing. Whether large or small, pacemaker spikes appear above or below the isoelectric line. This illustration shows an atrial pacemaker spike and a ventricular pacemaker spike.

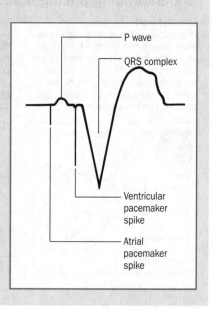

P wave

QRS complex

Ventricular pacemaker spike

Atrial pacemaker spike

Understanding pacemaker codes

A permanent pacemaker's three-letter (or sometimes five-letter) code refers to how it's programmed.

First letter
(chamber that's paced)
A atrium
V ventricle
D dual (both chambers)
O not applicable

Second letter
(chamber that's sensed)
A atrium
V ventricle
D dual (both chambers)
O not applicable

Third letter
(pulse generator's response)
I inhibited
T triggered
D dual (inhibited and triggered)
O not applicable

Fourth letter
(pacemaker's programmability)
P programmable basic functions
M multiple programmable parameters
C communicating functions such as telemetry rate responsiveness
N none

Fifth letter
(pacemaker's response to tachycardia)
P pacing ability
S shock
D dual ability to shock and pace
O none

Pacemaker malfunctions

Failure to pace
Electrocardiogram (ECG) shows no pacemaker activity when activity should be present.

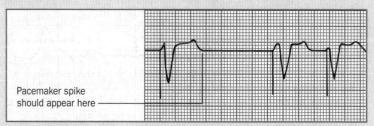

Pacemaker spike should appear here ——

Nursing interventions
If temporary pacemaker:
• Check connections to cable and position of pacing electrode in the patient (by X-ray).
• If the pulse generator is on but indicators aren't flashing, change the battery. If that doesn't help, change the pulse generator.
• Adjust the sensitivity setting.

If permanent pacemaker:
• Assess the patient's condition; if unstable, follow advanced cardiac life support (ACLS) protocol.
• If the patient's condition is stable, notify the cardiologist and expect a pacemaker evaluation to be performed.

Failure to capture
ECG shows pacemaker spikes but the heart isn't responding.

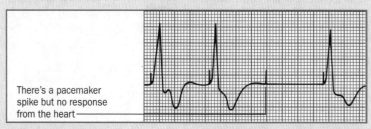

There's a pacemaker spike but no response from the heart ——

Nursing interventions
If temporary pacemaker:
• If the patient's condition has changed, notify the cardiologist and ask for new settings.
• If pacemaker settings are altered, return them to their correct positions.
• If the heart isn't responding, check all connections; increase milliamperes slowly (according to policy or cardiologist's order); turn the patient onto his

left side, then onto his right side; and schedule an anteroposterior or lateral chest X-ray to determine the position of the electrode.
If permanent pacemaker:
• Assess the patient's condition and follow ACLS protocol for resuscitation.
• If the patient's condition is stable, notify the cardiologist and expect a pacemaker evaluation to be performed.

(continued)

Pacemaker malfunctions *(continued)*

Failure to sense intrinsic beats (undersensing)
ECG shows pacemaker spikes anywhere in the cycle (the pacemaker fires, but at the wrong times for the wrong reasons).

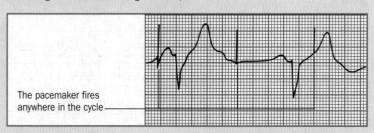

The pacemaker fires anywhere in the cycle——

Nursing interventions
If temporary pacemaker:
• If the pacemaker is undersensing, turn the sensitivity control completely to the right.
• If the pacemaker isn't functioning correctly, change the battery or pulse generator.
• Remove items in the room causing electromechanical interference (such as electric razors, radios, and cautery devices). Check ground wires on the bed and other equipment for damage. Unplug each piece and see if interference stops. When you locate the cause, ask a staff engineer to check it out.
• If the pacemaker is still firing on the T-wave, notify the cardiologist and turn off the pacemaker. Have atropine available in case the heart rate drops. Initiate cardiopulmonary resuscitation if needed.

If permanent pacemaker:
• Assess the patient's condition and follow ACLS protocol for resuscitation.
• If the patient's condition is stable, notify the cardiologist and expect a pacemaker evaluation to be performed.

Assessing pacemaker function

When you apply a magnet to a patient's permanent pacemaker, the device reverts to a predefined (asynchronous) response mode that allows you to assess various aspects of pacemaker function. Specifically, you can:
• determine which chambers are being paced
• assess capture
• provide emergency pacing if the device malfunctions
• ensure pacing despite electromagnetic interference
• assess battery life by checking the magnet rate—a predetermined rate that indicates the need for battery replacement.

You must know which implanted device the patient has before you consider using a magnet. The patient might have an implantable cardioverter-defibrillator (ICD), which is rarely an appropriate target for magnet application.

Because pacemakers and ICDs are similar in generator size and implant location, it isn't easy to differentiate between the two. In addition, a single device may perform multiple functions.

In general, you shouldn't apply a magnet to an ICD or a pacemaker-ICD combination. Applying a magnet to an ICD can cause an unexpected response because various responses can be programmed or determined by the manufacturer. When directed, applying a magnet to an ICD usually suspends therapies for ventricular tachycardia and fibrillation while leaving bradycardia pacing active, which may be helpful in patients who receive multiple, inappropriate shocks. Some models may beep when exposed to a magnetic field.

Implantable cardioverter-defibrillator placement

A specially trained cardiologist implants the pulse generator and leadwires in the cardiac catheterization laboratory with the patient under local anesthesia. Occasionally, a patient who requires other surgery, such as coronary artery bypass, may have the device implanted in the operating room.

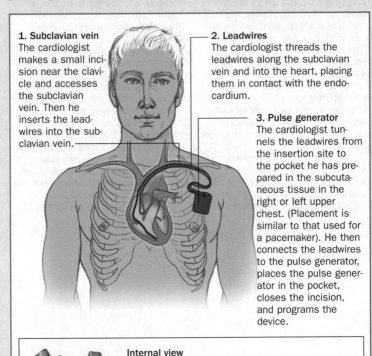

1. Subclavian vein
The cardiologist makes a small incision near the clavicle and accesses the subclavian vein. Then he inserts the leadwires into the subclavian vein.

2. Leadwires
The cardiologist threads the leadwires along the subclavian vein and into the heart, placing them in contact with the endocardium.

3. Pulse generator
The cardiologist tunnels the leadwires from the insertion site to the pocket he has prepared in the subcutaneous tissue in the right or left upper chest. (Placement is similar to that used for a pacemaker). He then connects the leadwires to the pulse generator, places the pulse generator in the pocket, closes the incision, and programs the device.

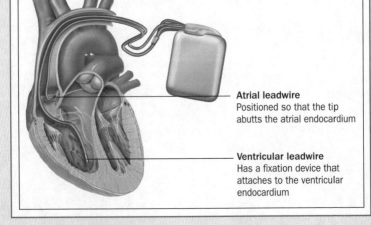

Internal view

Atrial leadwire
Positioned so that the tip abutts the atrial endocardium

Ventricular leadwire
Has a fixation device that attaches to the ventricular endocardium

Types of ICD therapies

Implantable cardioverter-defibrillators (ICDs) can deliver a range of therapies depending on the arrhythmia detected and how the device is programmed. Some ICDs can also detect and treat atrial arrhythmias or provide biventricular pacing. Therapies include antitachycardia pacing, cardioversion, defibrillation, and bradycardia pacing.

Therapy	Description
Antitachycardia pacing	A series of small, rapid, electrical pacing pulses are used to interrupt ventricular tachycardia (VT) and return the heart to its normal rhythm.
Cardioversion	A low- or high-energy shock (up to 35 joules) is timed to the R wave to terminate VT and return the heart to its normal rhythm.
Defibrillation	A high-energy shock (up to 35 joules) to the heart is used to terminate ventricular fibrillation and return the heart to its normal rhythm.
Bradycardia pacing	Electrical pacing pulses are used when the heart's natural electrical signals are too slow. ICD systems can pace one chamber (VVI pacing) of the heart at a preset rate or sense and pace both chambers (DDD pacing).

Managing an ICD

Keep these factors in mind when caring for a patient with an implantable cardioverter-defibrillator (ICD).

Device
• Know the device and how it's programmed, including:
 – type and model of ICD
 – status of the device (on or off)
 – detection rates
 – types of therapies that will be delivered and when.

Appropriateness
• Evaluate the appropriateness of ICD shocks, including:
 – number of isolated and multiple shocks
 – situation and activity related to shocks
 – patient symptoms
 – electrocardiogram rhythm
 – drugs taken.

Shocks
• Shocks may not occur despite ventricular tachycardia (VT) or ventricular fibrillation (VF) under certain circumstances, such as:
 – if the heart rate is less than the detection rate
 – if there's a lead or circuitry problem
 – if therapy is suspended or turned off
 – if the battery is depleted.
• Shocks can occur without VT or VF under certain circumstances, such as:
 – when the rate in sinus tachycardia ventures into the VT zone
 – when noise is detected on the sensing lead (from electromagnetic interference or lead dysfunction)
 – when the patient develops atrial fibrillation.

• Multiple shocks may occur in certain circumstances, such as:
 – when the patient has persistent or recurrent VT or VF
 – when the device malfunctions.
• Multiple shocks indicate a medical emergency, and the patient may require adjunct treatment, such as:
 – cardiopulmonary resuscitation (CPR)
 – external defibrillation
 – drugs, such as amiodarone, lidocaine, procainamide
 – suspension of tachyarrhythmia therapy by magnet application or reprogramming of device.

Problems
• If cardiac arrest occurs in a patient with an ICD, CPR and advanced cardiac life support should be used immediately.
• If the patient needs external defibrillation, take these steps:
 – Position the paddles as far from the device as possible or use anterior-posterior position.
 – Anticipate that defibrillation will result in "power on reset" and reversion to nominal settings.
 – Programming of the device should be verified with the programmer.
• Look for evidence of problems, including:
 – decreased cardiac output (hypotension, chest pain, dyspnea, syncope)
 – infection
 – pneumothorax
 – misplaced electrode (abnormal electrical stimulation occurring in synchrony with the pacemaker, such as pectoral muscle twitching)
 – stimulation of diaphragm (hiccups)
 – cardiac tamponade.

Laboratory tests

Crisis values of laboratory tests

Test	Low value	Common causes and effects	High value	Common causes and effects
Ammonia	< 15 mcg SI, < 8.8 µmol/L	Renal failure	> 50 mcg/dl SI, > 29.3 µmol/L	Severe hepatic disease: hepatic coma, Reye's syndrome, GI hemorrhage, heart failure
Calcium, serum	< 6 mg/dl SI, < 1.75 mmol/L	Vitamin D or parathyroid hormone deficiency: tetany, seizures	> 13 mg/dl SI, > 0.3 mmol/L	Hyperparathyroidism: coma
Carbon dioxide and bicarbonate blood	< 10 mEq/L SI, < 10 mmol/L	Complex pattern of metabolic and respiratory factors	> 40 mEq/L SI, > 40 mmol/L	Complex pattern of metabolic and respiratory factors
Creatine kinase (CK-MB)	—	—	> 5%	Acute myocardial infarction (MI)
Creatinine, serum	—	—	> 4 mg/dl SI, > 353.6 µmol/L	Renal failure: coma
Glucose, blood	< 40 mg/dl SI, < 2.22 mmol/L	Excessive insulin administration, brain damage	> 300 mg/dl SI, > 16.6 mmol/L (with ketonemia and electrolyte imbalance)	Diabetes: diabetic coma
Hemoglobin	< 8 g/dl SI, < 80 g/L	Hemorrhage or vitamin B_{12} or iron deficiency: heart failure	> 18 g/dl SI, > 180 g/L	Chronic obstructive pulmonary disease: thrombosis, polycythemia vera

(continued)

Crisis values of laboratory tests (continued)

Test	Low value	Common causes and effects	High value	Common causes and effects
International Normalized Ratio	—	—	> 3.0	Disseminated intravascular coagulation, un-controlled oral-anticoagulation
Platelet count	< 50 × 10^3/mm^3 SI, < 50 × 10^9/L	Bone marrow suppression: hemorrhage	> 500 × 10^3/mm^3 SI, > 500 × 10^9/L	Leukemia, re-action to acute bleeding: hemor-rhage
Potassium, serum	< 3 mEq/L SI, < 3 mmol/L	Vomiting and diarrhea, diuretic thera-py: cardiotoxici-ty, arrhythmia, cardiac arrest	> 6 mEq/L SI, > 6 mmol/L	Renal disease, diuretic therapy: cardiotoxicity, arrhythmia
PT	—	—	> 14 sec (> 20 sec for patient on war-farin)	Anticoagulant therapy, anticoag-ulation factor defi-ciency: hemor-rhage
PTT	—	—	> 40 sec (> 70 sec for patient on heparin)	Anticoagulation factor deficiency: hemorrhage
Sodium, serum	< 120 mEq/L SI, < 120 mmol/L	Diuretic thera-py: cardiac failure	> 160 mEq/L SI, > 160 mmol/L	Dehydration: vascular collapse
Troponin I	—	—	> 2 mcg/ml SI, > 2 mcg/L	Acute MI
White blood cell (WBC) count	< 2,000/ cells/mm^3 SI, < 2 × 10^9/L	Bone marrow suppression: infection	> 20,000 cells/mm^3 SI, > 20 × 10^9/L	Leukemia: infection
WBC count, CSF	—	—	> 10 cells/mm^3 SI, > 5 × 10^6/L	Meningitis, encephalitis: infection

Comprehensive metabolic panel

Test	Conventional units	SI units
Albumin	3.5 to 5 g/dl	35 to 50 g/L
Alkaline phosphatase	45 to 115 units/L	45 to 115 units/L
ALT	Male: 10 to 40 units/L	0.17 to 0.68 µkat/L
	Female: 7 to 35 units/L	0.12 to 0.60 µkat/L
AST	12 to 31 units/L	0.21 to 0.53 µkat/L
Bilirubin, total	0.2 to 1 mg/dl	3.5 to 17 µmol/L
BUN	8 to 20 mg/dl	2.9 to 7.5 mmol/L
Calcium	8.2 to 10.2 mg/dl	2.05 to 2.54 mmol/L
Carbon dioxide	22 to 26 mEq/L	22 to 26 mmol/L
Chloride	100 to 108 mEq/L	100 to 108 mmol/L
Creatinine	Male: 0.8 to 1.2 mg/dl	62 to 115 µmol/L
	Female: 0.6 to 0.9 mg/dl	53 to 97 µmol/L
Glucose	70 to 100 mg/dl	3.9 to 6.1 mmol/L
Potassium	3.5 to 5 mEq/L	3.5 to 5 mmol/L
Protein, total	6.3 to 8.3 g/dl	64 to 83 g/L
Sodium	135 to 145 mEq/L	135 to 145 mmol/L

Lipid panel

Test	Conventional units	SI units
Total cholesterol	< 200 mg/dl	< 5.18 mmol/L
HDL cholesterol	≥ 60 mg/dl	≥ 1.55 mmol/L
LDL cholesterol	< 130 mg/dl	< 3.36 mmol/L
VLDL cholesterol	< 130 mg/dl	< 3.4 mmol/L
Triglycerides	< 150 mg/dl	< 1.7 mmol/L

Thyroid panel

Test	Conventional units	SI units
T_3	80 to 200 ng/dl	1.2 to 3 nmol/L
T_4, free	0.9 to 2.3 ng/dl	10 to 30 nmol/L
T_4, total	5 to 13.5 mcg/dl	60 to 165 mmol/L
TSH	0.4 to 4.2 mIU/L	0.4 to 4.2 mIU/L

Other chemistry tests

Test	Conventional units	SI units
A/G ratio	3.4 to 4.8 g/dl	34 to 38 g/dl
Ammonia	< 50 ng/dl	< 36 µmol/L
Amylase	26 to 102 units/L	0.4 to 1.74 µkat/L
Anion gap	8 to 14 mEq/L	8 to 14 mmol/L
Bilirubin, direct	< 0.5 mg/dl	< 6.8 µmol/L
Calcitonin	Male: < 16 pg/ml	< 16 ng/L
	Female: < 8 pg/ml	< 8 ng/L
Calcium, ionized	4.65 to 5.28 mg/dl	1.1 to 1.25 mmol/L
Cortisol	a.m.: 7 to 25 mcg/dl	0.2 to 0.7 µmol/L
	p.m.: 2 to 14 mcg/dl	0.06 to 0.39 µmol/L
C-reactive protein	< 0.8 mg/dl	< 8 mg/L
Ferritin	Male: 20 to 300 ng/ml	20 to 300 mcg/L
	Female: 20 to 120 ng/ml	20 to 120 mcg/L
Folate	1.8 to 20 ng/ml	4.45 to 3 nmol/L
GGT	Male: 7 to 47 units/L	0.12 to 1.80 µkat/L
	Female: 5 to 25 units/L	0.08 to 0.42 µkat/L
HbA_{1c}	4% to 7%	0.04 to 0.07
Homocysteine	< 12 µmol/L	< 12 µmol/L
Iron	Male: 65 to 175 mcg/dl	11.6 to 31.3 µmol/L
	Female: 50 to 170 mcg/dl	9 to 30.4 µmol/L
Iron-binding capacity	250 to 400 mcg/dl	45 to 72 µmol/L
Lactic acid	0.5 to 2.2 mEq/L	0.5 to 2.2 mmol/L
Lipase	10 to 73 units/L	0.17 to 1.24 µkat/L
Magnesium	1.3 to 2.2 mg/dl	0.65 to 1.05 mmol/L
Osmolality	275 to 295 mOsm/kg	275 to 295 mOsm/kg
Phosphate	2.7 to 4.5 mg/dl	0.87 to 1.45 mmol/L
Prealbumin	19 to 38 mg/dl	190 to 380 mg/L
Uric acid	Male: 3.4 to 7 mg/dl	202 to 416 µmol/L
	Female: 2.3 to 6 mg/dl	143 to 357 µmol/L

Tumor markers

Test	Conventional units	SI units
Alpha-fetoprotein	< 40 ng/ml	< 40 mcg/L
CA 15-3	< 30 units/ml	< 30 kU/L
CA 19-9	< 37 units/ml	< 37 kU/L
CA 27-29	≤ 38 units/ml	≤ 38 kU/L
CA 125	< 35 units/ml	< 35 kU/L
Carcinoembryonic antigen	< 2.5 to 5 ng/ml	< 2.5 to 5 mcg/L
Human chorionic gonadotropin	< 2 ng/ml	< 2 mcg/L
Neuron-specific enolase	< 12.5 mcg/ml	—
PSA	Age 40 to 49: ≤ 2.5 ng/ml	≤ 2.5 mcg/L
	Age 50 to 59: ≤ 3.5 ng/ml	≤ 3.5 mcg/L
	Age 60 to 69: ≤ 4.5 ng/ml	≤ 4.5 mcg/L
	Age 70+: ≤ 6.5 ng/ml	≤ 6.5 mcg/LL

Complete blood count with differential

Test	Conventional units	SI units
Hemoglobin	Male: 14 to 17.4 g/dl	140 to 174 g/L
	Female: 12 to 16 g/dl	120 to 160 g/L
Hematocrit	Male: 42% to 52%	0.42 to 0.52
	Female: 36% to 48%	0.36 to 0.48
RBC	Male: 4.2 to 5.4 $\times$ 10^6/mm^3	4.2 to 5.4 $\times$ 10^{12}/L
	Female: 3.6 to 5 $\times$ 10^6/mm^3	3.6 to 5 $\times$ 10^{12}/L
MCH	26 to 34 pg/cell	0.40 to 0.53 fmol/cell
MCHC	32 to 36 g/dl	320 to 360 g/L
MCV	82 to 98 mm^3	82 to 98 fL
WBC	4,000 to 10,000/cells/mm^3	4 to 10 $\times$ 10^9/L
Bands	0% to 5%	0.03 to 0.08
Basophils	0% to 1%	0 to 0.01
Eosinophils	1% to 4%	0.01 to 0.04
Lymphocytes	25% to 40%	0.25 to 0.40
Monocytes	2% to 8%	0.02 to 0.08
Neutrophils	54% to 75%	0.54 to 0.75
Platelets	140,000 to 400,000/mm^3	140 to 400 $\times$ 10^9/L

Comparative red cell indices in anemias

	Normal findings (Normocytic, normochromic)	Iron deficiency anemia (Microcytic, hypochromic)	Pernicious anemia (Macrocytic, normochromic)
MCV	84 to 90 µm³	60 to 80 µm³	96 to 150 µm³
MCH	26 to 32 pg/cell	5 to 25 pg/cell	33 to 53 pg/cell
MCHC	30 to 36 g/dl	20 to 30 g/dl	33 to 38 g/dl

KEY
MCV = Mean corpuscular volume
MCH = Mean corpuscular hemoglobin
MCHC = Mean corpuscular hemoglobin concentration

Variations of hemoglobin type and distribution

Hemoglobin	Percentage of total hemoglobin	Clinical implications
Hb A	95% to 100% (SI, 0.95 to 1.0)	Normal
Hb A$_2$	4% to 5.8% (SI, 0.04 to 0.058)	ß-thalassemia minor
	1.5% to 3% (SI, 0.015 to 0.03)	Normal
	Less than 1.5% (SI, < 0.015)	Hb H disease
Hb F	Less than 1% (SI, < 0.01)	Normal
	2% to 5% (SI, 0.02 to 0.05)	ß-thalassemia minor
	10% to 90% (SI, 0.1 to 0.9)	ß-thalassemia major
	5% to 15% (SI, 0.05 to 0.15)	ß-d-thalassemia minor
	5% to 35% (SI, 0.05 to 0.35)	Heterozygous hereditary persistence of fetal Hb (HPFH)
	100% (SI, 1.0)	Homozygous HPFH
	15% (SI, 0.15)	Homozygous Hb S
Homozygous Hb S	70% to 98% (SI, 0.7 to 0.98)	Sickle cell disease
Homozygous Hb C	90% to 98% (SI, 0.9 to 0.98)	Hb C disease
Heterozygous Hb C	24% to 44% (SI, 0.24 to 0.44)	Hb C trait

Interpreting WBC differential values

The differential count measures the types of white blood cells (WBCs) as a percentage of the total WBC count (the relative value). The absolute value is obtained by multiplying the relative value of each cell type by the total WBC count. The relative and absolute values must be considered to obtain an accurate diagnosis.

For example, consider a patient whose WBC count is 6,000/µl (SI, 6×10^9/L) and whose differential shows 30% (SI, 0.3) neutrophils and 70% (SI, 0.7) lymphocytes. His relative lymphocyte count seems to be quite high (lymphocytosis), but when this figure is multiplied by his WBC count (6,000 × 70% = 4,200 lymphocytes/µl), (SI, [6×10^9/L] × 9.79 = 4.2 × 10^9/L lymphocytes), it's well within the normal range.

However, this patient's neutrophil count (30%; SI, 0.3) is low; when this figure is multiplied by the WBC count (6,000 × 30% = 1,800 neutrophils/ml) (SI, [6×10^9/L] × 0.30 = 1.8 × 10^9/L neutrophils), the result is a low absolute number, which may mean depressed bone marrow.

The normal percentages of WBC type in adults are:
Neutrophils: 54% to 75% (SI, 0.54 to 0.75)
Eosinophils: 1% to 4% (SI, 0.01 to 0.04)
Basophils: 0% to 1% (SI, 0 to 0.01)
Monocytes: 2% to 8% (SI, 0.02 to 0.08)
Lymphocytes: 25% to 40% (SI, 0.25 to 0.4).

Influence of disease on blood cell count

The white blood cell (WBC) differential aids diagnosis because some disorders affect only one WBC type. Below, each type is listed as well as its corresponding effect and cause.

Cell type	How affected
Neutrophils	*Increased by:* • Infections: osteomyelitis, otitis media, salpingitis, septicemia, gonorrhea, endocarditis, smallpox, chickenpox, herpes, Rocky Mountain spotted fever • Ischemic necrosis due to myocardial infarction, burns, carcinoma • Metabolic disorders: diabetic acidosis, eclampsia, uremia, thyrotoxicosis • Stress response due to acute hemorrhage, surgery, excessive exercise, emotional distress, third trimester of pregnancy, childbirth • Inflammatory diseases: rheumatic fever, rheumatoid arthritis, acute gout, vasculitis, myositis *Decreased by:* • Bone marrow depression due to radiation or cytotoxic drugs • Infections: typhoid, tularemia, brucellosis, hepatitis, influenza, measles, mumps, rubella, infectious mononucleosis • Hypersplenism: hepatic disease and storage diseases • Collagen vascular disease such as systemic lupus erythematosus (SLE) • Folic acid or vitamin B_{12} deficiency

(continued)

Influence of disease on blood cell count *(continued)*

Cell type	How affected
Eosinophils	*Increased by:* • Allergic disorders: asthma, hay fever, food or drug sensitivity, serum sickness, angioneurotic edema • Parasitic infections: trichinosis, hookworm, roundworm, amebiasis • Skin diseases: eczema, pemphigus, psoriasis, dermatitis, herpes • Neoplastic diseases: chronic myelocytic leukemia (CML), Hodgkin's disease, metastases and necrosis of solid tumors *Decreased by:* • Stress response • Cushing's syndrome
Basophils	*Increased by:* • CML, Hodgkin's disease, ulcerative colitis, chronic hypersensitivity states *Decreased by:* • Hyperthyroidism • Ovulation, pregnancy • Stress
Lymphocytes	*Increased by:* • Infections: tuberculosis (TB), hepatitis, infectious mononucleosis, mumps, rubella, cytomegalovirus • Thyrotoxicosis, hypoadrenalism, ulcerative colitis, immune diseases, lymphocytic leukemia *Decreased by:* • Severe debilitating illnesses: heart failure, renal failure, advanced TB • Defective lymphatic circulation, high levels of adrenal corticosteroids, immunodeficiency due to immunosuppressives
Monocytes	*Increased by:* • Infections: subacute bacterial endocarditis, TB, hepatitis, malaria • Collagen vascular disease: SLE, rheumatoid arthritis • Carcinomas • Monocytic leukemia • Lymphomas

Coagulation studies

Test	Conventional units	SI units
ACT	107 sec ± 13 sec	107 sec ± 13 sec
Bleeding time	3 to 6 min	3 to 6 min
D-dimer	< 250 mcg/L	< 1.37 nmol/L
Fibrinogen	200 to 400 mg/dl	2 to 4 g/L
INR (target therapeutic)	2.0 to 3.0	2.0 to 3.0
Plasminogen	80% to 130%	—
PT	10 to 14 sec	10 to 14 sec
PTT	21 to 35 sec	21 to 35 sec
Thrombin time	10 to 15 sec	10 to 15 sec

Collecting specimens for coagulation testing

Proper specimen collection and handling is especially important when collecting blood samples for coagulation testing. Damage to the vessel wall during venipuncture can cause coagulation to begin, thus affecting test results. Keep in mind the following guidelines for venipuncture and specimen collection.

Timing
Collect samples for coagulation testing at approximately the same time each day, if possible, to eliminate the circadian variations of the different coagulation proteins.

Venipuncture equipment
Avoid using small-bore (large-gauge [> 21G]) needles to collect coagulation test samples because this size needle may mechanically disrupt platelets and activate the coagulation cascade.

Collection technique
A clean venipuncture with a minimum of tissue trauma is essential to obtain a good quality plasma specimen for coagulation testing. Any trauma to the tissue can stimulate the release of tissue thromboplastin, which can contaminate the needle. Therefore, when drawing blood for several laboratory tests, don't draw the coagulation test sample first. If no other tests will be performed, first draw a *red-top* discard tube to negate the effect of tissue thromboplastin on test results. If you're drawing from an intermittent access device, discard 20 ml of blood before collecting the coagulation test sample (for a heparinized line, discard 30 ml). Make sure that the coagulation test tube is filled with blood to the appropriate level to achieve a whole blood–anticoagulant ratio of 9:1.

In addition, avoid prolonged application of the tourniquet because this can stimulate the release of tissue thromboplastin and elevate levels of coagulation factor VII, fibrin monomer, and tissue plasminogen activator.

Specimen handling and transport
Coagulation specimens should be kept capped during transport and storage before testing because uncapped specimens lose carbon dioxide. Loss of carbon dioxide would result in a pH increase, which would affect coagulation test results.

Blood coagulation factors

Factor	Synonym
I	Fibrinogen
II	Prothrombin
III	Tissue thromboplastin
IV	Calcium ion
V	Proaccelerin
VI	Accelerin
VII	Serum prothrombin (proconvertin)
VIII	Antihemophilic factor (hemophilic factor A)
IX	Christmas factor (hemophilic factor B, plasma thromboplastin component)
X	Stuart-Prower factor
XI	Plasma thromboplastin antecedent
XII	Hageman factor
XIII	Fibrin-stabilizing factor

Cardiac biomarkers

Protein	Conventional units	SI units	Initial evaluation
Troponin-I	< 0.35 mcg/L	< 0.35 mcg/L	4 to 6 hours
Troponin-T	< 0.1 mcg/L	< 0.1 mcg/L	4 to 8 hours
Myoglobin	< 55 ng/ml	< 55 mcg/L	2 to 4 hours
Hs-CRP	0.020 to 0.800 mg/dl	0.2 to 0.8 mg/L	—
Enzyme			
CK	Male: 55 to 170 units/L	0.94 to 2.89 µkat/L	—
	Female: 30 to 135 units/L	0.51 to 2.3 µkat/L	—
CK-MB	< 5%	< 0.05	4 to 8 hours
LD	135 to 280 units/L	2.34 to 4.68 µkat/L	2 to 5 days
Hormone			
BNP	< 100 pg/ml	< 100 ng/L	—

Profile	Site of synthesis
Precursor of fibrin	Liver
Precursor of thrombin	Liver
Activator of prothrombin	All tissues
Essential for prothrombin activation and formation of fibrin	From diet
Accelerates conversion of prothrombin to thrombin	Liver
Cofactor in the activation of thrombin by factor Xa	Liver
Accelerates conversion of prothrombin to thrombin	Liver
Associated with factors IX, XI, and XII; aids in forming activated factor X via intrinsic system and conversion of prothrombin to thrombin	Reticuloendothelial system
Activated by factor XI; essential to formation of activated factor X through intrinsic system; associated with factors VIII, XI, and XII	Liver
Triggers prothrombin conversion; requires vitamin K	Liver
Activated by factor XII; associated with factors VIII, IX, and XII in formation of activated factor X through intrinsic system	Unknown
First factor activated in the intrinsic pathway; activates factor XI	Unknown
Produces stronger urea-insoluble fibrin clot	Unknown

Peak	Time to return to normal
12 hours	3 to 10 days
12 to 48 hours	7 to 10 days
8 to 10 hours	24 hours
—	Depends on degree of inflammation
—	—
—	—
12 to 24 hours	72 to 96 hours
—	10 days
—	Depends on severity of heart failure

Release of cardiac enzymes and proteins

Because they're released by damaged tissue, serum proteins and isoenzymes (catalytic proteins that vary in concentration in specific organs) can help identify the compromised organ and assess the extent of damage. After an acute myocardial infarction, cardiac enzymes and proteins rise and fall in a characteristic pattern, as shown in this graph.

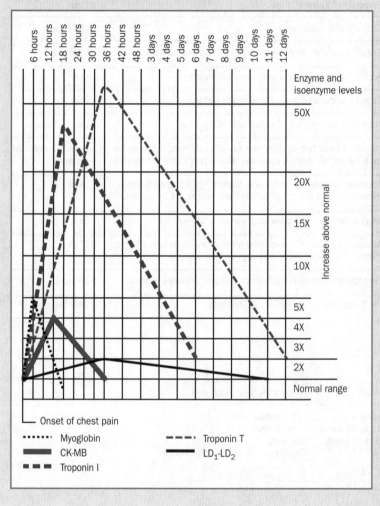

LD isoenzyme variations in disease

Disease	LD$_1$	LD$_2$	LD$_3$	LD$_4$	LD$_5$
Cardiovascular					
Myocardial infarction (MI)					
MI with hepatic congestion					
Rheumatic carditis					
Myocarditis					
Heart failure (decompensated)					
Shock					
Angina pectoris					
Pulmonary					
Pulmonary embolism					
Pulmonary infarction					
Hematologic					
Pernicious anemia					
Hemolytic anemia					
Sickle cell anemia					
Hepatobiliary					
Hepatitis					
Active cirrhosis					
Hepatic congestion					

Normal   Diagnostic   Not diagnostic

Adapted with permission from information from Helena Laboratories, 1513 Lindberg Drive, Beaumont, Tex.

Arterial blood gas results

Disorder	ABG findings	Possible causes
Respiratory acidosis (excess CO_2 retention)	• pH < 7.35 • HCO_3^- > 26 mEq/L (if compensating) • $Paco_2$ > 45 mm Hg	• Central nervous system depression from drugs, injury, or disease • Hypoventilation from respiratory, cardiac, musculoskeletal, or neuromuscular disease
Respiratory alkalosis (excess CO_2 loss)	• pH > 7.45 • HCO_3^- < 22 mEq/L (if compensating) • $Paco_2$ < 35 mm Hg	• Hyperventilation due to anxiety, pain, or improper ventilator settings • Respiratory stimulation from drugs, disease, hypoxia, fever, or high room temperature • Gram-negative bacteremia
Metabolic acidosis (HCO_3^- loss or acid retention)	• pH < 7.35 • HCO_3^- < 22 mEq/L • $Paco_2$ < 35 mm Hg (if compensating)	• Depletion of HCO_3^- from renal disease, diarrhea, or small-bowel fistulas • Excessive production of organic acids from hepatic disease, endocrine disorders such as diabetes mellitus, hypoxia, shock, or drug toxicity • Inadequate excretion of acids due to renal disease
Metabolic alkalosis (HCO_3^- retention or acid loss)	• pH > 7.45 • HCO_3^- > 26 mEq/L • $Paco_2$ > 45 mm Hg (if compensating)	• Loss of hydrochloric acid from prolonged vomiting or gastric suctioning • Loss of potassium from increased renal excretion (as in diuretic therapy) or corticosteroid overdose • Excessive alkali ingestion

Linking BNP levels to heart failure symptom severity

This table shows the level of B-type natriuretic peptide (BNP) levels and the correlation with symptoms of heart failure. The higher the level of BNP, the more severe the symptoms.

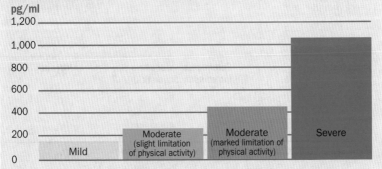

Adapted with permission of Biosite Diagnostics. © 2001 Biosite Diagnostics.

Two-hour postprandial plasma glucose levels by age

The greatest difference in normal and diabetic insulin responses, and thus in plasma glucose concentration, occurs about 2 hours after a glucose challenge. Test values can fluctuate according to the patient's age. After age 50, for example, normal levels rise markedly and steadily, sometimes reaching 160 mg/dl (SI, 8.82 mmol/L) or higher. In a younger patient, a glucose concentration of more than 145 mg/dl (SI, > 8 mmol/L) suggests incipient diabetes and requires further evaluation.

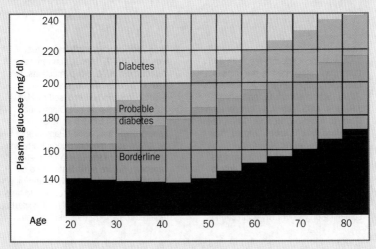

HIV testing

Test type	Specimen (mode of collection)	Test complexity*
Standard human immunodeficiency virus (HIV) test	Serum or plasma (phlebotomy)	High
Rapid test	Serum, plasma, or whole blood (phlebotomy, fingerstick)	Moderate§
Home sample collection test††	Dried blood spot (fingerstick)	High
Oral fluid test	Oral mucosal transudate (oral fluid collection device)	High
Urine-based test	Urine (urine cup)	High

Key:
* Complexity of specimen culture and testing as categorized by the Clinical Laboratory Improvements Amendments (CLIA) (Schochetman, G., and George, J.R., eds. *AIDS Testing: A Comprehensive Guide to Technical, Medical, Social, Legal, and Management Issues,* 2nd ed. New York: Springer-Verlag, 1994).
† All licensed enzyme immunoassays (EIAs) detect HIV-1, but not all detect HIV-2. EIAs that can detect HIV-1 and HIV-2 are required for blood donor screening and are recommended for diagnostic screening only where HIV-2 infection is likely. No licensed confirmatory test exists for HIV-2. Although current tests detect most HIV-1 group infections, few detect all such infections.
§ The one rapid test licensed by FDA, Abbott Murex Single Use Diagnostic System (SUDS) HIV-1 test (Abbott Laboratories, Inc., Abbott Park, Ill.), is classified as a moderate-complexity test and requires on-site laboratory testing capability. Future rapid tests could be classified by CLIA as "waived" and may not require the capability for on-site laboratory testing, depending on the expertise required to perform this test correctly.

Screening information	Strains detected†	Results
Enzyme immunoassay (EIA); Western blot or immunofluorescence assay (IFA)	HIV-1 and HIV-2	HIV negative: Test result at return visit (typically a few days to 1 to 2 weeks) HIV positive: Confirmed result at return visit
Rapid EIA: Western blot or IFA¶	HIV-1	HIV negative: Test result at time of testing (typically 10 to 60 minutes) HIV positive: Preliminary positive test result at time of testing**; confirmed result at return visit
EIA; Western blot or IFA	HIV-1	HIV negative: Test result when patient calls (typically 3 to 7 days) HIV positive: Confirmed result when patient calls
EIA; oral mucosal transudate Western blot	HIV-1	HIV negative: Test result at return visit (typically 1 to 2 weeks) HIV positive: Confirmed result at return visit
EIA; urine Western blot	HIV-1	HIV negative: Test result at return visit (typically 1 to 2 weeks) HIV positive: Test result at return visit; further confirmation by blood sample recommended because of lower specificity of urine Western blot compared with serum-based Western blot or IFA

¶ Future rapid tests may be able to be confirmed with a second rapid test to provide an immediate test result with high sensitivity, specificity, and predictive value comparable with EIA or Western blot (Stetter H.C., et al. "Field Evaluation of Rapid HIV Serologic tests for Screening and Confirming HIV-1 Infection in Honduras," *AIDS* 11:369-375, 1997).
** Information on providing "preliminary" positive test results from a single rapid test is available elsewhere (CDC. "Update: HIV Counseling and Testing using Rapid Tests—United States, 1995," *MMWR* 47:15-21, 1998).

†† Home sample collection is different from home-use testing. FDA has approved home sample collection, but not home-use HIV test kits (Kassler, W.J. "Advances in HIV Testing Technology and Their Potential Impact on Prevention," *AIDS Education Preview* 9 [suppl B]:27-40, 1997).

Viral hepatitis test panel

The six types of viral hepatitis produce similar symptoms, but differ in transmission mode, course of treatment, prognosis, and carrier status. When the clinical history is insufficient for differentiation, serologic tests can aid in diagnosis. Testing helps to identify antibodies specific to the causative virus and establish the type of hepatitis.

· Type A: Detection of an antibody to hepatitis A, confirming the diagnosis
· Type B: The presence of hepatitis B surface antigens and hepatitis B antibodies, confirming the diagnosis
· Type C: Diagnosis depends on serologic testing for the specific antibody one or more months after the onset of acute illness: until then, diagnosis principally established by obtaining negative test results for hepatitis A, B, and D
· Type D: Detection of intrahepatic delta antigens or immunoglobulin (Ig) M antidelta antigens in acute disease (or IgM and IgG in chronic disease), establishing the diagnosis
· Type E: Detection of hepatitis E antigens supports the diagnosis; however, possibly ruling out hepatitis C
· Type G: Detection of hepatitis G ribonucleic acid supporting the diagnosis (serologic assays are being developed)

Additional findings from liver function studies supporting the diagnosis include:
· increased serum aspartate aminotransferase and serum alanine aminotransferase levels in the prodromal stage of acute viral hepatitis
· slightly increased serum alkaline phosphatase levels
· elevated serum bilirubin levels; levels possibly remaining elevated late in the disease, especially with severe disease
· prolonged prothrombin time (more than 3 seconds longer than normal, indicating severe liver damage).

Serodiagnosis of acute viral hepatitis

This chart helps evaluate positive test results in acute viral hepatitis.

Test results			Interpretation
HBsAg	Anti-HBC IgM	Anti-HAV IgM	
−	−	+	Recent acute hepatitis A infection
+	+	−	Acute hepatitis B infection
+	−	−	Early acute hepatitis B infection or chronic hepatitis B
−	+	−	Confirms acute or recent infection with hepatitis B virus
−	−	−	Possible hepatitis C infection, other viral infection, or liver toxin
+	+	+	Recent probable hepatitis A infection and superimposed acute hepatitis B infection; uncommon profile

Key: + = positive   − = negative
Reprinted with permission of Abbott Laboratories, Abbott Park, Ill.

Antibiotic peaks and troughs

Test	Conventional units	SI units
Amikacin		
Peak	20 to 30 mcg/ml	34 to 52 µmol/L
Trough	1 to 4 mcg/ml	2 to 7 µmol/L
Chloramphenicol		
Peak	15 to 25 mcg/ml	46.4 to 77 µmol/L
Trough	5 to 15 mcg/ml	15.5 to 46.4 µmol/L
Gentamycin		
Peak	4 to 8 mcg/ml	8.4 to 16.7 µmol/L
Trough	1 to 2 mcg/ml	2.1 to 4.2 µmol/L
Tobramycin		
Peak	4 to 8 mcg/ml	8.6 to 17.1 µmol/L
Trough	1 to 2 mcg/ml	2.1 to 4.3 µmol/L
Vancomycin		
Peak	25 to 40 mcg/ml	14 to 27 µmol/L
Trough	5 to 10 mcg/ml	3.4 to 6.8 µmol/L

Urine tests

Test	Conventional units	SI units
Urinalysis		
Appearance	Clear to slightly hazy	–
Color	Straw to dark yellow	–
pH	4.5 to 8	–
Specific gravity	1.005 to 1.035	–
Glucose	None	–
Protein	None	–
RBCs	None or rare	–
WBCs	None or rare	–
Osmolality	50 to 1,400 mOsm/kg	–

Key facts about urine hormones

This chart lists the secretion sites and methods of measuring the major hormones and their metabolites.

Hormone or metabolite	Laboratory tests
Aldosterone	24-hour urine hormone analysis, urinary androgen evaluation, urinary thyroid panel
Free cortisol	24-hour urine hormone analysis, urinary adrenal steroid evaluation, urinary cortisol or thyroid analysis
Catecholamines	Urine catecholamines, HVA, VMA, adrenalin urine test, dopamine urine test
Total estrogens	24-hour urine steroid hormone panel
Estriol	24-hour urine steroid hormone panel
Human chorionic gonadotropin (hCG)	Urine hCG
Pregnanetriol	24-hour urine hormone analysis
17-hydroxycorticosteroids	24-hour urine hormone and steroid analysis
17-ketosteroids	24-hour urine hormone and steroid analysis
17-ketogenic steroids	24-hour urine hormone and steroid analysis
Vanillylmandelic acid (VMA)	Urine VMA
Homovanillic acid (HVA)	Urine HVA
5-hydroxyindoleacetic acid	Urine 5-hydroxyindoleacetic acid
Pregnanediol	24-hour urine hormone analysis

Reference values

3 to 19 mcg/24 hours (SI, 8 to 51 nmol/d)

Less than 50 mcg/24 hours

Epinephrine: 0 to 20 mcg/24 hours
Norepinephrine: 15 to 80 mcg/24 hours
Dopamine: 65 to 400 mcg/24 hours

Nonpregnant females: 40 to 60 mcg/24 hours
Pregnant females: First trimester—0 to 800 mcg/24 hours, second trimester—800 to 5,000 mcg/24 hours, third trimester—5,000 to 50,000 mcg/24 hours

Postmenopausal females: Less than 10 mcg/24 hours
Males: 4 to 25 mcg/24 hours

Values vary, but should show steady rise during pregnancy

Nonpregnant women/men: None measured
First trimester: 500,000 International Units/24 hours
Second trimester: 10,000 to 25,000 International Units/24 hours
Third trimester: 5,000 to 15,000 International Units/24 hours
Males (16 years and older): 0.4 to 2.5 mg/24 hours
Females (16 years and older): 0.1 to 1.8 mg/24 hours

Males: 4.5 to 12 mg/24 hours
Females: 2.5 to 10 mg/24 hours

Males: 10 to 25 mg/24 hours
Females: 4 to 6 mg/24 hours

Males: 4 to 14 mg/24 hours
Females: 2 to 12 mg/24 hours

1.4 to 6.5 mg/24 hours

Less than 10 mg/24 hours

Qualitative results: Negative
Quantitative results: 2 to 7 mg/24 hours

First trimester: 10 to 30 mg/24 hours
Second trimester: 35 to 70 mg/24 hours
Third trimester: 70 to 100 mg/24 hours
Postmenopausal women: 0.2 to 1mg/24 hours
Males: 0 to 1 mg/24 hours

CSF analysis

Test	Normal	Abnormal
Pressure	50 to 180 mm H_2O	Increase Decrease
Appearance	Clear, colorless	Cloudy Xanthochromic or bloody Brown, orange, or yellow
Protein	15 to 50 mg/dl (SI, 0.15 to 0.5 g/L)	Marked increase Marked decrease
Gamma globulin	3% to 12% of total protein	Increase
Glucose	50 to 80 mg/dl (SI, 2.8 to 4.4 mmol/L)	Increase Decrease
Cell count	0 to 5 white blood cells No RBCs	Increase RBCs
VDRL	Nonreactive	Positive
Chloride	118 to 130 mEq/L (SI, 118 to 130 mmol/L)	Decrease
Gram stain	No organisms	Gram-positive or gram-negative organisms

---

Implications

Increased intracranial pressure
Spinal subarachnoid obstruction above
puncture site

Infection
Subarachnoid, intracerebral, or intraventricular hemorrhage; spinal cord obstruction; traumatic lumbar puncture (only in initial specimen)
Elevated protein levels, red blood cell (RBC) breakdown (blood present for at least 3 days)

Tumors, trauma, hemorrhage, diabetes mellitus, polyneuritis, blood in cerebrospinal fluid (CSF)
Rapid CSF production

Demyelinating disease, neurosyphilis, Guillain-Barré syndrome

---

Systemic hyperglycemia
Systemic hypoglycemia, bacterial or fungal infection, meningitis, mumps, postsubarachnoid hemorrhage

---

Active disease: meningitis, acute infection, onset of chronic illness, tumor, abscess, infarction, demyelinating disease
Hemorrhage or traumatic lumbar puncture

Neurosyphilis

Infected meninges

Bacterial meningitis

4 Medications

Drug administration guidelines

Precautions for drug administration

Whenever you administer medication, observe these precautions to ensure that you're giving the right drug in the right dose to the right patient.

Check the order

Check the order on the patient's medication record against the physician's order.

Check the label

Check the label on the medication three times before administering it to the patient to ensure that you're administering the prescribed medication in the prescribed dose. Check it when you take the container from the shelf or drawer, right before pouring the medication into the medication cup or drawing it into the syringe, and before returning the container to the shelf or drawer. If you're administering a unit-dose medication, check the label for the third time immediately after pouring the medication and again before discarding the wrapper. Don't open a unit-dose medication until you're at the patient's bedside.

Confirm the patient's identity

Before giving the medication, confirm the patient's identity by checking two patient identifiers. Then make sure that you have the correct medication.

Explain the procedure to the patient and provide privacy.

Have a written order

Make sure that you have a written order for every medication that's to be given. If the order is verbal, make sure that the physician signs for it within the specified time.

Give labeled medication

Don't give medication from a poorly labeled or unlabeled container. Furthermore, don't attempt to label drugs or reinforce drug labels yourself; a pharmacist must do that.

Monitor medication

Never give a medication that someone else has poured or prepared. Never allow your medication cart or tray out of your sight. Never return unwrapped or prepared medications to stock containers. Instead, dispose of them and notify the pharmacy.

Respond to the patient's questions

If the patient questions you about his medication or the dosage, check his medication record again. If the medication is correct, reassure him that it's correct. Make sure to tell him about changes in his medication or dosage. Instruct him, as appropriate, about possible adverse reactions and encourage him to report any that he experiences.

Enteral drug administration

Oral drugs

Most drugs are administered orally because this route is usually the safest, most convenient, and least expensive. Drugs for oral administration are available in many forms, including tablets, enteric-coated tablets, capsules, syrups, elixirs, oils, liquids, suspensions, powders, and granules. Some require special preparation before administration, such as mixing with juice to make them more palatable.

• Assess the patient's condition, including his level of consciousness, ability to swallow, and vital signs, as needed. Changes in his condition may warrant withholding medication.

• Give the patient his medication and, as needed, liquid to aid swallowing, minimize adverse effects, or promote absorption. If appropriate, crush the medication to facilitate swallowing.

• Stay with the patient until he has swallowed the drug.

Drug delivery through a nasogastric tube or gastric tube

A nasogastric (NG) tube allows direct instillation of medication into the GI system for the patient who can't ingest it orally. A gastric tube is inserted through the abdominal wall and medications may be administered through it.

• After unclamping the tube, attach the catheter-tip syringe and gently draw back on the piston of the syringe to check for residual gastric contents. If the residual content is within an acceptable amount, prepare the medication for administration.

• Reattach the syringe, without the piston, to the end of the tube. Holding the tube upright at a level slightly above the patient's nose or abdomen, open the clamp and pour in the medication slowly and steadily, as shown here.

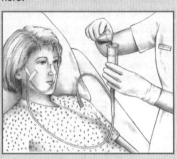

• After the medication is instilled, irrigate the tube by adding 30 to 50 ml of water (15 to 30 ml for a child).

• Then reclamp the tube.

Buccal and sublingual medications

Certain drugs are given buccally (between the patient's cheek and teeth) or sublingually (under the patient's tongue) to bypass the digestive tract and facilitate their absorption into the bloodstream.

• For buccal administration, place the tablet in the patient's buccal pouch, between his cheek and his teeth.

• For sublingual administration, place the tablet under the patient's tongue.

• Instruct the patient to keep the medication in place until it dissolves completely to ensure absorption.

• To prevent accidental swallowing, caution the patient against chewing the tablet or touching it with his tongue.

Respiratory drug administration

Handheld oropharyngeal inhalers

Handheld inhalers include the metered-dose inhaler and the turbo-inhaler. These devices deliver topical medications to the respiratory tract, producing local and systemic effects.

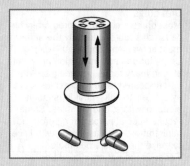

To use a metered-dose inhaler

• Shake the inhaler bottle. Remove the cap and insert the stem into the small hole on the flattened portion of the mouthpiece, as shown below.

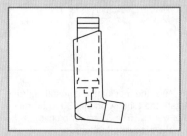

• Have the patient exhale. Place the inhaler about 1" (2.5 cm) in front of his open mouth.
• As you push the bottle down against the mouthpiece, instruct the patient to inhale slowly through his mouth and to continue inhaling until his lungs feel full. Compress the bottle against the mouthpiece only once.
• Remove the inhaler and tell the patient to hold his breath for several seconds. Then instruct him to exhale slowly through pursed lips to keep the distal bronchioles open, allowing increased absorption and diffusion of the drug.

To use a turbo-inhaler

• Hold the mouthpiece in one hand. With the other hand, slide the sleeve away from the mouthpiece as far as possible, as shown top of next column.
• Unscrew the tip of the mouthpiece by turning it counterclockwise.
• Press the colored portion of the medication capsule into the propeller stem of the mouthpiece. Screw the inhaler together again.

• Holding the inhaler with the mouthpiece at the bottom, slide the sleeve all the way down and then up again to puncture the capsule and release the medication. Do this only once.
• Have the patient exhale completely and tilt his head back. Instruct him to place the mouthpiece in his mouth, close his lips around it, and inhale once. Tell him to hold his breath for several seconds.
• Remove the inhaler from the patient's mouth and tell him to exhale as much air as possible.
• Repeat the procedure until all of the medication in the device has been inhaled.

To use a holding chamber (InspirEase)

• Insert the inhaler into the mouthpiece of the holding chamber and shake the inhaler. Then place the mouthpiece into the opening of the holding device and twist the mouthpiece to lock it in place.
• Extend the holding device, have the patient exhale, and place the mouthpiece into his mouth.
• Press down on the inhaler once. Then have the patient inhale slowly and deeply, collapsing the bag completely. If he breathes incorrectly, the bag will make a whistling sound. Tell the patient to hold his breath for 5 to 10 seconds and then to exhale slowly into the bag. Then repeat the inhaling and exhaling steps.
• Have the patient wait 1 to 2 minutes and repeat the procedure, if ordered.

Nasal drug administration

Nasal drugs may be instilled through drops, a spray (using an atomizer), or an aerosol (using a nebulizer). Most produce local rather than systemic effects. Nasal drugs include vasoconstrictors, antiseptics, anesthetics, hormones, vaccines, and corticosteroids.

To instill nose drops
• To reach the ethmoidal and sphenoidal sinuses, have the patient lie on his back, with his neck hyperextended and his head tilted back over the edge of the bed. Support his head with one hand to prevent neck strain.
• To reach the maxillary and frontal sinuses, have the patient lie on his back, with his head toward the affected side and hanging slightly over the edge of the bed. Ask him to rotate his head laterally after hyperextension. Support his head with one hand to prevent neck strain.
• To relieve ordinary nasal congestion, help the patient into a reclining or supine position, with his head tilted slightly toward the affected side. Aim the dropper upward, toward the patient's eye, rather than downward, toward his ear.
• Insert the dropper about ⅓" (8.5 mm) into the nostril. Make sure that it doesn't touch the sides of the nostril to avoid contaminating the dropper or making the patient sneeze.

To use a nasal spray
• Have the patient sit upright, with his head erect.
• Occlude one of the patient's nostrils, and insert the atomizer tip about ½" (1.5 cm) into the open nostril. Position the tip straight up, toward the inner canthus of the eye.
• Depending on the drug, have the patient hold his breath or inhale. Squeeze the atomizer once quickly and firmly—just enough to coat the inside of the nose. Excessive force may propel the medication into the patient's sinuses and cause a headache. Repeat the procedure in the other nostril, as ordered.

To use a nasal aerosol
• Shake the aerosol and hold it between your thumb and index finger, with the index finger on top of the cartridge.
• Tilt the patient's head back slightly, and carefully insert the adapter tip into one nostril. Depending on the medication, tell the patient to hold his breath or to inhale.
• Press your fingers together firmly to release one measured dose of medication.
• Shake the aerosol and repeat the procedure to instill medication into the other nostril.

Topical drug administration

Topical drugs, such as lotions and ointments, are applied directly to the patient's skin. They're commonly used for local, rather than systemic, effects. Typically, they must be applied two or three times per day to achieve a full therapeutic effect.

· Apply medication to the affected area with long, smooth strokes that follow the direction of hair growth, as below left.

· When applying medication to the patient's face, use a cotton-tipped applicator for small areas such as under the eyes. For larger areas, use a sterile gauze pad and follow the directions shown below right.

· To apply a shampoo, follow package directions. Apply medication with your fingertips, or instruct the patient to do so, as shown bottom right. Massage it into the scalp, if appropriate.

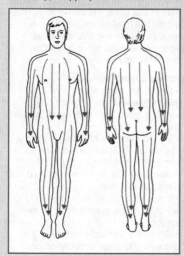

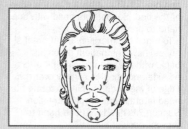

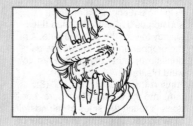

Eye and ear drug administration

Eyedrops or ointments serve diagnostic and therapeutic purposes. During an eye examination, these medications can be used to anesthetize the eye, dilate the pupil, and stain the cornea to identify anomalies. Therapeutic uses include lubrication of the eye and treatment of such conditions as glaucoma and infections.

Eye medication

To instill eyedrops

· Steady the hand that's holding the dropper by resting it against the patient's forehead. With your other hand, pull down the lower lid of the affected eye and instill the drops in the conjunctival sac. Never instill eyedrops directly onto the eyeball.

To apply eye ointment

· Squeeze a small ribbon of medication on the edge of the conjunctival sac, from the inner to the outer canthus, as shown below. Cut off the ribbon by turning the tube.

Eardrops

Eardrops may be instilled to treat infection or inflammation, to soften cerumen for later removal, to produce local anesthesia, or to facilitate the removal of an insect trapped in the ear.

To instill eardrops

· To avoid damaging the ear canal with the dropper, gently rest the hand that's holding the dropper against the patient's head. Straighten the patient's ear canal and instill the ordered number of drops. To avoid patient discomfort, aim the dropper so that the drops fall against the sides of the ear canal, not on the eardrum. Hold the ear canal in position until you see the medication disappear down the canal. After instilling the drops, lightly massage the tragus of the ear or apply gentle pressure.

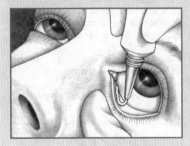

Vaginal and rectal drug administration

Vaginal drugs are suppositories, creams, gels, and ointments that can be inserted as topical treatment for infection (particularly *Trichomonas vaginalis* and candidal vaginitis) or inflammation or as a contraceptive. Suppositories melt when they come in contact with the warm vaginal mucosa, and their medication diffuses topically—as effectively as creams, gels, and ointments.

Vaginal suppositories or ointment

To insert a suppository
· Put on gloves and expose the vagina by spreading the labia. While the labia are still separated, insert the suppository 3″ to 4″ (7.5 to 10 cm) into the vagina.

To insert an ointment, a cream, or a gel
· Fit the applicator to the tube of medication and gently squeeze the tube to fill the applicator with the prescribed amount of medication. Lubricate the applicator tip.
· Put on gloves and expose the vagina.
· Insert the applicator about 2″ (5 cm) into the patient's vagina and administer the medication by depressing the plunger on the applicator.

Rectal suppositories or ointment

A rectal suppository is a small, solid, medicated mass, usually cone-shaped, with a cocoa butter or glycerin base. It may be inserted to stimulate peristalsis and defecation or to relieve pain, vomiting, and local irritation. An ointment is a semisolid medication that's used to produce local effects. It may be applied externally to the anus or internally to the rectum.

To insert a rectal suppository
· Lift the patient's upper buttock with your nondominant hand to expose the anus.
· Using the index finger of your dominant hand, insert the suppository—tapered end first—about 3″ (7.5 cm) until you feel it pass the internal anal sphincter, as shown here.
· Direct the tapered end of the suppository toward the side of the rectum so that it touches the membranes.

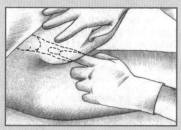

To apply an ointment
· For internal application
· Lift the patient's upper buttock with your nondominant hand to expose the anus.
· Gently insert the applicator, directing it toward the umbilicus, as shown here.
· Squeeze the tube to eject medication.

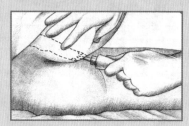

I.M. injection sites

An I.M. injection deposits medication deep into well-vascularized muscle for rapid systemic action and absorption of up to 5 ml.

Deltoid
If the volume to be administered is greater than 2 ml, don't use this site.

Ventrogluteal
This is the preferred injection site for adults and children older than 7 months.

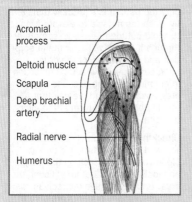

Acromial process
Deltoid muscle
Scapula
Deep brachial artery
Radial nerve
Humerus

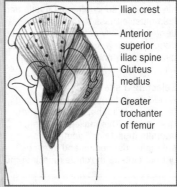

Iliac crest
Anterior superior iliac spine
Gluteus medius
Greater trochanter of femur

Dorsogluteal
If the site isn't identified properly, damage to the sciatic nerve can occur.

Vastus lateralis
The use of the middle third of this muscle is the preferred site for the neonate.

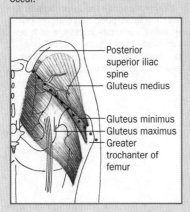

Posterior superior iliac spine
Gluteus medius
Gluteus minimus
Gluteus maximus
Greater trochanter of femur

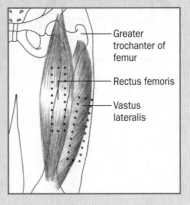

Greater trochanter of femur
Rectus femoris
Vastus lateralis

Modifying I.M. injections

Before you give an I.M. injection to an elderly patient, consider the physical changes that accompany aging and choose your equipment, site, and technique accordingly.

Choosing a needle
Remember that an elderly patient usually has less subcutaneous tissue and less muscle mass than a younger patient—especially in the buttocks and deltoids. As a result, you may need to use a shorter needle than you would for a younger adult.

Selecting a site
An elderly patient typically has more fat around the hips, abdomen, and thigh areas. This makes the vastus lateralis muscle and ventrogluteal area (gluteus medius and minimus, but not gluteus maximus muscles) the

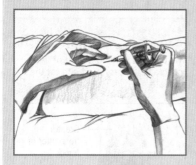

primary injection sites. If the patient can stand, instruct him to point the toes inward (foot inversion) to decrease pain felt with I.M. gluteus injections.

You should be able to palpate the muscle in these areas easily. However, if the patient is extremely thin, gently pinch the muscle to elevate it and to avoid putting the needle completely through it (which will alter the absorption and distribution of the drug).

Caution: Never give an I.M. injection in an immobile limb because of poor drug absorption and the risk that a sterile abscess will form at the injection site.

Checking technique
To avoid inserting the needle in a blood vessel, pull back on the plunger and look for blood before injecting the drug. Because of age-related vascular changes, elderly patients are also at greater risk for hematomas. To check bleeding after an I.M. injection, you may need to apply direct pressure over the puncture site for a longer time than usual.

Gently massage the injection site to aid drug absorption and distribution. However, avoid site massage with certain drugs given by the Z-track injection technique, such as iron dextran and hydroxyzine hydrochloride.

Displacing the skin for Z-track injection

By blocking the needle pathway after an injection, the Z-track technique allows I.M. injection while minimizing the risk of subcutaneous irritation and staining from such drugs as iron dextran. The illustrations here show how to perform a Z-track injection.

Before the procedure begins, the skin, subcutaneous fat, and muscle lie in their normal positions.

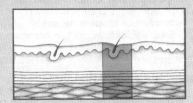

To begin, place your finger on the skin surface and pull the skin and subcutaneous layers out of alignment with the underlying muscle. You should move the skin about ½″ (1.5 cm).

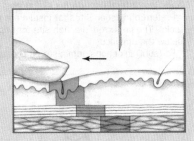

Insert the needle at a 90-degree angle at the site where you initially placed your finger. Inject the drug and withdraw the needle.

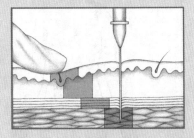

Finally, remove your finger from the skin surface, allowing the layers to return to their normal positions. The needle track (shown by the dotted line) is now broken at the junction of each tissue layer, trapping the drug in the muscle.

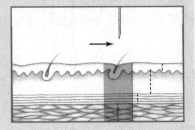

Subcutaneous drug administration

Before giving the injection, elevate the subcutaneous tissue at the site by grasping it firmly, as shown at right. Insert the needle at a 45- or 90-degree angle to the skin surface, depending on needle length and the amount of subcutaneous tissue at the site.

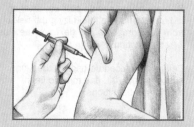

Some medications, such as heparin, should always be injected at a 90-degree angle.

Subcutaneous injection sites

Potential subcutaneous (subQ) injection sites (as indicated by the dotted areas in the illustration below) include the fat pads on the abdomen, upper hips, upper back, and lateral upper arms and thighs.

Preferred injection sites for insulin are the arms, abdomen, thighs, and buttocks. The preferred injection site for heparin is the lower abdomen fat pad, just below the umbilicus.

For subQ injections administered repeatedly, such as insulin, rotate sites.

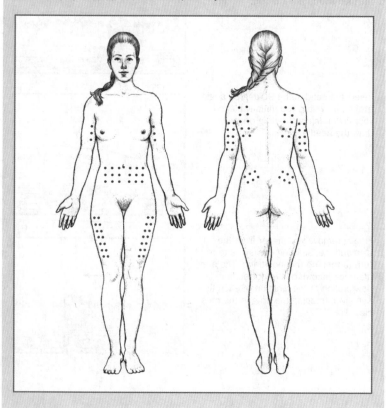

Intradermal drug administration

Used primarily for diagnostic purposes, as in allergy or tuberculin testing, an intradermal injection is administered in small amounts (usually 0.5 ml or less) into the outer layers of the skin. Because little systemic absorption takes place, this type of injection is used primarily to produce a local effect.

The ventral forearm is the most commonly used site because of its easy access and lack of hair.
· Locate an injection site from those shown below.

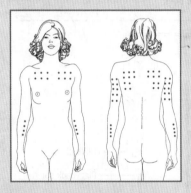

· With an alcohol pad, clean the surface of the ventral forearm about two or three fingerbreadths distal to the antecubital space. Make sure that the test site is free from hair and blemishes. Allow the skin to dry completely before administering the injection.
·While holding the patient's forearm in your hand, stretch the skin taut with your thumb.
· With your free hand, hold the needle at a 15-degree angle to the patient's arm, with its bevel up.
· Insert the needle about ⅛″ (3 mm) below the epidermis. Stop when the bevel tip of the needle is under the skin and inject the antigen slowly. You should feel some resistance as you do this, and a wheal should form as you inject the antigen, as shown below.

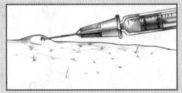

If no wheal forms, you have injected the antigen too deeply. Withdraw the needle, and administer another test dose at least 2″ (5 cm) from the first site.
· Withdraw the needle at the same angle at which it was inserted. Don't rub the site. This could irritate the underlying tissue, which may affect the test results.

I.V. drug administration

A secondary I.V. line is a complete I.V. set that's connected to the lower Y-port (secondary port) of a primary line instead of to the I.V. catheter or needle. It features an I.V. container, long tubing, and either a microdrip or macrodrip system. It can be used for continuous or intermittent drug infusion. When used continuously, it permits drug infusion and titration while the primary line maintains a constant total infusion rate.

I.V. bolus injection

The I.V. bolus injection method allows rapid I.V. drug administration to quickly achieve peak levels in the bloodstream. It may be used for drugs that can't be given I.M. because they're toxic or for a patient with a reduced ability to absorb these drugs. This method may also be used to deliver drugs that can't be diluted.

Bolus doses may be injected directly into a vein, through an existing I.V. line, or through an implanted vascular access port.

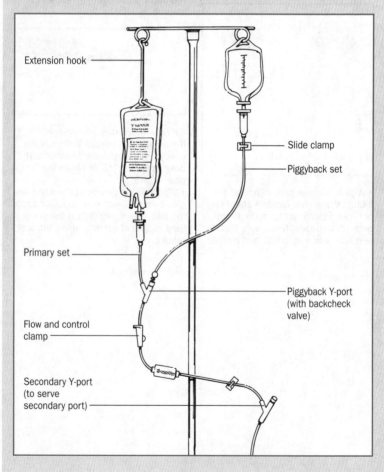

Extension hook

Slide clamp

Piggyback set

Primary set

Piggyback Y-port (with backcheck valve)

Flow and control clamp

Secondary Y-port (to serve secondary port)

Starting an I.V. infusion

Getting ready

- Use the largest vein and the appropriate gauge catheter for the type of infusion.
- Apply a tourniquet 4″ to 6″ (10 to 15 cm) above the puncture site.
- Leave the tourniquet in place for no more than 3 minutes.
- Lower the patient's arm below the heart and have him pump his fist (not make a fist).
- Try the cephalic and basilic veins first. (They have large lumens and the best blood flow, and are more durable and comfortable.)
- Lightly palpate the vein with the index and middle fingers of your nondominant hand.
- Stretch the skin to anchor the vein.
- Put on gloves and clean the site with a facility-approved antimicrobial solution using a vigorous side-to-side motion.
- If you're using 2% chlorhexidine gluconate swabs, use a vigorous back-and-forth motion, then allow 30 seconds for the solution to dry.
- If you're using 70% isopropyl alcohol or 10% povidone-iodine, use concentric circles, starting in the center and cleaning a diameter 2″ to 3″ (5 to 7.5 cm).
- The drying time is 30 seconds for 70% isopropyl alcohol and 2 minutes for povidone-iodine.
- Lightly press the skin with the thumb of your nondominant hand about 1½″ (4 cm) from the intended insertion site.

Inserting the device

- Open the I.V. catheter package and inspect the catheter for flaws or contamination. If any are found, discard it and obtain another catheter.
- Apply traction to the skin and anchor the vein with your nondominant hand, but don't touch the area just beside or directly over the vein.
- Insert the needle bevel up, and advance it until blood appears in the flashback chamber.
- Lower the catheter or needle angle so that it's parallel with the skin and then insert it a little bit more to ensure that the catheter tip is in the vein.
- Verify that blood continues to flow into the flashback chamber.
- If flashback stops and the chamber isn't full, slowly and carefully back out the catheter until flashback returns.
- Holding the needle or stylet steady, use your index finger or nondominant hand to gently slide the catheter over the needle and into the vein up to the hub.
- Follow the manufacturer's instructions for catheter advancement and activation of the safety feature.
- Stop immediately if you meet resistance or if the patient complains of severe pain.
- Release the tourniquet and apply digital pressure proximal to the insertion site on the vein to minimize blood backflow.
- Hold the primed extension set; remove the stylet from the catheter hub, activating the safety feature.
- Attach the extension set to the hub of the catheter and flush to verify patency.
- Secure the catheter with tape per your facility's policy.
- Apply a transparent dressing over the site.
- Document which arm was used; anatomic name of vein; catheter gauge, length, and brand; and number of attempts. Quote the patient regarding how the I.V. feels.

Common veins

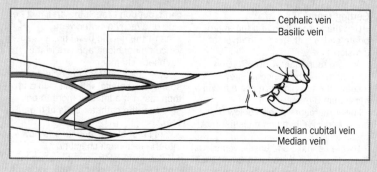

Local complications of peripheral veins

Type	Finding	Intervention
Phlebitis	• Tenderness at site • Redness at tip of catheter and along vein	• Remove device. • Apply warm soaks. • Notify physician.
Infiltration (nonvesicant solution)	• Coolness at site • Skin taut • Slowing of rate	• Remove device. • Apply cold compresses.
Extravasation (vesicant solution)	• Swelling at site • Discomfort (pain, burning) at site • Blanching	• Remove device. • Notify physician. • Treat site per I.V. solution recommendations.
Catheter dislodgment	• Catheter backed out of vein • Solution infiltrating	• Remove device.

Local complications of peripheral veins *(continued)*

Type	Finding	Intervention
Severed catheter	• Leakage from catheter shaft	• Notify physician. • If part of catheter enters bloodstream, place tourniquet above I.V. site to prevent progression of broken part.
Hematoma	• Tenderness at site • Bruised area around site	• Remove device. • Apply pressure, cold compresses. • Apply warm soaks.
Venous spasm	• Pain along vein; blanched skin • Flow rate sluggish with clamp open	• Decrease flow rate.
Vasovagal reaction	• Sudden collapse of vein during venipuncture • Sudden pallor, sweating, faintness, dizziness, nausea and hypotension	• Lower head of bed. • Check vital signs. • Have patient take deep breaths.
Thrombosis	• Painful, red, swollen vein • Sluggish or stopped I.V. flow	• Remove device. • Apply warm soaks. • Notify physician.
Thrombophlebitis	• Severe discomfort at site • Reddened, swollen, hardened vein	• Follow interventions for thrombosis.
Nerve, tendon, or ligament damage	• Extreme pain (like electric shock when nerve is punctured), numbness, and muscle contraction • Delayed effects: paralysis, numbness, and deformity	• Stop procedure. • Notify physician.

Antidotes for extravasation

Antidote	Extravasated drug
Ascorbic acid injection	• dactinomycin
Edetate calcium disodium (calcium EDTA)	• cadmium • copper • manganese • zinc
Hyaluronidase 15 units/ml	• aminophylline • calcium solutions • contrast media • dextrose solutions (concentrations of 10% or more) • nafcillin • potassium solutions • total parenteral nutrition solutions • vinblastine • vincristine • vindesine
Hydrocortisone sodium succinate 100 mg/ml Usually followed by topical application of hydrocortisone cream 1%	• doxorubicin • vincristine
Phentolamine	• dobutamine • dopamine • epinephrine • metaraminol bitartrate • norepinephrine
Sodium bicarbonate 8.4%	• carmustine • daunorubicin • doxorubicin • vinblastine • vincristine
Sodium thiosulfate 10%	• cisplatin • dactinomycin • mechlorethamine • mitomycin

Dosage calculation formulas and common conversions

Common calculations

$$\text{Body surface area in m}^2 = \sqrt{\frac{\text{height in cm} \times \text{weight in kg}}{3{,}600}}$$

$$\text{mcg/ml} = \text{mg/ml} \times 1{,}000$$

$$\text{ml/minute} = \frac{\text{ml/hour}}{60}$$

$$\text{gtt/minute} = \frac{\text{volume in ml to be infused} \times \text{drip factor in gtt/ml}}{\text{time in minutes}}$$

$$\text{mg/minute} = \frac{\text{mg in bag} \times \text{flow rate} \div 60}{\text{ml in bag}}$$

$$\text{mcg/minute} = \frac{\text{mg in bag} \div 0.06 \times \text{flow rate}}{\text{ml in bag}}$$

$$\text{mcg/kg/minute} = \frac{\text{mcg/ml} \times \text{ml/minute}}{\text{weight in kg}}$$

Common conversions

1 kg	=	1,000 g
1 g	=	1,000 mg
1 mg	=	1,000 mcg
1″	=	2.54 cm
1 L	=	1,000 ml
1 ml	=	1,000 microliters
1 tsp	=	5 ml
1 tbs	=	15 ml
2 tbs	=	30 ml
8 oz	=	240 ml
1 oz	=	30 g
1 lb	=	454 g
2.2 lb	=	1 kg

Body surface area nomogram

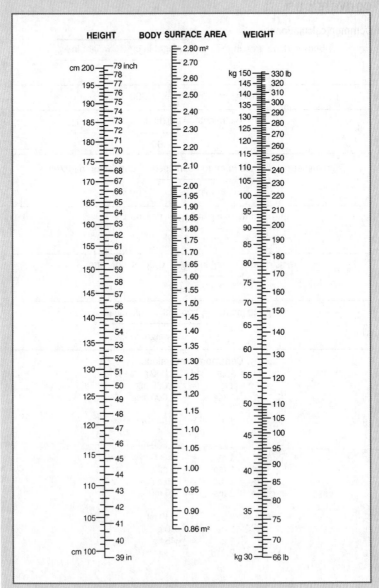

Reprinted with permission from Geigy Scientific Tables, 8th ed., vol. 5, p. 105 ©
Novartis, 1990.

Insulin overview

Insulin type	Onset	Peak (hours)	Usual effective duration (hours)	Usual maximum duration (hours)
Animal				
Regular	0.5 to 2 hours	3 to 4	4 to 6	6 to 8
NPH	4 to 6 hours	8 to 14	16 to 20	20 to 24
Human				
Insulin aspart	5 to 10 minutes	1 to 3	3 to 5	4 to 6
Insulin lispro	< 15 minutes	0.5 to 1.5	2 to 4	4 to 6
Regular	0.5 to 1 hour	2 to 3	3 to 6	6 to 10
NPH	2 to 4 hours	4 to 10	10 to 16	14 to 18
Lente	3 to 4 hours	4 to 12	12 to 18	16 to 20
Ultralente	6 to 10 hours	—	18 to 20	20 to 24
Insulin glargine	1 hour	—	24	24

Mixing insulin

When mixing insulin, always draw up clear insulin first, then cloudy.

To mix insulin, follow these steps:
• Wipe the rubber top of the insulin vials with alcohol.
• Gently roll the cloudy insulin between your palms.
• Remove the needle cap.
• Pull out the plunger until the end of the plunger in the barrel aligns with the number of units of cloudy insulin that you need.
• Push the needle through the rubber top of the cloudy insulin bottle.
• Inject air into the bottle.
• Remove the needle.
• Pull out the plunger until the end of the plunger in the barrel aligns with the units of clear insulin that you need.
• Push the needle through the rubber top of the clear insulin bottle.
• Inject the air into the bottle.
• Without removing the needle, turn the bottle upside down.
• Withdraw the plunger until it aligns with the number of units of clear regular insulin that you need.
• Gently pull the needle out of the bottle.
• Push the needle into the cloudy insulin bottle without injecting the clear insulin into the bottle.
• Withdraw the plunger until you reach your total dosage of insulin in units (clear combined with cloudy).

Insulin infusion pumps

A subcutaneous (subQ) insulin infusion pump provides continuous, long-term insulin therapy for patients with type 1 diabetes mellitus. Complications include site infection, catheter clogging, and insulin loss from loose reservoir-catheter connections. Insulin pumps work on either an open-loop or a closed-loop system.

Open-loop system
• Is the most common.
• Infuses insulin but can't respond to changes in patient's serum glucose levels.
• Delivers insulin in small (basal) doses every few minutes; large (bolus) doses are set by patient.
• Consists of reservoir-containing insulin syringe, small pump, infusion-rate selector that allows insulin release adjustments, battery, and plastic catheter with attached needle leading from syringe to subQ injection site.
• Needle is held in place with waterproof tape.
• Pump is worn on a belt or in a pocket.
• Infusion line must have clear path to injection site.
• Infusion-rate selector releases about one-half the total daily insulin.
• Patient releases the remainder in bolus doses before meals and snacks.

• Patient must change syringe daily.
• Patient must change needle, catheter, and injection site every other day.

Closed-loop system
• Self-contained; detects and responds to changing serum glucose levels.
• Includes glucose sensor, programmable computer, power supply, pump, and insulin reservoir.
• The computer triggers continuous insulin delivery in appropriate amounts.

Nonneedle catheter system
• Uses tiny plastic catheter inserted into the skin over a needle using a special insertion device.
• The needle is withdrawn, leaving the catheter in place (in the abdomen, thigh, or flank).
• Catheter is changed every 2 to 3 days.

Troubleshooting I.V. pump alarms

A number of electronic devices are available that assist the nurse in controlling the rate and volume of solution infusion. The most common device is an I.V. pump. Safe use of an I.V. requires an understanding of potential device alarms.

Alarm	Possible cause	Intervention
Air in tubing	• Empty I.V. bag	• Spike new I.V. bag and reprime tubing.
	• Hole in I.V. tubing	• Change I.V. tubing.
Low battery power	• Unplugged for extended period	• Plug in device.
	• Loss of power to outlet	• Move plug to another outlet. • Move plug to emergency outlet.
Downstream occlusion alarm	• Clotted catheter	• Flushing will determine clotting; select new site.
	• I.V. dressing too tight	• Change dressing.
	• Infiltration	• Remove catheter and change site.
	• Kinked tubing	• Locate and remove kink.
	• Filter or extension tubing added	• Stop infusions before adding filters or extensions to tubing and allow pump to establish a new baseline resistance.
	• Addition of a viscous solution	• Allow pump to establish a new baseline pressure.
	• Catheter gauge and tubing length	• Select the smallest catheter that will accept the desired flow rate and the largest vein available.

Calculating drip rates

When calculating the flow rate of I.V. solutions, remember that the number of drops required to deliver 1 ml varies with the type of administration set. To calculate the drip rate, you must know the calibration of the drip rate for each specific manufacturer's product. As a quick guide, refer to the chart below. Use this formula to calculate specific drip rates:

$$\frac{\text{volume of infusion (in ml)}}{\text{time of infusion (in minutes)}} \times \text{drip factor (in drops/ml)} = \text{drops/minute}$$

	Ordered volume					
	500 ml/24 hr or 21 ml/hr	1,000 ml/24 hr or 42 ml/hr	1,000 ml/20 hr or 50 ml/hr	1,000 ml/10 hr or 100 ml/hr	1,000 ml/8 hr or 125 ml/hr	1,000 ml/6 hr or 167 ml/hr
Drops/ml	**Drops/minute to infuse**					
Macrodrip						
10	4	7	8	17	21	28
15	5	11	13	25	31	42
20	7	14	17	33	42	56
Microdrip						
60	21	42	50	100	125	167

Tips for high-risk drips

Patient-controlled analgesia (PCA), heparin, and insulin infusions can be especially dangerous if administered incorrectly. If possible, have another nurse independently check the practitioner's order, your calculations, and the pump settings for these drugs before starting them.

PCA
Be sure to note:
• strength of the drug solution in the syringe
• number of drug administrations during assessment period
• basal dose patient received, if any
• amount of solution received (number of injections × volume of injections + basal doses)
• total amount of drug received (amount of solution × solution strength).

Heparin
Be sure to:
• determine the solution's concentration (Divide the units of drug added by the amount of the solution in milliliters.)
• state as a fraction: the desired dose over the unknown flow rate
• cross-multiply to find the flow rate.

Insulin
Be sure to:
• remember that regular insulin is the only type given by I.V. route
• always use an infusion pump
• use concentrations of 1 unit/ml.

Infusion flow rates

Epinephrine infusion rates
Mix 1 mg in 250 ml (4 mcg/ml).

Dose *(mcg/minute)*	Infusion rate *(ml/hour)*
1	15
2	30
3	45
4	60
5	75
6	90
7	105
8	120
9	135
10	150
15	225
20	300
25	375
30	450
35	525
40	600

Isoproterenol infusion rates
Mix 1 mg in 250 ml (4 mcg/ml).

Dose *(mcg/minute)*	Infusion rate *(ml/hour)*
1	15
2	30
3	45
4	60
5	75
6	90
7	105
8	120
9	135
10	150
15	225
20	300
25	375
30	450

Nitroglycerin infusion rates
Determine the infusion rate in ml/hour using the ordered dose and the concentration of the drug solution.

Dose *(mcg/minute)*	25 mg/250 ml *(100 mcg/ml)*	50 mg/250 ml *(200 mcg/ml)*	100 mg/250 ml *(400 mcg/ml)*
5	3	2	1
10	6	3	2
20	12	6	3
30	18	9	5
40	24	12	6
50	30	15	8
60	36	18	9
70	42	21	10
80	48	24	12
90	54	27	14
100	60	30	15
150	90	45	23
200	120	60	30

Dobutamine infusion rates

Mix 250 mg in 250 ml of D_5W (1,000 mcg/ml). Determine the infusion rate in ml/hr using the ordered dose and the patient's weight in pounds or kilograms.

Dose (mcg/kg/min)	Patient's weight								
	lb 88 *kg* 40	99 45	110 50	121 55	132 60	143 65	154 70	165 75	176 80
2.5	6	7	8	8	9	10	11	11	12
5	12	14	15	17	18	20	21	23	24
7.5	18	20	23	25	27	29	32	34	36
10	24	27	30	33	36	39	42	45	48
12.5	30	34	38	41	45	49	53	56	60
15	36	41	45	50	54	59	63	68	72
20	48	54	60	66	72	78	84	90	96
25	60	68	75	83	90	98	105	113	120
30	72	81	90	99	108	117	126	135	144
35	84	95	105	116	126	137	147	158	168
40	96	108	120	132	144	156	168	180	192

| 187 | 198 | 209 | 220 | 231 | 242 |
85	90	95	100	105	110
13	14	14	15	16	17
26	27	29	30	32	33
38	41	43	45	47	50
51	54	57	60	63	66
64	68	71	75	79	83
77	81	86	90	95	99
102	108	114	120	126	132
128	135	143	150	158	165
153	162	171	180	189	198
179	189	200	210	221	231
204	216	228	240	252	264

Dopamine infusion rates

Mix 400 mg in 250 ml of D_5W (1,600 mcg/ml). Determine the infusion rate in ml/hour using the ordered dose and the patient's weight in pounds or kilograms.

Dose (mcg/kg/min)	Patient's weight							
	lb *kg*	*88* *40*	*99* *45*	*110* *50*	*121* *55*	*132* *60*	*143* *65*	*154* *70*	*165* *75*
2.5		4	4	5	5	6	6	7	7
5		8	8	9	10	11	12	13	14
7.5		11	13	14	15	17	18	20	21
10		15	17	19	21	23	24	26	28
12.5		19	21	23	26	28	30	33	35
15		23	25	28	31	34	37	39	42
20		30	34	38	41	45	49	53	56
25		38	42	47	52	56	61	66	70
30		45	51	56	62	67	73	79	84
35		53	59	66	72	79	85	92	98
40		60	68	75	83	90	98	105	113
45		68	76	84	93	101	110	118	127
50		75	84	94	103	113	122	131	141

| 176 | 187 | 198 | 209 | 220 | 231 |
80	85	90	95	100	105
8	8	8	9	9	10
15	16	17	18	19	20
23	24	25	27	28	30
30	32	34	36	38	39
38	40	42	45	47	49
45	48	51	53	56	59
60	64	68	71	75	79
75	80	84	89	94	98
90	96	101	107	113	118
105	112	118	125	131	138
120	128	135	143	150	158
135	143	152	160	169	177
150	159	169	178	188	197

Nitroprusside infusion rates

Mix 50 mg in 250 ml of D$_5$W (200 mcg/ml). Determine the infusion rate in ml/hour using the ordered dose and the patient's weight in pounds or kilograms.

Dose (mcg/kg/min)	Patient's weight								
	lb 88 *kg* 40	99 45	110 50	121 55	132 60	143 65	154 70	165 75	176 80
0.3	4	4	5	5	5	6	6	7	7
0.5	6	7	8	8	9	10	11	11	12
1	12	14	15	17	18	20	21	23	24
1.5	18	20	23	25	27	29	32	34	36
2	24	27	30	33	36	39	42	45	48
3	36	41	45	50	54	59	63	68	72
4	48	54	60	66	72	78	84	90	96
5	60	68	75	83	90	98	105	113	120
6	72	81	90	99	108	117	126	135	144
7	84	95	105	116	126	137	147	158	168
8	96	108	120	132	144	156	168	180	192
9	108	122	135	149	162	176	189	203	216
10	120	135	150	165	180	195	210	225	240

187 85	198 90	209 95	220 100	231 105	242 110
8	8	9	9	9	10
13	14	14	15	16	17
26	27	29	30	32	33
38	41	43	45	47	50
51	54	57	60	63	66
77	81	86	90	95	99
102	108	114	120	126	132
128	135	143	150	158	165
153	162	171	180	189	198
179	189	200	210	221	231
204	216	228	240	252	264
230	243	257	270	284	297
255	270	285	300	315	330

Dangerous effects of drug combinations

If possible, avoid administering these drug combinations to prevent dangerous drug interactions.

Drug	Interacting drug	Possible effect
Aminoglycosides amikacin gentamicin kanamycin neomycin netilmicin streptomycin tobramycin	Parenteral cephalosporins • Ceftazidime • Ceftizoxime	Possible enhanced nephrotoxicity
	Loop diuretics • Bumetanide • Ethacrynic acid • Furosemide	Possible enhanced ototoxicity
Amphetamines amphetamine benzphetamine dextroamphetamine methamphetamine	Urine alkalinizers • Potassium citrate • Sodium acetate • Sodium bicarbonate • Sodium citrate • Sodium lactate • Tromethamine	Decreased urinary excretion of amphetamine
Angiotensin-converting enzyme (ACE) inhibitors benazepril captopril enalapril fosinopril lisinopril quinapril ramipril	Indomethacin Nonsteroidal anti-inflammatory drugs (NSAIDs)	Decreased or abolished effectiveness of antihypertensive action of ACE inhibitors
Barbiturate anesthetics methohexital thiopental	Opiate analgesics	Enhanced central nervous system and respiratory depression
Barbiturates amobarbital aprobarbital butabarbital mephobarbital pentobarbital phenobarbital primidone secobarbital	Valproic acid	Increased serum barbiturate levels

Dangerous effects of drug combinations *(continued)*

Drug	Interacting drug	Possible effect
Beta-adrenergic blockers acebutolol atenolol betaxolol carteolol esmolol levobunolol metoprolol nadolol penbutolol pindolol propranolol timolol	Verapamil	Enhanced pharmacologic effects of both beta-adrenergic blockers and verapamil
Carbamazepine	Erythromycin	Increased risk of carbamazepine toxicity
Carmustine	Cimetidine	Enhanced risk of bone marrow toxicity
Ciprofloxacin	Antacids that contain magnesium or aluminum hydroxide, iron supplements, sucralfate, multivitamins that contain iron or zinc	Decreased plasma levels and effectiveness of ciprofloxacin
Clonidine	Beta-adrenergic blockers	Enhanced rebound hypertension following rapid clonidine withdrawal
Cyclosporine	Carbamazepine, isoniazid, phenobarbital, phenytoin, rifabutin, rifampin	Reduced plasma levels of cyclosporine
Cardiac glycosides	Loop and thiazide diuretics	Increased risk of cardiac arrhythmias due to hypokalemia
	Thiazide-like diuretics	Increased therapeutic or toxic effects
Digoxin	Amiodarone	Decreased renal clearance of digoxin
	Quinidine	Enhanced clearance of digoxin
	Verapamil	Elevated serum digoxin levels
Dopamine	Phenytoin	Hypertension and bradycardia

(continued)

Dangerous effects of drug combinations *(continued)*

Drug	Interacting drug	Possible effect
Epinephrine	Beta-adrenergic blockers	Increased systolic and diastolic pressures; marked decrease in heart rate
Erythromycin	Carbamazepine	Decreased carbamazepine clearance
	Theophylline	Decreased hepatic clearance of theophylline
Ethanol	Disulfiram Furazolidone Metronidazole	Acute alcohol intolerance reaction
Furazolidone	Amine-containing foods Anorexiants	Inhibits monoamine oxidase (MAO), possibly leading to hypertensive crisis
Heparin	Salicylates NSAIDs	Enhanced risk of bleeding
Levodopa	Furazolidone	Enhanced toxic effects of levodopa
Lithium	Thiazide diuretics NSAIDs	Decreased lithium excretion
Meperidine	MAO inhibitors	Cardiovascular instability and increased toxic effects
Methotrexate	Probenecid	Decreased methotrexate elimination
	Salicylates	Increased risk of methotrexate toxicity
MAO inhibitors	Amine-containing foods Anorexiants Meperidine	Risk of hypertensive crisis
Nondepolarizing muscle relaxants	Aminoglycosides Inhaled anesthetics	Enhanced neuromuscular blockade
Potassium supplements	Potassium-sparing diuretics	Increased risk of hyperkalemia
Quinidine	Amiodarone	Increased risk of quinidine toxicity
Sympathomimetics	MAO inhibitors	Increased risk of hypertensive crisis
Tetracyclines	Antacids containing magnesium, aluminum, or bismuth salts Iron supplements	Decreased plasma levels and effectiveness of tetracyclines

Dangerous effects of drug combinations *(continued)*

Drug	Interacting drug	Possible effect
Theophylline	Carbamazepine	Reduced theophylline levels
	Cimetidine	Increased theophylline levels
	Ciprofloxacin	Increased theophylline levels
	Erythromycin	Increased theophylline levels
	Phenobarbital	Reduced theophylline levels
	Rifampin	Reduced theophylline levels
Warfarin	Testosterone	Possible enhanced bleeding caused by increased hypoprothrombinemia
	Barbiturates Carbamazepine	Reduced effectiveness of warfarin
	Amiodarone Cephalosporins (certain ones) Chloral hydrate Cholestyramine Cimetidine Clofibrate Co-trimoxazole Dextrothyroxine Disulfiram	Increased risk of bleeding
	Erythromycin Glucagon Metronidazole Phenylbutazone Quinidine Quinine Salicylates Sulfinpyrazone Thyroid drugs Tricyclic antidepressants	Increased risk of bleeding
	Chlordiazepoxide Carbamazepine Vitamin K	Decreased pharmacologic effect
	Rifampin Trazodone	Decreased risk of bleeding
	Methimazole Propylthiouracil	Increased or decreased risk of bleeding

(continued)

Herb-drug interactions

Herb	Drug	Possible effects
Aloe	Cardiac glycosides, antiarrhythmics	May lead to hypokalemia, which may potentiate cardiac glycosides and antiarrhythmics
	Thiazide diuretics, licorice, and other potassium-wasting drugs	Increases the effects of potassium wasting
	Orally administered drugs	Causes potential for decreased absorption of drugs because of more rapid GI transit time
Bilberry	Antiplatelets, anticoagulants	Decreases platelet aggregation
	Insulin, hypoglycemics	May increase serum insulin levels, causing hypoglycemia; increases effect with diabetes drugs
Capsicum	Antiplatelets, anticoagulants	Decreases platelet aggregation and increases fibrinolytic activity, prolonging bleeding time
	Nonsteroidal anti-inflammatory drugs (NSAIDs)	Stimulates GI secretions to help protect against NSAID-induced GI irritation
	Angiotensin-converting enzyme inhibitors	May cause cough
	Theophylline	Increases absorption of theophylline, possibly leading to higher serum levels or toxicity
	Monoamine oxidase (MAO) inhibitors	Decreases the effects resulting from the increased catecholamine secretion
	Central nervous system (CNS) depressants, such as opioids, benzodiazepines, barbiturates	Increases sedative effect
	Histamine-2 blockers, proton pump inhibitors	Causes potential for decreased effectiveness because of increased acid secretion
Chamomile	Drugs requiring GI absorption	May delay drug absorption
	Anticoagulants	May enhance anticoagulant therapy and prolong bleeding time (if warfarin constituents)
	Iron	May reduce iron absorption because of tannic acid content

Herb-drug interactions *(continued)*

Herb	Interacting drug	Possible effect
Echinacea	Immunosuppressants	May counteract immunosuppressant drugs
	Hepatotoxics	May increase hepatotoxicity with drugs known to elevate liver enzyme levels
	Warfarin	Increases bleeding time without an increased International Normalized Ratio (INR)
Evening primrose	Anticonvulsants	Lowers seizure threshold
Feverfew	Antiplatelets, anticoagulants	May decrease platelet aggregation and increase fibrinolytic activity
Garlic	Antiplatelets, anticoagulants	Enhances platelet inhibition, leading to increased anticoagulation
	Insulin, other drugs causing hypoglycemia	May increase serum insulin levels, causing hypoglycemia, an additive effect with antidiabetics
	Antihypertensives	Causes potential for additive hypotension
	Antihyperlipidemics	May have additive lipid-lowering properties
Ginger	Chemotherapy	May reduce nausea associated with chemotherapy
	H_2-blockers, proton pump inhibitors	Causes potential for decreased effectiveness because of increased acid secretion by ginger
	Antiplatelets, anticoagulants	Inhibits platelet aggregation by antagonizing thromboxane synthase and enhancing prostacyclin, leading to prolonged bleeding time
	Calcium channel blockers	May increase calcium uptake by myocardium, leading to altered drug effects
	Antihypertensives	May antagonize antihypertensive effect

(continued)

Herb-drug interactions *(continued)*

Herb	Interacting drug	Possible effect
Ginkgo	Antiplatelets, anticoagulants	May enhance platelet inhibition, leading to increased anticoagulation
	Anticonvulsants	May decrease effectiveness of anticonvulsants
	Drugs known to lower seizure threshold	May further reduce seizure threshold
Ginseng	Stimulants	May potentiate stimulant effects
	Warfarin	May antagonize warfarin, resulting in a decreased INR
	Antibiotics	May enhance the effects of some antibiotics (Siberian ginseng)
	Anticoagulants, antiplatelets	Decreases platelet adhesiveness
	Digoxin	May falsely elevate digoxin levels
	MAO inhibitors	Potentiates action of MAO inhibitors
	Hormones, anabolic steroids	May potentiate effects of hormone and anabolic steroid therapies (estrogenic effects of ginseng may cause vaginal bleeding and breast nodules)
	Alcohol	Increases alcohol clearance, possibly by increasing activity of alcohol dehydrogenase
	Furosemide	May decrease diuretic effect of furosemide
	Antipsychotics	May stimulate CNS activity
Goldenseal	Heparin	May counteract anticoagulant effect of heparin
	Diuretics	Increases diuretic effect
	H_2-blockers, proton pump inhibitors	Causes potential for decreased effectiveness because of increased acid secretion by goldenseal
	General anesthetics	May potentiate hypotensive action of general anesthetics

Herb-drug interactions *(continued)*

Herb	Interacting drug	Possible effect
Goldenseal *(continued)*	CNS depressants, such as opioids, barbiturates, benzodiazepines	Increases sedative effect
Grapeseed	Warfarin	Increases the effects and INR caused by tocopherol content of grapeseed
Green tea	Warfarin	Decreases effectiveness resulting from vitamin content of green tea
Hawthorn berry	Digoxin	Causes additive positive inotropic effect, with potential for digoxin toxicity
Kava	CNS stimulants or depressants	May hinder therapy with CNS stimulants
	Benzodiazepines	May result in comalike states
	Alcohol	Potentiates the depressant effect of alcohol and other CNS depressants
	Levodopa	Decreases the effectiveness of levodopa
Licorice	Digoxin	Causes hypokalemia, which predisposes to digoxin toxicity
	Hormonal contraceptives	Increases fluid retention and potential for increased blood pressure resulting from fluid overload
	Corticosteroids	Causes additive and enhanced effects of the corticosteroids
	Spironolactone	Decreases the effects of spironolactone
Ma huang	MAO inhibitors	Potentiates MAO inhibitors
	CNS stimulants, caffeine, theophylline	Causes CNS stimulation
	Digoxin	Increases the risk of arrhythmias
	Hypoglycemics	Decreases hypoglycemic effect because of hyperglycemia caused by ma huang
Melatonin	CNS depressants (such as opioids, barbiturates, benzodiazepines)	Increases sedative effects

(continued)

Herb-drug interactions *(continued)*

Herb	Interacting drug	Possible effect
Milk thistle	Drugs causing diarrhea	Increases bile secretion and often causes loose stools; may increase effect of other drugs commonly causing diarrhea; also causes liver membrane-stabilization and antioxidant effects leading to protection from liver damage from various hepatotoxic drugs such as acetaminophen, phenytoin, ethanol, phenothiazines, butyrophenones
Nettle	Anticonvulsants	May increase sedative adverse effects and risk of seizure
	Opioids, anxiolytics, hypnotics	May increase sedative adverse effects
	Warfarin	Decreases effectiveness resulting from vitamin K content of aerial parts of nettle
	Iron	May reduce iron absorption because of tannic acid content
Passion flower	CNS depressants (such as opioids, barbiturates, benzodiazepines)	Increases sedative effect
St. John's wort	Selective serotonin reuptake inhibitors (SSRIs), MAO inhibitors, nefazodone, trazodone	Causes additive effects with SSRIs, MAO inhibitors, and other antidepressants, potentially leading to serotonin syndrome, especially when combined with SSRIs
	Indinavir; HIV protease inhibitors (PIs); nonnucleoside reverse transcriptase inhibitors (NNRTIs)	Induces cytochrome P450 metabolic pathway, which may decrease therapeutic effects of drugs using this pathway for metabolism (use of St. John's wort and PIs or NNRTIs should be avoided because of the potential for subtherapeutic antiretroviral levels and insufficient virologic response that could lead to resistance or class cross-resistance)
	Opioids, alcohol	Enhances the sedative effect of opioids and alcohol
	Photosensitizing drugs	Increases photosensitivity
	Sympathomimetic amines (such as pseudoephedrine)	Causes additive effects

Herb-drug interactions *(continued)*

Herb	Interacting drug	Possible effect
St. John's wort *(continued)*	Digoxin	May reduce serum digoxin concentrations, decreasing therapeutic effects
	Reserpine	Antagonizes the effects of reserpine
	Hormonal contraceptives	Increases breakthrough bleeding when taken with hormonal contraceptives; also decreases the contraceptive's effectiveness
	Theophylline	May decrease serum theophylline levels, making the drug less effective
	Anesthetics	May prolong the effect of anesthesia drugs
	Cyclosporine	Decreases cyclosporine levels below therapeutic levels, threatening transplanted organ rejection
	Iron	May reduce iron absorption because of tannic acid content
	Warfarin	Has the potential to alter INR; reduces the effectiveness of anticoagulant, requiring increased dosage of drug
Valerian	Sedative hypnotics, CNS depressants	Enhances the effects of sedative hypnotic drugs
	Alcohol	Increases sedation with alcohol (although debated)
	Iron	May reduce iron absorption because of tannic acid content

Pharmacokinetics in older adults

Differences in the way older people absorb, distribute, metabolize, and eliminate drugs can alter the effects of medications. The age-related differences are listed below.

Absorption

- Change in quality and quantity of digestive enzymes
- Increased gastric pH
- Decreased number of absorbing cells
- Decreased GI motility
- Decreased intestinal blood flow
- Decreased GI emptying time

Distribution

- Decreased cardiac output and reserve
- Decreased blood flow to target tissues, liver, and kidneys
- Decreased distribution space and area
- Decreased lean body mass
- Increased adipose stores
- Decreased plasma protein (decreases protein-binding drugs)
- Decreased total body water

Metabolism

- Decreased microsomal metabolism of drug
- Decreased hepatic biotransformation

Elimination

- Decreased renal excretion of drug
- Decreased glomerular filtration
- Decreased renal tubular secretion

Drugs causing confusion in older adults

These drug classes can cause confusion in older adults:

- antiarrhythmics
- anticholinergics
- antiemetics
- antihistamines
- antihypertensives
- antiparkinsonian agents
- antipsychotics
- diuretics
- histamine blockers
- opioid analgesics
- sedative-hypnotics
- tranquilizers.

Medications associated with falls

This chart highlights some classes of drugs that are commonly prescribed for older patients and the possible adverse effects of each that may increase a patient's risk of falling.

Drug class	Adverse effects
Alcohol	• Intoxication • Motor incoordination • Agitation • Sedation • Confusion
Antidiabetic drugs	• Acute hypoglycemia
Antihypertensives	• Hypotension
Antipsychotics	• Orthostatic hypotension • Muscle rigidity • Sedation
Benzodiazepines and antihistamines	• Excessive sedation • Confusion • Paradoxical agitation • Loss of balance
Diuretics	• Hypovolemia • Orthostatic hypotension • Electrolyte imbalance
Hypnotics	• Excessive sedation • Ataxia • Poor balance • Confusion • Paradoxical agitation
Opioids	• Hypotension • Sedation • Motor incoordination • Agitation
Tricyclic antidepressants	• Orthostatic hypotension

Adverse reactions misinterpreted as age-related changes

Some conditions result from aging, others from drug therapy; however, some can result from aging and drug therapy. This chart indicates drug classes and their associated adverse reactions.

Adverse reactions

Drug classifications	Agitation	Anxiety	Arrhythmias	Ataxia	Changes in appetite	Confusion	Constipation	Depression	Difficulty breathing	Disorientation	Dizziness	Drowsiness	Edema	Fatigue	Hypotension	Insomnia	Memory loss	Muscle weakness	Restlessness	Sexual dysfunction	Tremors	Urinary dysfunction	Vision changes
Alpha$_1$-adrenergic blockers		•				•	•				•	•	•	•	•	•				•		•	•
Angiotensin-converting enzyme inhibitors						•	•	•			•			•	•	•				•			•
Antianginals	•	•	•			•					•		•	•	•	•		•	•			•	•
Antiarrhythmics			•				•	•		•		•		•	•								
Anticholinergics	•	•	•		•	•	•			•	•			•	•		•	•	•			•	•
Anticonvulsants	•		•	•	•	•	•	•		•	•	•	•	•	•	•					•	•	•
Antidepressants, tricyclic	•	•	•		•	•	•	•	•	•	•			•	•					•	•	•	•
Antidiabetics, oral											•			•									
Antihistamines					•	•	•			•	•	•		•							•	•	•
Antilipemics							•				•			•		•	•		•		•	•	•
Antiparkinsonians	•	•		•	•	•	•	•		•	•		•	•	•	•		•			•	•	•
Antipsychotics	•	•	•	•	•	•	•	•		•	•		•	•	•			•	•	•	•	•	•
Barbiturates	•	•	•		•			•	•			•		•	•			•					
Benzodiazepines	•		•		•	•	•	•	•	•	•	•		•		•	•	•			•	•	•
Beta-adrenergic blockers		•	•			•	•			•			•	•		•			•	•	•	•	•
Calcium channel blockers		•	•			•		•		•		•	•	•	•	•				•		•	•
Corticosteroids	•				•		•				•	•		•		•		•					•
Diuretics							•			•			•	•		•			•			•	
Nonsteroidal anti-inflammatory drugs		•			•	•	•			•	•	•		•		•		•					•
Opioids	•	•			•	•	•	•	•	•	•		•	•	•			•	•			•	•
Skeletal muscle relaxants	•	•		•	•		•			•	•		•	•	•						•		
Thyroid hormones			•		•									•							•		

Preventing adverse drug reactions in older patients

A drug's action in the body and its interaction with body tissues (pharmacodynamics) both change significantly in older people. In this chart, you'll find the information you need to help prevent adverse drug reactions in your elderly patients.

Pharmacology	Indications	Special considerations
Adrenergics, direct- and indirect-acting • Exert excitatory actions on the heart, glands, and vascular smooth muscle and peripheral inhibitory actions on smooth muscles of the bronchial tree	• Hypotension • Cardiac stimulation • Bronchodilation • Shock	• An elderly patient may be more sensitive to therapeutic and adverse effects of some adrenergics and may require lower doses.
Adrenocorticoids, systemic • Stimulate enzyme synthesis needed to decrease the inflammatory response	• Inflammation • Immunosuppression • Adrenal insufficiency • Rheumatic and collagen diseases • Acute spinal cord injury	• These drugs may aggravate hyperglycemia, delay wound healing, or contribute to edema, insomnia, or osteoporosis in an elderly patient. • Decreased metabolic rate and elimination may cause increased plasma levels and increase the risk of adverse effects. Monitor the elderly patient carefully.
Alpha-adrenergic blockers • Block the effects of peripheral neurohormonal transmitters (norepinephrine, epinephrine) on adrenergic receptors in various effector systems	• Peripheral vascular disorders • Hypertension • Benign prostatic hyperplasia	• Hypotensive effects may be more pronounced in an elderly patient. • These drugs should be administered at bedtime to reduce potential for dizziness or light-headedness.
Aminoglycosides • Inhibit bacterial protein synthesis	• Infection caused by susceptible organisms	• The elderly patient may have decreased renal function and thus be at greater risk for nephrotoxicity, ototoxicity, and superinfection (common).

(continued)

Preventing adverse drug reactions in older patients (continued)

Pharmacology	Indications	Special considerations
Angiotensin-converting enzyme (ACE) inhibitors • Prevent the conversion of angiotensin I to angiotensin II • Decrease vasoconstriction and adrenocortical secretion of aldosterone	• Hypertension • Heart failure	• Diuretic therapy should be discontinued before ACE inhibitors are started to reduce the risk of hypotension. • An elderly patient may need lower doses because of impaired drug clearance.
Anticholinergics • Exert antagonistic action on acetylcholine and other cholinergic agonists within the parasympathetic nervous system	• Hypersecretory conditions • GI tract disorders • Sinus bradycardia • Dystonia and Parkinsonism • Perioperative use • Motion sickness	• These drugs should be used cautiously in an elderly adult, who may be more sensitive to the effects of these drugs; a lower dosage may be indicated.
Antihistamines • Prevent access and subsequent activity of histamine	• Allergy • Pruritus • Vertigo • Nausea and vomiting • Sedation • Cough suppression • Dyskinesia	• An elderly patient is usually more sensitive to the adverse effects of antihistamines; he's especially likely to experience a greater degree of dizziness, sedation, hypotension, and urine retention.
Barbiturates • Decrease presynaptic and postsynaptic excitability, producing central nervous system (CNS) depression	• Seizure disorders • Sedation (including preanesthesia) • Hypnosis	• An elderly patient and a patient receiving subhypnotic doses may experience hyperactivity, excitement, or hyperanalgesia. Use with caution.
Benzodiazepines • Act selectively on polysynaptic neuronal pathways throughout the CNS; synthetically produced sedative-hypnotic	• Seizure disorders • Anxiety, tension, insomnia • Surgical adjuncts for conscious sedation or amnesia • Skeletal muscle spasm, tremor	• These drugs should be used cautiously in an elderly patient, who's sensitive to the drugs' CNS effects; parenteral administration is more likely to cause apnea, hypotension, bradycardia, and cardiac arrest.

Preventing adverse drug reactions in older patients (continued)

Pharmacology	Indications	Special considerations
Beta-adrenergic blockers • Compete with beta agonists for available beta-receptor sites; individual agents differ in their ability to affect beta receptors	• Hypertension • Angina • Arrhythmias • Glaucoma • Myocardial infarction (MI) • Migraine prophylaxis	• Increased bioavailability or delayed metabolism in the elderly patient may require a lower dosage; an elderly patient may also experience enhanced adverse effects.
Calcium channel blockers • Inhibit calcium influx across the slow channels of myocardial and vascular smooth muscle cells, causing dilation of coronary arteries, peripheral arteries, and arterioles and slowing cardiac conduction	• Angina • Arrhythmias • Hypertension	• These drugs should be used cautiously in an elderly patient because the half-life of calcium channel blockers may be increased as a result of decreased clearance.
Cardiac glycosides • Directly increase myocardial contractile force and velocity, atrioventricular node refractory period, and total peripheral resistance • Indirectly depress sinoatrial node and prolong conduction to the atrioventricular node	• Heart failure • Arrhythmias • Paroxysmal atrial tachycardia or atrioventricular junctional rhythm • MI • Cardiogenic shock • Angina	• These drugs should be used cautiously in an elderly patient with renal or hepatic dysfunction or with electrolyte imbalance that may predispose him to toxicity.
Cephalosporins • Inhibit bacterial cell wall synthesis, causing rapid cell lysis	• Infection caused by susceptible organisms	• Because the elderly patient commonly has impaired renal function, he may require a lower dosage. • An older adult is more susceptible to superinfection and coagulopathies.
Coumadin derivatives • Interfere with the hepatic synthesis of vitamin K-dependent clotting factors II, VII, IX, and X, decreasing the blood's coagulation potential	• Treatment for or prevention of thrombosis or embolism	• An older adult has an increased risk of hemorrhage because of altered hemostatic mechanisms or age-related hepatic and renal deterioration.

(continued)

Preventing adverse drug reactions in older patients *(continued)*

Pharmacology	Indications	Special considerations
Diuretics, loop • Inhibit sodium and chloride reabsorption in the ascending loop of Henle and increase excretion of potassium, sodium, chloride, and water	• Edema • Hypertension	• An elderly or debilitated patient is more susceptible to drug-induced diuresis and can quickly develop dehydration, hypovolemia, hypokalemia, and hyponatremia, which may cause circulatory collapse.
Diuretics, potassium-sparing • Act directly on the distal renal tubules, inhibiting sodium reabsorption and potassium excretion	• Edema • Hypertension • Diagnosis of primary hyperaldosteronism	• An older patient may need a smaller dosage because of his susceptibility to drug-induced diuresis and hyperkalemia.
Diuretics, thiazide and thiazide-like • Interfere with sodium transport, thereby increasing renal excretion of sodium, chloride, water, potassium, and calcium	• Edema • Hypertension • Diabetes insipidus	• Age-related changes in cardiovascular and renal function make the elderly patient more susceptible to excessive diuresis, which may lead to dehydration, hypovolemia, hyponatremia, hypomagnesemia, and hypokalemia.
Estrogens • Promote development and maintenance of the female reproductive system and secondary sexual characteristics; inhibition of the release of pituitary gonadotropins	• Moderate to severe vasomotor symptoms of menopause • Atrophic vaginitis • Carcinoma of the breast and prostate • Prophylaxis of postmenopausal osteoporosis	• A postmenopausal woman on long-term estrogen therapy has an increased risk of developing endometrial cancer.
Histamine-2 (H_2) receptor antagonists • Inhibit histamine's action at H_2 receptors in gastric parietal cells, reducing gastric acid output and concentration, regardless of the stimulatory agent or basal conditions	• Duodenal ulcer • Gastric ulcer • Hypersecretory states • Reflux esophagitis • Stress ulcer prophylaxis	• These drugs should be used cautiously in an elderly patient because of his increased risk of developing adverse reactions, particularly those affecting the CNS.

Preventing adverse drug reactions in older patients *(continued)*

Pharmacology	Indications	Special considerations
Insulin		
• Increases glucose transport across muscle cells and fat-cell membranes to reduce blood glucose levels • Promotes conversion of glucose to glycogen • Stimulates amino acid uptake and conversion to protein in muscle cells • Inhibits protein degradation • Stimulates triglyceride formation and lipoprotein lipase activity; inhibits free fatty acid release from adipose tissue	• Diabetic ketoacidosis • Diabetes mellitus • Diabetes mellitus inadequately controlled by diet and oral antidiabetic agents • Hyperkalemia	• Insulin is available in many forms that differ in onset, peak, and duration of action; the physician will specify the individual dosage and form. • Blood glucose measurement is an important guide to dosage and management. • The elderly patient's diet and his ability to recognize hypoglycemia are important. • A source of diabetic teaching should be provided, especially for the elderly patient, who may need follow-up home care.
Iron supplements, oral		
• Are needed in adequate amounts for erythropoiesis and efficient oxygen transport; essential component of hemoglobin	• Iron deficiency anemia	• Iron-induced constipation is common among elderly patients; stress proper diet to minimize constipation. • An elderly patient may also need higher doses due to reduced gastric secretions and because achlorhydria may lower his capacity for iron absorption.
Nitrates		
• Relax smooth muscle; generally used for vascular effects (vasodilatation)	• Angina pectoris • Acute MI	• Severe hypotension and cardiovascular collapse may occur if nitrates are combined with alcohol. • Transient dizziness, syncope, or other signs of cerebral ischemia may occur; instruct the elderly patient to take nitrates while sitting.
Nonsteroidal anti-inflammatory drugs (NSAIDs)		
• Interfere with prostaglandins involved with pain; anti-inflammatory action that contributes to analgesic effect	• Pain • Inflammation • Fever	• A patient older than age 60 may be more susceptible to the toxic effects of NSAIDs because of decreased renal function; these drugs' effects on renal prostaglandins may cause fluid retention and edema, a drawback for a patient with heart failure.

(continued)

Preventing adverse drug reactions in older patients *(continued)*

Pharmacology	Indications	Special considerations
Opioid agonists • Act at specific opiate receptor–binding sites in the CNS and other tissues; alteration of pain perception without affecting other sensory functions	• Analgesia • Pulmonary edema • Preoperative sedation • Anesthesia • Cough suppression • Diarrhea	• Lower doses are usually indicated for elderly patients, who tend to be more sensitive to the therapeutic and adverse effects of these drugs.
Opioid agonists-antagonists • Act, in theory, on different opiate receptors in the CNS to a greater or lesser degree, thus yielding slightly different effects	• Pain	• Lower doses may be indicated in patients with renal or hepatic dysfunction to prevent drug accumulation.
Opioid antagonists • Act differently, depending on whether an opioid agonist has been administered previously, the actions of that opioid, and the extent of physical dependence on it	• Opioid-induced respiratory depression • Adjunct in treating opiate addiction	• These drugs are contraindicated for opioid addicts, in whom they may produce an acute abstinence syndrome.
Penicillins • Inhibit bacterial cell-wall synthesis, causing rapid cell lysis; most effective against fast-growing susceptible organisms	• Infection caused by susceptible organisms	• An elderly patient (and others with low resistance from immunosuppressants or radiation therapy) should be taught the signs and symptoms of bacterial and fungal superinfection.
Phenothiazine • Believed to function as dopamine antagonists, blocking postsynaptic dopamine receptors in various parts of the CNS; antiemetic effects resulting from blockage of the chemoreceptor trigger zones	• Psychosis • Nausea and vomiting • Anxiety • Severe behavior problems • Tetanus • Porphyria • Intractable hiccups • Neurogenic pain • Allergies and pruritus	• An older adult needs a lower dosage because he's more sensitive to these drugs' therapeutic and adverse effects, especially cardiac toxicity, tardive dyskinesia, and other extrapyramidal effects. • Dosage should be titrated to patient response.

Preventing adverse drug reactions in older patients *(continued)*

Pharmacology	Indications	Special considerations
Salicylates • Decrease formation of prostaglandins involved in pain and inflammation	• Pain • Inflammation • Fever	• A patient older than age 60 with impaired renal function may be more susceptible to these drugs' toxic effects. • The effect of salicylates on renal prostaglandins may cause fluid retention and edema, a significant disadvantage for a patient with heart failure.
Serotonin-reuptake inhibitors • Inhibit reuptake of serotonin; have little or no effect on other neurotransmitters	• Major depression • Obsessive-compulsive disorder • Bulimia nervosa	• These drugs should be used cautiously in a patient with hepatic impairment.
Sulfonamides • Inhibit folic acid biosynthesis needed for cell growth	• Bacterial and parasitic infections • Inflammation	• These drugs should be used cautiously in an elderly patient, who's more susceptible to bacterial and fungal superinfection, folate deficiency anemia, and renal and hematologic effects because of diminished renal function.
Tetracyclines • Inhibit bacterial proteinsynthesis	• Bacterial, protozoal, rickettsial, and fungal infections • Sclerosing agent	• Some elderly patients have decreased esophageal motility; administer tetracyclines with caution and monitor for local irritation from slowly passing oral forms.
Thrombolytic enzymes • Convert plasminogen to plasmin for promotion of clot lysis	• Thrombosis, thromboembolism	• Patients age 75 and older are at greater risk for cerebral hemorrhage because they're more apt to have preexisting cerebrovascular disease.

(continued)

Preventing adverse drug reactions in older patients *(continued)*

Pharmacology	Indications	Special considerations
Thyroid hormones • Have catabolic and anabolic effects • Influence normal metabolism, growth and development, and every organ system; vital to normal CNS function	• Hypothyroidism • Nontoxic goiter • Thyrotoxicosis • Diagnostic use	• In a patient older than age 60, the initial hormone replacement dose should be 25% less than the recommended dose.
Thyroid hormones antagonists • Inhibit iodine oxidation in the thyroid gland through a block of iodine's ability to combine with tyrosine to form thyroxine	• Hyperthyroidism • Preparation for thyroidectomy • Thyrotoxic crisis • Thyroid carcinoma	• Serum thyroid-stimulating hormone should be monitored as a sensitive indicator of thyroid hormone levels. Dosage adjustment may be required.
Tricyclic antidepressants • Inhibit neurotransmitter reuptake, resulting in increased concentration and enhanced activity of neurotransmitters in the synaptic cleft	• Depression • Obsessive-compulsive disorder • Enuresis • Severe, chronic pain	• Lower doses are indicated in an elderly patient because he's more sensitive to both the therapeutic and adverse effects of tricyclic antidepressants.

Drugs that shouldn't be crushed

Many drug forms, such as slow-release, enteric-coated, encapsulated beads, wax-matrix, sublingual, and buccal forms, are designed to release their active ingredients over a certain period or at preset intervals after administration. The disruptions caused by crushing these drug forms can dramatically affect the absorption rate and increase the risk of adverse reactions.

Other reasons not to crush these drug forms include such considerations as taste, tissue irritation, and unusual formulation—for example, a capsule within a capsule, a liquid within a capsule, or a multiple-compressed tablet. Avoid crushing the following drugs, listed by brand name, for the reasons noted beside them.

Accutane (irritant)
Aciphex (delayed release)
Adalat CC (sustained release)
Advicor (extended release)
Aggrenox (extended release)
Allegra D (extended release)
Altocor (extended release)
Amnesteem (irritant)
Arthrotec (delayed release)
Asacol (delayed release)
Augmentin XR (extended release)
Avinza (extended release)
Azulfidine EN-tabs (enteric coated)
Bellergal-S (slow release)
Biaxin XL (extended release)
Bisacodyl (enteric coated)
Bontril Slow-Release (slow release)
Breonesin (liquid filled)
Brexin L.A. (slow release)
Bromfed (slow release)
Bromfed-PD (slow release)
Calan SR (sustained release)
Carbatrol (extended release)
Cardizem CD, LA, SR (slow release)
Cartia XT (extended release)
Ceclor CD (slow release)
Ceftin (strong, persistent taste)
Charcoal Plus DS (enteric coated)
Chloral Hydrate (liquid within a capsule, taste)
Chlor-Trimeton Allergy 8-hour and 12-hour (slow release)
Choledyl SA (slow release)
Cipro XR (extended release)
Claritin-D 12-hour (slow release)
Claritin-D 24-hour (slow release)
Colace (liquid within a capsule)
Colazal (granules within capsules must reach the colon intact)
Colestid (protective coating)
Compazine Spansules (slow release)
Concerta (extended release)

Congess SR (sustained release)
Contac 12-Hour, Maximum Strength 12-Hour (slow release)
Cotazym-S (enteric coated)
Covera-HS (extended release)
Creon (enteric coated)
Cytovene (irritant)
Dallergy, Dallergy-Jr (slow release)
Deconamine SR (slow release)
Depakene (slow release, mucous membrane irritant)
Depakote (enteric coated)
Depakote ER (extended release)
Desyrel (taste)
Dexedrine Spansule (slow release)
Diamox Sequels (slow release)
Dilacor XR (extended release)
Dilatrate-SR (slow release)
Diltia XT (extended release)
Dimetapp Extentabs (slow release)
Ditropan XL (slow release)
Dolobid (irritant)
Drisdol (liquid filled)
Dristan (protective coating)
Drixoral (slow release)
Dulcolax (enteric coated)
DynaCirc CR (slow release)
Easprin (enteric coated)
Ecotrin (enteric coated)
Ecotrin Maximum Strength (enteric coated)
E.E.S. 400 Filmtab (enteric coated)
Effexor XR (extended release)
Emend (hard gelatin capsule)
E-Mycin (enteric coated)
Entex LA (slow release)
Entex PSE (slow release)
Eryc (enteric coated)
Ery-Tab (enteric coated)
Erythrocin Stearate (enteric coated)
Erythromycin Base (enteric coated)

(continued)

Drugs that shouldn't be crushed *(continued)*

Eskalith CR (slow release)
Extendryl JR, SR (slow release)
Feldene (mucous membrane irritant)
Feosol (enteric coated)
Feratab (enteric coated)
Fergon (slow release)
Fero-Folic 500 (slow release)
Fero-Grad-500 (slow release)
Ferro-Sequel (slow release)
Feverall Children's Capsules, Sprinkle (taste)
Flomax (slow release)
Fumatinic (slow release)
Geocillin (taste)
Glucophage XR (extended release)
Glucotrol XL (slow release)
Guaifed (slow release)
Guaifed-PD (slow release)
Guaifenex LA (slow release)
Guaifenex PSE (slow release)
Humibid DM, LA, Pediatric (slow release)
Hydergine LC (liquid within a capsule)
Hytakerol (liquid filled)
Iberet (slow release)
ICAPS Plus (slow release)
ICAPS Time Release (slow release)
Imdur (slow release)
Inderal LA (slow release)
Indocin SR (slow release)
InnoPran XL (extended release)
Ionamin (slow release)
Isoptin SR (sustained release)
Isordil Sublingual (sublingual)
Isordil Tembid (slow release)
Isosorbide Dinitrate Sublingual (sublingual)
Kaon-Cl (slow release)
K-Dur (slow release)
Klor-Con (slow release)
Klotrix (slow release)
K-Tab (slow release)
Levbid (slow release)
Levsinex Timecaps (slow release)
Lithobid (slow release)
Macrobid (slow release)
Mestinon Timespans (slow release)
Metadate CD, ER (extended release)
Methylin ER (extended release)
Micro-K Extencaps (slow release)
Motrin (taste)
MS Contin (slow release)
Mucinex (extended release)

Naprelan (slow release)
Nexium (sustained release)
Niaspan (extended release)
Nitroglyn (slow release)
Nitrong (slow release)
Nitrostat (sublingual)
Norflex (slow release)
Norpace CR (slow release)
Oramorph SR (slow release)
Oruvail (extended release)
OxyContin (slow release)
Pancrease (enteric coated)
Pancrease MT (enteric coated)
Paxil CR (controlled release)
PCE (slow release)
Pentasa (controlled release)
Phazyme (slow release)
Phazyme 95 (slow release)
Phenytex (extended release)
Plendil (slow release)
Prelu-2 (slow release)
Prevacid, Prevacid SoluTab (delayed release)
Prilosec (slow release)
Prilosec OTC (delayed release)
Pro-Banthine (taste)
Procanbid (slow release)
Procardia (delayed absorption)
Procardia XL (slow release)
Protonix (delayed release)
Proventil Repetabs (slow release)
Prozac Weekly (slow release)
Quibron-T/SR (slow release)
Quinidex Extentabs (slow release)
Respaire SR (slow release)
Respbid (slow release)
Risperdal M-Tab (delayed release)
Ritalin-LA, -SR (slow release)
Rondec-TR (slow release)
Sinemet CR (slow release)
Slo-Bid Gyrocaps (slow release)
Slo-Niacin (slow release)
Slo-Phyllin GG, Gyrocaps (slow release)
Slow FE (slow release)
Slow-K (slow release)
Slow-Mag (slow release)
Sorbitrate (sublingual)
Sotret (irritant)
Sudafed 12-Hour (slow release)
Sustaire (slow release)
Tegretol-XR (extended release)
Ten-K (slow release)

Drugs that shouldn't be crushed *(continued)*

Tenuate Dospan (slow release)
Tessalon Perles (slow release)
Theobid Duracaps (slow release)
Theochron (slow release)
Theoclear LA (slow release)
Theolair-SR (slow release)
Theo-Sav (slow release)
Theospan-SR (slow release)
Theo-24 (slow release)
Theovent (slow release)
Theo-X (slow release)
Thorazine Spansules (slow release)
Tiazac (sustained release)
Topamax (taste)
Toprol XL (extended release)
T-Phyl (slow release)

Trental (slow release)
Trinalin Repetabs (slow release)
Tylenol Extended Relief (slow release)
Uniphyl (slow release)
Vantin (taste)
Verelan, Verelan PM (slow release)
Volmax (slow release)
Voltaren (enteric coated)
Voltaren-XR (extended release)
Wellbutrin SR (sustained release)
Xanax XR (extended release)
Zerit XR (extended release)
Zomig-ZMT (delayed release)
ZORprin (slow release)
Zyban (slow release)
Zyrtec-D 12-hour (extended release)

Identifying the most dangerous drugs

Almost any drug can cause an adverse reaction in some patients, but the following drugs cause about 90% of all reported reactions.

Anticoagulants
- Heparin
- Warfarin

Antimicrobials
- Cephalosporins
- Penicillins
- Sulfonamides

Bronchodilators
- Sympathomimetics
- Theophylline

Cardiac drugs
- Antihypertensives
- Digoxin
- Diuretics
- Quinidine

Central nervous system drugs
- Analgesics
- Anticonvulsants
- Neuroleptics
- Sedative-hypnotics

Diagnostic agents
- X-ray contrast media

Hormones
- Corticosteroids
- Estrogens
- Insulin

Common antidotes

Drug or toxin	Antidote
Acetaminophen	Acetylcysteine (Mucomyst)
Anticholinergics	Physostigmine (Antilirium)
Benzodiazepines	Flumazenil (Romazicon)
Calcium channel blockers	Calcium chloride
Cyanide	Amyl nitrate, sodium nitrite, and sodium thiosulfate (Cyanide Antidote Kit); methylene blue
Digoxin, cardiac glycosides	Digoxin immune Fab (Digibind)
Ethylene glycol	Ethanol
Heparin	Protamine sulfate
Insulin-induced hypoglycemia	Glucagon
Iron	Deferoxamine mesylate (Desferal)
Lead	Edetate calcium disodium (Calcium Disodium Versenate)
Opioids	Naloxone (Narcan), nalmefene (Revex), naltrexone (ReVia)
Organophosphates, anticholinesterases	Atropine, pralidoxime (Protopam)
Warfarin	Vitamin K

Therapeutic drug monitoring guidelines

Drug	Laboratory test monitored	Therapeutic ranges of test
Aminoglycoside antibiotics (amikacin, gentamicin, tobramycin)	Amikacin peak Amikacin trough Gentamicin/tobramycin peak Gentamicin/tobramycin trough Creatinine	20 to 30 mcg/ml 1 to 8 mcg/ml 4 to 12 mcg/ml < 2 mcg/ml 0.6 to 1.3 mg/dl
Angiotensin-converting enzyme (ACE) inhibitors (benazepril, captopril, enalapril, enalaprilat, fosinopril, lisinopril, moexipril, quinapril, ramipril, trandolapril)	White blood cell (WBC) count with differential Creatinine Blood urea nitrogen (BUN) Potassium	***** 0.6 to 1.3 mg/dl 5 to 20 mg/dl 3.5 to 5 mEq/L
Amphotericin B	Creatinine BUN Electrolytes (especially potassium and magnesium) Liver function Complete blood count (CBC) with differential and platelets	0.6 to 1.3 mg/dl 5 to 20 mg/dl Potassium: 3.5 to 5 mEq/L Magnesium: 1.5 to 2.5 mEq/L Sodium: 135 to 145 mEq/L Chloride: 98 to 106 mEq/L * *****
Antibiotics	WBC with differential Cultures and sensitivities	*****
Biguanides (metformin)	Creatinine Fasting glucose Glycosylated hemoglobin CBC	0.6 to 1.3 mg/dl 70 to 110 mg/dl 5.5% to 8.5% of total hemoglobin *****
Carbamazepine	Carbamazepine CBC with differential Liver function BUN Platelet count	4 to 12 mcg/ml ***** * 5 to 20 mg/dl 150 to 450 $\times$ 10^3/mm^3

Note: ***** For those areas marked with asterisks, the following values can be used:

Hemoglobin: Women: 12 to 16 g/dl; Men: 13 to 18 g/dl
Hematocrit: Women 37% to 48%; Men: 42% to 52%
Red blood cell count (RBC): 4 to 5.5 $\times$ 10^6/mm^3
WBC count: 5 to 10 $\times$ 10^3/mm^3

Differential: Neutrophils: 45% to 74%
Bands: 0% to 8%
Lymphocytes: 16% to 45%
Monocytes: 4% to 10%
Eosinophils: 0% to 7%
Basophils: 0% to 2%

Monitoring guidelines

Wait until the administration of the third dose to check drug levels. Obtain blood for peak level 30 minutes after I.V. infusion ends or 60 minutes after I.M. administration. For trough levels, draw blood just before the next dose. Dosage may need to be adjusted accordingly. Recheck after three doses. Monitor creatinine and BUN levels and urine output for signs of decreasing renal function. Monitor urine for increased proteins, cells, and casts.

Monitor the WBC count with differential before therapy, monthly during the first 3 to 6 months, and then periodically for the first year. Monitor renal function and potassium level periodically.

Monitor creatinine, BUN, and electrolyte levels at least weekly during therapy. Monitor blood counts and liver function test results regularly during therapy.

Results of specimen cultures and sensitivities will determine the cause of the infection and the best treatment. Monitor the WBC count with differential weekly during therapy.

Check renal function and hematologic values before starting therapy and at least annually thereafter. If the patient has impaired renal function, don't use metformin because it may cause lactic acidosis. Monitor response to therapy by evaluating fasting glucose and glycosylated hemoglobin levels periodically. A patient's home monitoring of glucose levels helps monitor compliance and response.

Monitor blood counts and platelet count before therapy, monthly during the first 2 months, and then yearly. Liver function, BUN, and urinalysis results should be checked before and periodically during therapy.

(continued)

* For those areas marked with one asterisk, the following values can be used:

Alanine aminotransferase: 7 to 56 units/L
Aspartate aminotransferase: 5 to 40 units/L
Alkaline phosphatase: 17 to 142 units/L
Lactate dehydrogenase: 60 to 220 units/L
Gamma glutamyl transferase (GGT): < 40 units/L
Total bilirubin: 0.2 to 1 mg/dl

Therapeutic drug monitoring guidelines *(continued)*

Drug	Laboratory test monitored	Therapeutic ranges of test
Clozapine	WBC with differential	*****
Corticosteroids (cortisone, hydrocortisone, prednisone, prednisolone, triamcinolone, methylprednisolone, dexamethasone, betamethasone)	Electrolytes (especially potassium) Fasting glucose	Potassium: 3.5 to 5 mEq/L Magnesium: 1.7 to 2.1 mEq/L Sodium: 135 to 145 mEq/L Chloride: 98 to 106 mEq/L Calcium: 8.6 to 10 mg/dl 70 to 110 mg/dl
Digoxin	Digoxin Electrolytes (especially potassium, magnesium, and calcium) Creatinine	0.8 to 2 ng/ml Potassium: 3.5 to 5 mEq/L Magnesium: 1.7 to 2.1 mEq/L Sodium: 135 to 145 mEq/L Chloride: 98 to 106 mEq/L Calcium: 8.6 to 10 mg/dl 0.6 to 1.3 mg/dl
Diuretics	Electrolytes Creatinine BUN Uric acid Fasting glucose	Potassium: 3.5 to 5 mEq/L Magnesium: 1.7 to 2.1 mEq/L Sodium: 135 to 145 mEq/L Chloride: 98 to 106 mEq/L Calcium: 8.6 to 10 mg/dl 0.6 to 1.3 mg/dl 5 to 20 mg/dl 2 to 7 mg/dl 70 to 110 mg/dl
Erythropoietin	Hematocrit Serum ferritin Transferrin saturation CBC with differential Platelet count	Women: 36% to 48% Men: 42% to 52% 10 to 383 mg/ml 220 to 400 mg/dl ***** 150 to 450 $\times$ 10^3/mm^3
Ethosuximide	Ethosuximide Liver function CBC with differential	40 to 100 mcg/ml * *****

Note: ***** For those areas marked with asterisks, the following values can be used:

Hemoglobin: Women: 12 to 16 g/dl; Men: 13 to 18 g/dl
Hematocrit: Women 37% to 48%; Men: 42% to 52%
Red blood cell count (RBC): 4 to 5.5 $\times$ 10^6/mm^3
WBC count: 5 to 10 $\times$ 10^3/mm^3

Differential: Neutrophils: 45% to 74%
Bands: 0% to 8%
Lymphocytes: 16% to 45%
Monocytes: 4% to 10%
Eosinophils: 0% to 7%
Basophils: 0% to 2%

Monitoring guidelines

Obtain a WBC count with differential before starting therapy, weekly during therapy, and 4 weeks after discontinuing the drug.

Monitor electrolyte and glucose levels regularly during long-term therapy.

Check digoxin levels just before the next dose or a minimum of 6 to 8 hours after the last dose. To monitor maintenance therapy, check drug levels at least 1 to 2 weeks after therapy is initiated or changed. Adjust therapy based on the entire clinical picture, not solely based on drug levels. Also, check electrolyte levels and renal function periodically during therapy.

To monitor fluid and electrolyte balance, perform baseline and periodic determinations of electrolyte, calcium, BUN, uric acid, and glucose levels.

After therapy is initiated or changed, monitor hematocrit twice weekly for 2 to 6 weeks until it's stabilized in the target range and a maintenance dose is determined. Monitor hematocrit regularly thereafter.

Check drug level 8 to 10 days after therapy is initiated or changed. Periodically monitor the CBC with differential and results of liver function tests and urinalysis.

(continued)

* For those areas marked with one asterisk, the following values can be used:

Alanine aminotransferase: 7 to 56 units/L
Aspartate aminotransferase: 5 to 40 units/L
Alkaline phosphatase: 17 to 142 units/L
Lactate dehydrogenase: 60 to 220 units/L
Gamma glutamyl transferase (GGT): < 40 units/L
Total bilirubin: 0.2 to 1 mg/dl

Therapeutic drug monitoring guidelines *(continued)*

Drug	Laboratory test monitored	Therapeutic ranges of test
Gemfibrozil	Lipids	Total cholesterol: < 200 mg/dl Low-density lipoprotein (LDL): < 130 mg/dl High-density lipoprotein (HDL): Women: 40 to 75 mg/dl Men: 37 to 70 mg/dl Triglycerides: 10 to 160 mg/dl
	Liver function	*
	Serum glucose	70 to 100 mg/dl
	CBC	*****
Heparin	Partial thromboplastin time (PTT)	1.5 to 2.5 times control
	Hematocrit	*****
	Platelet count	150 to 450 × 10^3/mm³
3-hydroxy-3-methylglutaryl coenzyme A (HMG-CoA) reductase inhibitors (fluvastatin, lovastatin, pravastatin, simvastatin)	Lipids	Total cholesterol: < 200 mg/dl LDL: < 130 mg/dl HDL: Women: 40 to 75 mg/dl Men: 37 to 70 mg/dl Triglycerides: 10 to 160 mg/dl
	Liver function	*
Insulin	Fasting glucose	70 to 110 mg/dl
	Glycosylated hemoglobin	5.5% to 8.5% of total hemoglobin
Isotretinoin	Pregnancy test	Negative
	Liver function	*
	Lipids	Total cholesterol: < 200 mg/dl LDL: < 130 mg/dl HDL: Women: 40 to 75 mg/dl Men: 37 to 70 mg/dl Triglycerides: 10 to 160 mg/dl
	CBC with differential	*****
	Platelet count	150 to 450 × 10^3/mm³

Note: ***** For those areas marked with asterisks, the following values can be used:

Hemoglobin: Women: 12 to 16 g/dl; Men: 13 to 18 g/dl

Hematocrit: Women 37% to 48%; Men: 42% to 52%

Red blood cell count (RBC): 4 to 5.5 × 10^6/mm³

WBC count: 5 to 10 × 10^3/mm³

Differential: Neutrophils: 45% to 74%
    Bands: 0% to 8%
    Lymphocytes: 16% to 45%
    Monocytes: 4% to 10%
    Eosinophils: 0% to 7%
    Basophils: 0% to 2%

Monitoring guidelines

Therapy is usually withdrawn after 3 months if response is inadequate. The patient must be fasting to measure triglyceride levels. Obtain blood counts periodically during the first 12 months.

When drug is given by continuous I.V. infusion, check PTT every 4 hours in the early stages of therapy, and daily thereafter. When drug is given by deep subcutaneous injection, check PTT 4 to 6 hours after injection, and daily thereafter.

Perform liver function tests at baseline, 6 to 12 weeks after therapy is initiated or changed, and approximately every 6 months thereafter. If adequate response isn't achieved within 6 weeks, consider changing therapy.

Monitor response to therapy by evaluating glucose and glycosylated hemoglobin levels. Glycosylated hemoglobin level is a good measure of long-term control. A patient's home monitoring of glucose levels helps measure compliance and response.

Use a serum or urine pregnancy test with a sensitivity of at least 25 International Units/ml. Perform one test before therapy and a second test during the second day of the menstrual cycle before therapy begins or at least 11 days after the last unprotected act of sexual intercourse, whichever is later. Repeat pregnancy tests monthly. Obtain baseline liver function tests and lipid levels; repeat every 1 to 2 weeks until a response is established (usually 4 weeks).

(continued)

---

* For those areas marked with one asterisk, the following values can be used:

Alanine aminotransferase: 7 to 56 units/L
Aspartate aminotransferase: 5 to 40 units/L
Alkaline phosphatase: 17 to 142 units/L
Lactate dehydrogenase: 60 to 220 units/L
Gamma glutamyl transferase (GGT): < 40 units/L
Total bilirubin: 0.2 to 1 mg/dl

Therapeutic drug monitoring guidelines *(continued)*

Drug	Laboratory test monitored	Therapeutic ranges of test
Linezolid	CBC with differential and platelets	*****
	Cultures and sensitivities	
	Platelet count	150 to 450 $\times$ $10^3/mm^3$
	Liver function	*
	Amylase	35 to 118 International Units/L
	Lipase	10 to 150 units/L
Lithium	Lithium	0.6 to 1.2 mEq/L
	Creatinine	0.6 to 1.3 mg/dl
	CBC	*****
	Electrolytes (especially potassium and sodium)	Potassium: 3.5 to 5 mEq/L Magnesium: 1.7 to 2.1 mEq/L Sodium: 135 to 145 mEq/L Chloride: 98 to 106 mEq/L
	Fasting glucose	70 to 110 mg/dl
	Thyroid function tests	Thyroid-stimulating hormone (TSH): 0.2 to 5.4 micro-units/ml T_3: 80 to 200 ng/dl T_4: 5.4 to 11.5 mcg/dl
Methotrexate	Methotrexate	Normal elimination: ~ 10 micromol 24 hours postdose ~ 1 micromol 48 hours postdose < 0.2 micromol 72 hours postdose
	CBC with differential	*****
	Platelet count	150 to 450 $\times$ $10^3/mm^3$
	Liver function	*
	Creatinine	0.6 to 1.3 mg/dl

Note: ***** For those areas marked with asterisks, the following values can be used:

Hemoglobin: Women: 12 to 16 g/dl; Men: 13 to 18 g/dl

Hematocrit: Women 37% to 48%; Men: 42% to 52%

Red blood cell count (RBC): 4 to 5.5 $\times$ $10^6/mm^3$

WBC count: 5 to 10 $\times$ $10^3/mm^3$

Differential: Neutrophils: 45% to 74%
Bands: 0% to 8%
Lymphocytes: 16% to 45%
Monocytes: 4% to 10%
Eosinophils: 0% to 7%
Basophils: 0% to 2%

Monitoring guidelines

Obtain a baseline CBC with differential and platelet count. Repeat weekly, especially if the patient receives more than 2 weeks of therapy. Monitor liver function test results and amylase and lipase levels during therapy.

Checking lithium levels is crucial to safe use of the drug. Obtain lithium levels immediately before the next dose. Monitor levels twice weekly until they are stable. When at a steady state, levels should be checked weekly; when the patient is receiving the appropriate maintenance dose, levels should be checked every 2 to 3 months. Monitor creatinine, electrolyte, and fasting glucose levels; CBC; and thyroid function test results before therapy is initiated and periodically during therapy.

Monitor methotrexate levels according to the dosing protocol. Monitor the CBC with differential, platelet count, and liver and renal function test results more frequently when therapy is initiated or changed and when methotrexate levels may be elevated, such as when the patient is dehydrated.

(continued)

* For those areas marked with one asterisk, the following values can be used:

Alanine aminotransferase: 7 to 56 units/L
Aspartate aminotransferase: 5 to 40 units/L
Alkaline phosphatase: 17 to 142 units/L
Lactate dehydrogenase: 60 to 220 units/L
Gamma glutamyl transferase (GGT): < 40 units/L
Total bilirubin: 0.2 to 1 mg/dl

■

Therapeutic drug monitoring guidelines *(continued)*

Drug	Laboratory test monitored	Therapeutic ranges of test
Nonnucleoside reverse transcriptase inhibitors (nevirapine, delavirdine, efavirenz)	Liver function	*
	CBC with differential and platelets	*****
	Lipids (efavirenz)	Total cholesterol: < 200 mg/dl LDL: < 130 mg/dl HDL: Women: 40 to 75 mg/dl Men: 37 to 70 mg/dl Triglycerides: 10 to 160 mg/dl
	Amylase	35 to 118 International Units/L
Phenytoin	Phenytoin	10 to 20 mcg/ml
	CBC	*****
Potassium chloride	Potassium	3.5 to 5 mEq/L
Procainamide	Procainamide N-acetylprocainamide (NAPA)	3 to 10 mcg/ml (procainamide) 10 to 30 mcg/ml (combined procainamide and NAPA)
	CBC	*****
	Liver function	*
	ANA titer	Negative
Protease inhibitors (amprenavir, indinavir, lopinavir, nelfinavir, ritonavir, saquinavir)	Fasting glucose	70 to 110 mg/dl
	Liver function	*
	CBC with differential	*****
	Lipids	Total cholesterol: < 200 mg/dl LDL: < 130 mg/dl HDL: Women: 40 to 75 mg/dl Men: 37 to 70 mg/dl Triglycerides: 10 to 160 mg/dl
	Amylase	35 to 118 International Units/L
	Creatine kinase (CK)	Women: 20 to 170 International Units/L Men: 30 to 220 International Units/L

Note: ***** For those areas marked with asterisks, the following values can be used:

Hemoglobin: Women: 12 to 16 g/dl; Men: 13 to 18 g/dl
Hematocrit: Women 37% to 48%; Men: 42% to 52%
Red blood cell count (RBC): 4 to 5.5 × 10^6/mm³
WBC count: 5 to 10 × 10^3/mm³

Differential: Neutrophils: 45% to 74%
  Bands: 0% to 8%
  Lymphocytes: 16% to 45%
  Monocytes: 4% to 10%
  Eosinophils: 0% to 7%
  Basophils: 0% to 2%

Monitoring guidelines

Obtain baseline liver function tests and monitor results closely during the first 12 weeks of therapy. Continue to monitor them regularly during therapy. Check the CBC with differential and platelet count before therapy and periodically during therapy. Monitor lipid levels during efavirenz therapy. Monitor the amylase level during efavirenz and delavirdine therapy.

Monitor phenytoin levels immediately before the next dose and 7 to 10 days after therapy is initiated or changed. Obtain a CBC at baseline and monthly early in therapy. Watch for toxic effects at therapeutic levels. Adjust the measured level for hypoalbuminemia or renal impairment, which can increase free drug levels.

After oral replacement therapy is initiated, check the level weekly until it's stable and every 3 to 6 months thereafter.

Measure procainamide levels 6 to 12 hours after a continuous infusion is started or immediately before the next oral dose. Combined (procainamide and NAPA) levels can be used as an index of toxicity in patients with renal impairment. Obtain a CBC periodically during longer-term therapy.

Obtain a baseline glucose level, liver function test results, a CBC with differential, and lipid, CK, and amylase levels. Monitor during therapy.

(continued)

* For those areas marked with one asterisk, the following values can be used:

Alanine aminotransferase: 7 to 56 units/L
Aspartate aminotransferase: 5 to 40 units/L
Alkaline phosphatase: 17 to 142 units/L
Lactate dehydrogenase: 60 to 220 units/L
Gamma glutamyl transferase (GGT): < 40 units/L
Total bilirubin: 0.2 to 1 mg/dl

Therapeutic drug monitoring guidelines *(continued)*

Drug	Laboratory test monitored	Therapeutic ranges of test
Quinidine	Quinidine CBC Liver function Creatinine Electrolytes (especially potassium)	2 to 6 mcg/ml ***** * 0.6 to 1.3 mg/dl Potassium: 3.5 to 5 mEq/L Magnesium: 1.7 to 2.1 mEq/L Sodium: 135 to 145 mEq/L Chloride: 98 to 106 mEq/L
Sulfonylureas	Fasting glucose Glycosylated hemoglobin	70 to 110 mg/dl 4% to 7% of total hemoglobin
Theophylline	Theophylline	10 to 20 mcg/ml
Thiazolidinediones (rosiglitazone, pioglita- zone)	Fasting glucose Glycosylated hemoglobin Liver function	70 to 110 mg/dl 4% to 7% of total hemoglobin *
Thyroid hormone	Thyroid function tests	TSH: 0.2 to 5.4 microunits/ml T_3: 80 to 200 ng/dl T_4: 5.4 to 11.5 mcg/dl
Valproate sodium, valproic acid, divalproex sodium	Valproic acid Liver function Ammonia PTT BUN Creatinine CBC with differential Platelet count	50 to 100 mcg/ml * 15 to 45 mcg/dl 10 to 14 seconds 5 to 20 mg/dl 0.6 to 1.3 mg/dl ***** 150 to 450 $\times$ 10^3/mm^3
Vancomycin	Vancomycin Creatinine	20 to 40 mcg/ml (peak) 5 to 15 mcg/ml (trough) 0.6 to 1.3 mg/dl

Note: ***** For those areas marked with asterisks, the following values can be used:

Hemoglobin: Women: 12 to 16 g/dl; Men: 13 to 18 g/dl
Hematocrit: Women 37% to 48%; Men: 42% to 52%
Red blood cell count (RBC): 4 to 5.5 $\times$ 10^6/mm^3
WBC count: 5 to 10 $\times$ 10^3/mm^3

Differential: Neutrophils: 45% to 74%
Bands: 0% to 8%
Lymphocytes: 16% to 45%
Monocytes: 4% to 10%
Eosinophils: 0% to 7%
Basophils: 0% to 2%

Monitoring guidelines

Obtain levels immediately before the next oral dose and 30 to 35 hours after therapy is initiated or changed. Obtain blood counts, liver and kidney function test results, and electrolyte levels periodically. With more specific assays, therapeutic levels are < 1 mcg/1 ml.

Monitor response to therapy by evaluating fasting glucose and glycosylated hemoglobin levels periodically. The patient should monitor glucose levels at home to help measure compliance and response.

Obtain theophylline levels immediately before the next dose of sustained-release oral drug and at least 2 days after therapy is initiated or changed.

Monitor response by evaluating fasting glucose and glycosylated hemoglobin levels. Obtain baseline liver function test results, and repeat the tests periodically during therapy.

Monitor thyroid function test results every 2 to 3 weeks until the appropriate maintenance dose is determined, and annually thereafter.

Monitor liver function test results, ammonia level, coagulation test results, renal function test results, CBC, and platelet count at baseline and periodically during therapy. Monitor liver function test results closely during the first 6 months of therapy.

Check vancomycin levels with the third dose administered, at the earliest. Obtain peak levels 1½ to 2½ hours after a 1-hour infusion or when I.V. infusion is complete. Obtain trough levels within 1 hour of the next dose administered. Renal function can be used to adjust dosing and intervals.

(continued)

* For those areas marked with one asterisk, the following values can be used:

Alanine aminotransferase: 7 to 56 units/L
Aspartate aminotransferase: 5 to 40 units/L
Alkaline phosphatase: 17 to 142 units/L
Lactate dehydrogenase: 60 to 220 units/L
Gamma glutamyl transferase (GGT): < 40 units/L
Total bilirubin: 0.2 to 1 mg/dl

■

Therapeutic drug monitoring guidelines *(continued)*

Drug	Laboratory test monitored	Therapeutic ranges of test
Warfarin	International Normalized Ratio (INR)	For acute myocardial infarction, atrial fibrillation, treatment of pulmonary embolism, prevention of systemic embolism, tissue heart valves, valvular heart disease, or prophylaxis or treatment of venous thrombosis: 2 to 3 For mechanical prosthetic valves or recurrent systemic embolism: 3 to 4.5

Note: ***** For those areas marked with asterisks, the following values can be used:

Hemoglobin: Women: 12 to 16 g/dl; Men: 13 to 18 g/dl
Hematocrit: Women 37% to 48%; Men: 42% to 52%
Red blood cell count (RBC): 4 to 5.5 × 10^6/mm^3
WBC count: 5 to 10 × 10^3/mm^3

Differential: Neutrophils: 45% to 74%
Bands: 0% to 8%
Lymphocytes: 16% to 45%
Monocytes: 4% to 10%
Eosinophils: 0% to 7%
Basophils: 0% to 2%

Monitoring guidelines

Check INR daily, beginning 3 days after therapy is initiated. Continue checking it until the therapeutic goal is achieved, and monitor it periodically thereafter. Also check levels 7 days after a change in the warfarin dose or concomitant, potentially interacting therapy.

* For those areas marked with one asterisk, the following values can be used:

Alanine aminotransferase: 7 to 56 units/L
Aspartate aminotransferase: 5 to 40 units/L
Alkaline phosphatase: 17 to 142 units/L
Lactate dehydrogenase: 60 to 220 units/L
Gamma glutamyl transferase (GGT): < 40 units/L
Total bilirubin: 0.2 to 1 mg/dl

Dialyzable drugs

The amount of a drug removed by dialysis differs among patients and depends on several factors, including the patient's condition, the drug's properties, length of dialysis and dialysate used, rate of blood flow or dwell time, and purpose of dialysis. This table shows the effect of hemodialysis on selected drugs.

Drug	Level reduced by hemodialysis	Drug	Level reduced by hemodialysis
acetaminophen	Yes (may not affect toxicity)	ceftizoxime	Yes
		ceftriaxone	No
acetazolamide	No	cefuroxime	Yes
acyclovir	Yes	cephalexin	Yes
allopurinol	Yes	cephalothin	Yes
alprazolam	No	cephradine	Yes
amikacin	Yes	chloral hydrate	Yes
amiodarone	No	chlorambucil	No
amitriptyline	No	chloramphenicol	Yes (very small amount)
amlodipine	No		
amoxicillin	Yes	chlordiazepoxide	No
amoxicillin and clavulanate potassium	Yes	chloroquine	No
		chlorpheniramine	No
		chlorpromazine	No
amphotericin B	No	chlorthalidone	No
ampicillin	Yes	cimetidine	Yes
ampicillin and sulbactam sodium	Yes	ciprofloxacin	Yes (only by 20%)
		cisplatin	No
aspirin	Yes	clindamycin	No
atenolol	Yes	clofibrate	No
azathioprine	Yes	clonazepam	No
aztreonam	Yes	clonidine	No
captopril	Yes	clorazepate	No
carbamazepine	No	cloxacillin	No
carbenicillin	Yes	codeine	No
carmustine	No	colchicine	No
cefaclor	Yes	cortisone	No
cefadroxil	Yes	co-trimoxazole	Yes
cefamandole	Yes	cyclophosphamide	Yes
cefazolin	Yes	diazepam	No
cefepime	Yes	diazoxide	Yes
cefonicid	Yes (only by 20%)	diclofenac	No
cefoperazone	Yes	dicloxacillin	No
cefotaxime	Yes	didanosine	Yes
cefotetan	Yes (only by 20%)	digoxin	No
cefoxitin	Yes	diltiazem	No
cefpodoxime	Yes	diphenhydramine	No
ceftazidime	Yes	dipyridamole	No
ceftibuten	Yes	disopyramide	Yes

Dialyzable drugs *(continued)*

Drug	Level reduced by hemodialysis	Drug	Level reduced by hemodialysis
doxazosin	No	irbesartan	No
doxepin	No	iron dextran	No
doxorubicin	No	isoniazid	Yes
doxycycline	No	isosorbide	Yes
enalapril	Yes	isradipine	No
erythromycin	Yes (only by 20%)	kanamycin	Yes
ethacrynic acid	No	ketoconazole	No
ethambutol	Yes (only by 20%)	ketoprofen	Yes
ethchlorvynol	Yes	labetalol	No
ethosuximide	Yes	levofloxacin	No
famciclovir	Yes	lidocaine	No
famotidine	No	lisinopril	Yes
fenoprofen	No	lithium	Yes
flecainide	No	lomefloxacin	No
fluconazole	Yes	lomustine	No
flucytosine	Yes	loracarbef	Yes
fluorouracil	Yes	loratadine	No
fluoxetine	No	lorazepam	No
flurazepam	No	mechlorethamine	No
foscarnet	Yes	mefenamic acid	No
fosinopril	No	meperidine	No
furosemide	No	mercaptopurine	Yes
gabapentin	Yes	meropenem	Yes
ganciclovir	Yes	methadone	No
gemfibrozil	No	methicillin	No
gemifloxacin	Yes	methotrexate	Yes
gentamicin	Yes	methyldopa	Yes
glipizide	No	methylprednisolone	No
glyburide	No	metoclopramide	No
guanfacine	No	metolazone	No
haloperidol	No	metoprolol	No
heparin	No	metronidazole	Yes
hydralazine	No	mexiletine	Yes
hydrochloro-thiazide	No	mezlocillin	Yes
		miconazole	No
hydroxyzine	No	midazolam	No
ibuprofen	No	minocycline	No
imipenem and cilastatin	Yes	minoxidil	Yes
		misoprostol	No
imipramine	No	morphine	No
indapamide	No	nabumetone	No
indomethacin	No	nadolol	Yes
insulin	No	nafcillin	No

(continued)

Dialyzable drugs *(continued)*

Drug	Level reduced by hemodialysis	Drug	Level reduced by hemodialysis
naproxen	No	pyridoxine	Yes
nelfinavir	Yes	quinapril	No
netilmicin	Yes	quinidine	Yes
nifedipine	No	quinine	Yes
nimodipine	No	ranitidine	Yes
nitrofurantoin	Yes	rifampin	No
nitroglycerin	No	rofecoxib	No
nitroprusside	Yes	salsalate	Yes
nizatidine	No	sertraline	No
norfloxacin	No	sotalol	Yes
nortriptyline	No	stavudine	Yes
ofloxacin	Yes	streptomycin	Yes
olanzapine	No	sucralfate	No
omeprazole	No	sulbactam	Yes
oxacillin	No	sulfamethoxazole	Yes
oxazepam	No	sulindac	No
paroxetine	No	temazepam	No
penicillin G	Yes	theophylline	Yes
pentamidine	No	ticarcillin	Yes
pentazocine	Yes	ticarcillin and	Yes
perindopril	Yes	clavulanate	
phenobarbital	Yes	timolol	No
phenylbutazone	No	tobramycin	Yes
phenytoin	No	tocainide	Yes
piperacillin	Yes	tolbutamide	No
piperacillin and	Yes	topiramate	Yes
tazobactam		trazodone	No
piroxicam	No	triazolam	No
prazosin	No	trimethoprim	Yes
prednisone	No	valacyclovir	Yes
primidone	Yes	valproic acid	No
procainamide	Yes	valsartan	No
promethazine	No	vancomycin	Yes
propoxyphene	No	verapamil	No
propranolol	No	warfarin	No
protriptyline	No	zolpidem	No

Procedures

Inserting a nasopharyngeal airway

First, hold the airway beside the patient's face to make sure it's the proper size (as shown below left). It should be slightly smaller than the patient's nostril diameter and slightly longer than the distance from the tip of his nose to his earlobe.

To insert the airway, hyperextend the patient's neck (unless contraindicated). Then push up the tip of his nose and pass the airway into his nostril (as shown below right). Avoid pushing against any resistance to prevent tissue trauma and airway kinking.

To check for correct airway placement, first close the patient's mouth. Then place your finger over the tube's opening to detect air exchange. Also, depress the patient's tongue with a tongue blade and look for the airway tip behind the uvula.

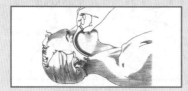
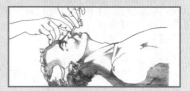

Inserting an oral airway

Unless this position is contraindicated, hyperextend the patient's head (as shown top right) before using either the cross-finger or tongue blade insertion method.

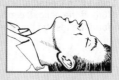

To insert an oral airway using the cross-finger method, place your thumb on the patient's lower teeth and your index finger on his upper teeth. Gently open his mouth by pushing his teeth apart (as shown middle right).

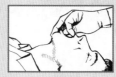

Insert the airway upside down to avoid pushing the tongue toward the pharynx, and slide it over the tongue toward the back of the mouth. Rotate the airway as it approaches the posterior wall of the pharynx so that it points downward (as shown below right).

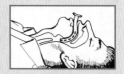

To use the tongue blade technique, open the patient's mouth and depress his tongue with the blade. Guide the airway over the back of the tongue as you did for the cross-finger technique.

Performing Allen's test

Rest the patient's arm on the mattress or bedside stand, and support his wrist with a rolled towel. Have him clench his fist. Then, using your index and middle fingers, press on the radial and ulnar arteries. Hold this position for a few seconds.

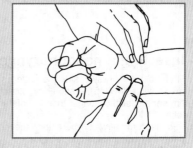

Without removing your fingers from the patient's arteries, ask him to unclench his fist and hold his hand in a relaxed position. The palm will be blanched because pressure from your fingers has impaired the normal blood flow.

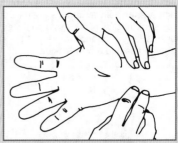

Release pressure on the patient's ulnar artery. If the hand becomes flushed, which indicates blood filling the vessels, you can safely proceed with the radial artery puncture. If the hand doesn't flush, perform the test on the other arm.

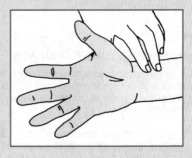

Arterial puncture technique

The angle of needle penetration in arterial blood gas sampling depends on which artery will be sampled. For the radial artery, which is used most commonly, the needle should enter bevel up at a 30- to 45-degree angle over the radial artery. After collecting the sample, apply pressure to the site for at least 5 minutes.

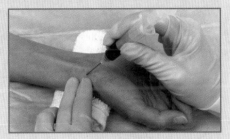

Using a bag-mask device

Place the mask over the patient's face so that the apex of the triangle covers the bridge of the nose and the base lies between the lower lip and chin.

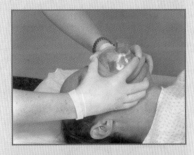

Make sure that the patient's mouth remains open underneath the mask. Attach the bag to the mask and to the tubing leading to the oxygen source.

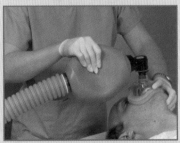

Or, if the patient has a tracheostomy or endotracheal tube in place, remove the mask from the bag and attach the device directly to the tube.

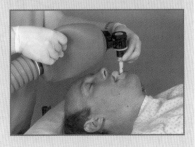

Bandaging techniques

Circular
Each turn encircles the previous one, covering it completely. Use this technique to anchor a bandage.

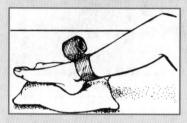

Spiral
Each turn partially overlaps the previous one. Use this technique to wrap a long, straight body part or one of increasing circumference.

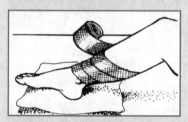

Spiral-reverse
Anchor the bandage, and then reverse direction halfway through each spiral turn. Use this technique to accommodate the increasing circumference of a body part.

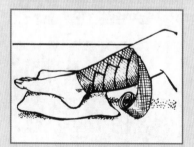

Figure eight
Anchor below the joint, and then use alternating ascending and descending turns to form a figure eight. Use this technique around joints.

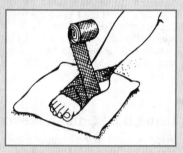

Recurrent
This technique includes a combination of recurrent and circular turns. Hold the bandage as you make each recurrent turn, and then use the circular turns as a final anchor. Use this technique for a stump, a hand, or the scalp.

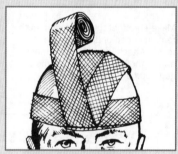

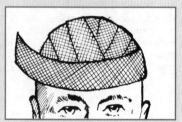

Monitoring blood glucose

• Before using a blood glucose meter, follow the manufacturer's instructions for calibration.

• Explain the procedure to the patient.

• Wash your hands and put on gloves.

• Select the puncture site—usually the lateral side of a fingertip.

• Avoid selecting cold, cyanotic, or swollen puncture sites to ensure an adequate blood sample. If you can't obtain a capillary sample, perform venipuncture and place a large drop of venous blood on the reagent strip.

• If necessary, dilate the capillaries by applying a warm, moist compress to the area for about 10 minutes.

• Wipe the puncture site with an alcohol pad, and dry it thoroughly with a gauze pad.

• To collect a sample from the fingertip with a disposable lancet, position the lancet on the side of the patient's fingertip perpendicular to the lines of the fingerprints. Pierce the skin sharply and quickly. Alternatively, you can use a mechanical blood-letting device, which uses a spring-loaded lancet.

• Don't squeeze the puncture site, to avoid diluting the sample with tissue fluid.

• Touch a drop of blood to the reagent patch on the strip; make sure you cover the entire patch.

• Briefly apply pressure to the puncture site. Ask the adult patient to hold a gauze pad firmly over the puncture site until bleeding stops.

• Insert the strip into the meter, and watch for the digital display of the resulting glucose level.

• Apply a small adhesive bandage to the puncture site, if needed.

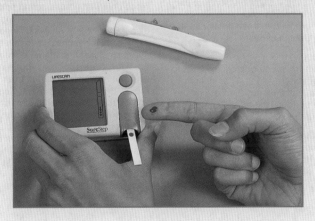

Transfusing blood: Check, verify, and inspect

The most common cause of a severe transfusion reaction is receiving the wrong blood. Before administering blood or blood products, take these steps.

Check

Check to make sure an informed consent form was signed. Then double-check the patient's name, medical record number, ABO blood group, Rh status (and other compatibility factors), and blood bank identification number against the label on the blood bag. Also check the expiration date on the bag. Then check and record the patient's vital signs.

Verify

Ask another nurse to verify all information, according to your facility's policy. (Most facilities require double identification.) Make sure that you and the nurse who checked the blood or blood product sign the blood confirmation slip. If even a slight discrepancy exists, don't administer the blood or blood product. Instead, immediately notify the blood bank.

Inspect

Inspect the blood or blood product to detect abnormalities. Then confirm the patient's identity by checking the name and medical record number on his wristband.

Transfusion don'ts

A blood transfusion requires extreme care. Here are some tips on what *not* to do when administering a transfusion:

• Don't add any medications to the blood bag.
• Never give blood products without checking the order against the blood bag label—the only way to tell whether the request form has been stamped with the wrong name. Most life-threatening reactions occur when this step is omitted.
• Don't transfuse the blood product if you discover a discrepancy in the blood number, blood slip type, or patient identification number.
• Don't piggyback blood into the port of an existing infusion set. Most solutions, including dextrose in water, are incompatible with blood. Administer blood only with normal saline solution.
• Don't hesitate to stop the transfusion if your patient shows changes in vital signs, is dyspneic or restless, or develops chills, hematuria, or pain in the flank, chest, or back. Your patient could go into shock, so don't remove the I.V. device that's in place. Keep it open with a slow infusion of normal saline solution; call the physician and the laboratory.
• Don't transfuse blood that has been nonrefrigerated for more than 4 hours. Once started, a transfusion must be infused within 4 hours.

Monitoring a blood transfusion

To help avoid transfusion reactions and safeguard your patient, follow these guidelines.

• Record vital signs before the transfusion, 15 minutes after the start of the transfusion, and just after the transfusion is complete, and more frequently if warranted by the patient's condition and transfusion history or the facility's policy. Most acute hemolytic reactions occur during the first 30 minutes of the transfusion, so watch your patient extra carefully during the first 30 minutes.
• Always have sterile normal saline solution—an isotonic solution—set up as a primary line along with the transfusion.
• Act promptly if your patient develops wheezing and bronchospasm. These signs may indicate an allergic reaction or anaphylaxis. If, after a few milliliters of blood are transfused, the patient becomes dyspneic and shows generalized flushing and chest pain (with or without vomiting and diarrhea), he could be having an anaphylactic reaction. Stop the blood transfusion immediately, start the normal saline solution, check and document vital signs, and call the physician and initiate anaphylaxis procedure.
• If the patient develops a transfusion reaction, return the remaining blood together with a posttransfusion blood sample and any other required specimens to the blood bank.

Transfusing plasma or plasma fractions

• Obtain baseline vital signs.
• Flush the patient's venous access device with normal saline solution.
• Attach the plasma, fresh frozen plasma, albumin, factor VIII concentrate, prothrombin complex, platelets, or cryoprecipitate to the patient's venous access device.
• Begin the transfusion, and adjust the flow rate as ordered.
• Take the patient's vital signs, and assess him frequently for signs or symptoms of a transfusion reaction, such as fever, chills, or nausea.
• After the infusion, flush the line with 20 to 30 ml of normal saline solution. Then disconnect the I.V. line. If therapy is to continue, resume the prescribed infusate and adjust the flow rate as ordered.
• Record the type and amount of plasma or plasma fraction administered, duration of the transfusion, baseline and posttransfusion vital signs, and any adverse reactions.

Performing hip-spica cast care

After a hip-spica cast is applied, turn the patient every 1 to 2 hours to speed drying time. Be sure to turn the patient to his unaffected side to prevent pressure to the affected side. If the patient is an infant, you can turn him by yourself. If the patient is an older child or an adolescent, seek assistance before attempting to turn him. When turning the patient, don't use the stabilizer bar between his legs for leverage. Excessive pressure to this bar may disrupt the cast. Handle a damp cast only with your palms to avoid misshaping the cast material.

• After the cast dries, inspect its inside edges for stray pieces of casting material that may irritate the skin. (A traditional hip-spica cast requires 24 to 48 hours to dry. However, a hip-spica cast made from newer, quick-drying substances takes only 8 to 10 hours to dry. If made of fiberglass, it will dry in less than 1 hour).

• Cut several petal-shaped pieces of moleskin and place them, overlapping, around the open edges of the cast to protect the patient's skin. Use waterproof adhesive tape around the perineal area.

• Give the patient a sponge bath to remove any cast fragments from the skin.

• Assess the patient's legs for coldness, swelling, cyanosis, or mottling. Also assess pulse strength, toe movement, sensation (numbness, tingling, or burning), and capillary refill. Perform these circulatory assessments every 1 to 2 hours while the cast is wet and every 3 to 4 hours after the cast dries.

• Check the patient's exposed skin for redness or irritation, and observe the patient for pain or discomfort caused by hot spots (pressure-sensitive areas under the cast). Also be alert for a foul odor. These signs and symptoms suggest a pressure ulcer or infection.

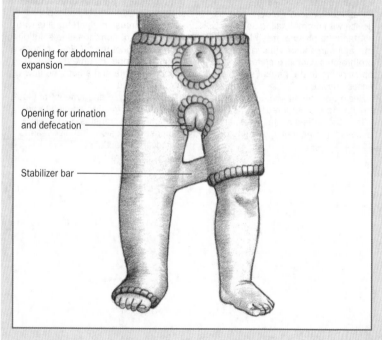

Opening for abdominal expansion

Opening for urination and defecation

Stabilizer bar

Petaling a cast

Rough cast edges can be cushioned by petaling them with adhesive tape or moleskin. To do this, first cut several 4″ × 2″ (10 × 5 cm) strips. Round off one end of each strip to keep it from curling. Make sure the rounded end of the strip is on the outside of the cast; then tuck the straight end just inside the cast edge.

Smooth the moleskin with your finger until you're sure it's secured inside and out. Repeat the procedure, overlapping the moleskin pieces until you've gone all the way around the cast edge.

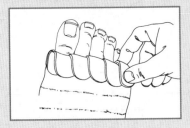
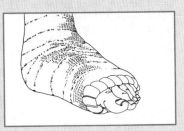

Removing a cast

Typically, a cast is removed when a fracture heals or requires further manipulation. Less common indications include cast damage, a pressure ulcer under the cast, excessive drainage or bleeding, and constriction.

Explain the procedure to the patient. Tell him he'll feel some heat and vibration as the cast is split with the cast saw. If the patient is a child, tell him that the saw is very noisy but won't cut the skin beneath. Warn the patient that when the padding is cut, he'll see discolored skin and signs of poor muscle tone. Reassure him that you'll stay with him. These illustrations show how a plaster cast is removed.

The practitioner cuts one side of the cast then the other. As he does so, closely monitor the patient's anxiety level.

Next, the practitioner opens the cast pieces with a spreader.

Lastly, using cast scissors, the practitioner cuts through the cast padding.

When the cast is removed, provide skin care to remove accumulated dead skin and to begin restoring the extremity's normal appearance.

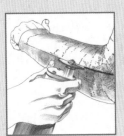
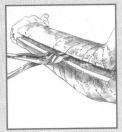
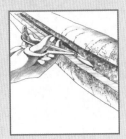

Applying a condom catheter

Apply an adhesive strip to the shaft of the penis about 1″ (2.5 cm) from the scrotal area. Roll the condom catheter onto the penis past the adhesive strip, leaving about ½″ (1.3 cm) clearance at the end. Press the sheath gently against the skin until it adheres. Using extension tubing, connect the condom catheter to the leg bag or drainage bag.

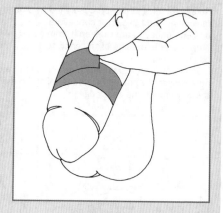

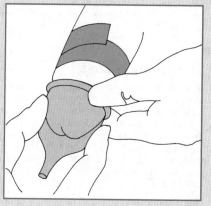

Removing a central venous catheter

· Place the patient in a supine position to prevent an air embolism.

· Wash your hands, and put on clean gloves and a mask.

· Turn off all infusions.

· Remove and discard the old dressing, and change to sterile gloves.

· Inspect the site for signs of drainage and inflammation.

· Clip the sutures and, using forceps, remove the catheter in a slow, even motion. Have the patient perform Valsalva's maneuver as the catheter is withdrawn to prevent an air embolism.

· Apply pressure to the site until bleeding stops.

· Apply povidone-iodine ointment to the insertion site to seal it. Cover the site with a gauze pad, and apply a transparent semipermeable dressing over the gauze. Label the dressing with the date and time of the removal and your initials.

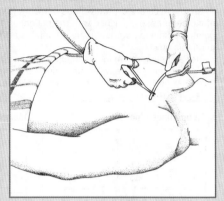

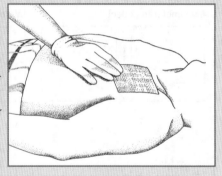

Measuring CVP with a manometer

To ensure accurate central venous pressure (CVP) readings, make sure the manometer base is aligned with the patient's right atrium (the zero reference point). The manometer set usually contains a leveling rod to allow you to determine this quickly.

After adjusting the manometer's position, examine the typical three-way stopcock. By turning it to any position shown here, you can control the direction of fluid flow. Four-way stopcocks also are available.

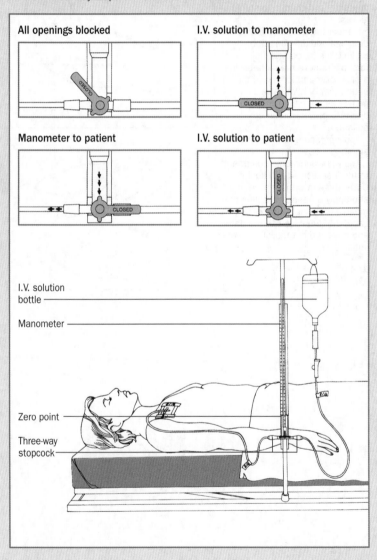

All openings blocked

I.V. solution to manometer

Manometer to patient

I.V. solution to patient

I.V. solution bottle

Manometer

Zero point

Three-way stopcock

Using a nasal balloon catheter

To control epistaxis, a balloon catheter may be inserted instead of nasal packing. Self-retaining and disposable, the catheter may have a single or double balloon to apply pressure to bleeding nasal tissues. If bleeding is still uncontrolled, arterial ligation, cryotherapy, or arterial embolization may be performed.

Assisting with insertion

To assist with inserting a single- or double-balloon catheter, prepare the patient as you would for nasal packing. Be sure to discuss the procedure thoroughly to alleviate the patient's anxiety and promote his cooperation.

Explain that the catheter tip will be lubricated with an antibiotic or a water-soluble lubricant to ease passage and prevent infection.

Providing routine care

The tip of the single-balloon catheter will be inserted in the nostrils until it reaches the posterior pharynx. Then the balloon will be inflated with normal saline solution, pulled gently into the posterior nasopharynx, and secured at the nostrils with the collapsible bulb.

With a double-balloon catheter, the posterior balloon is inflated with normal saline solution; then the anterior balloon is inflated.

To check catheter placement, mark the catheter at the nasal vestibule; then inspect for that mark and observe the oropharynx for the posteriorly placed balloon. Assess the nostrils for irritation or erosion. Remove secretions by gently suctioning the airway of a double-balloon catheter or by dabbing away crusted external secretions if the patient has a catheter with no airway.

To prevent damage to nasal tissue, the balloon may be deflated for 10 minutes every 24 hours. If bleeding recurs or remains uncontrolled, packing may be added.

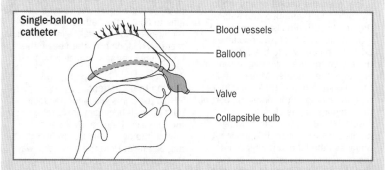

Single-balloon catheter — Blood vessels, Balloon, Valve, Collapsible bulb

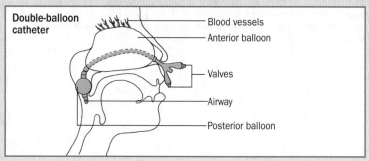

Double-balloon catheter — Blood vessels, Anterior balloon, Valves, Airway, Posterior balloon

Inserting a urinary catheter

· Place the female patient in the supine position, with her knees flexed and separated and her feet flat on the bed, about 2′ (61 cm) apart.

· Place the male patient in the supine position with his legs extended and flat on the bed.

· Ask the patient to hold the position to give you a clear view of the urinary meatus.

· Place the linen-saver pads on the bed between the patient's legs and under the hips.

· To create the sterile field, open the prepackaged kit and place it between the female patient's legs or next to the male patient's hip. Put on the sterile gloves.

· Place the sterile drape under the patient's hips.

· Cover the patient's lower abdomen with the sterile fenestrated drape so that only the genital area remains exposed. Take care not to contaminate your gloves.

· Tear open the packet of antiseptic cleaning agent, and use it to saturate the sterile cotton balls or applicators.

· Open the packet of water-soluble lubricant, and apply it to the catheter tip; attach the drainage bag to the other end of the catheter. Make sure all tubing ends remain sterile, and make sure the clamp at the emptying port of the drainage bag is closed.

Note: Some nurses use a syringe prefilled with water-soluble lubricant and instill the lubricant directly into the male urethra, instead of on the catheter tip. This method helps prevent trauma to the urethral lining and possible urinary tract infection. Check your facility's policy.

· Before inserting the catheter, inflate the balloon with sterile water to inspect it for function and leaks and then aspirate the solution to deflate the balloon.

For the female patient

· Separate the labia majora and labia minora as widely as possible with the thumb, middle, and index fingers of your nondominant hand so you have a full view of the urinary meatus. Keep the labia well-separated throughout the procedure.

· With your dominant hand, pick up a sterile saturated cotton ball with the plastic forceps and wipe one side of the urinary meatus with a single downward motion. Discard the cotton ball.

· Wipe the other side with another sterile saturated cotton ball in the same way. Then wipe directly over the meatus with still another sterile applicator or cotton ball.

· Insert and advance the catheter 2″ to 3″ (5 to 8 cm)—while continuing to hold the labia apart—until urine begins to flow. If the catheter is inadvertently inserted into the vagina, leave it there as a landmark. Then begin the procedure over again using new supplies.

For the male patient

· Hold the penis with your nondominant hand. If uncircumcised, retract the foreskin. Then gently lift and stretch the penis to a 60- to 90-degree angle. Hold the penis this way throughout the procedure to straighten the urethra.

· Use your dominant hand to clean the glans with a sterile saturated cotton ball held in forceps. Clean in a circular motion, starting at the urinary meatus and working outward. Discard the cotton ball.

· Repeat the procedure using another sterile applicator or cotton ball.

· Pick up the catheter with your dominant hand, and prepare to insert the lubricated tip into the urinary meatus. Tell the patient to breathe deeply and slowly. Hold the catheter close to its tip.

· Never force a catheter during insertion. Maneuver it gently as the patient bears down or coughs. If you still meet resistance, stop and notify the physician.

· Advance the catheter to the bifurcation 5" to 7½" (13 to 19 cm), and check for urine flow.

After insertion

· When urine stops flowing, attach the prefilled syringe to the luer-lock syringe and inflate the balloon to keep the catheter in place in the bladder. If the male patient's foreskin was retracted, replace it.

· Hang the collection bag below bladder level to prevent urine reflux into the bladder, which can cause infection, and to facilitate gravity drainage of urine. Make sure the tubing doesn't get tangled in the bed's side rails.

· Secure the catheter to the female patient's thigh to prevent possible tension on the urogenital trigone.

· Secure the catheter to the male patient's abdomen or anterior thigh to prevent pressure on the urethra at the penoscrotal junction, which can lead to formation of urethrocutaneous fistulas.

Assessing chest drainage system leaks

When attempting to locate a leak in a chest drainage system, try:
• clamping the chest tube momentarily at various points along its length, beginning at the tube's proximal end and working down toward the drainage system
• checking the seal around the connections
• pushing any loose connections back together and taping them securely.
   The bubbling will stop when a clamp is placed between the air leak and the water seal. If you clamp along the tube's entire length and the bubbling doesn't stop, you may need to replace the drainage unit because it may be cracked.

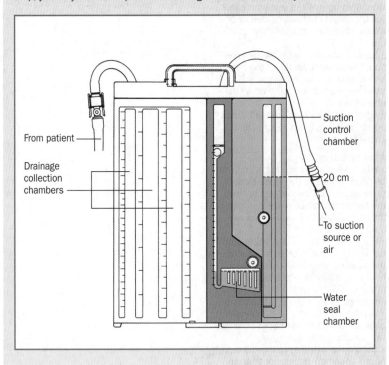

Troubleshooting chest drains

Problem	Interventions
Patient rolling over on drainage tubing, causing obstruction	• Reposition the patient, and remove kinks in the tubing. • Auscultate for decreased breath sounds, and percuss for dullness, which indicates a fluid accumulation, or for hyperresonance, which indicates an air accumulation.
Dependent loops in tubing trapping fluids and preventing effective drainage	• Make sure the chest drainage unit is positioned below the patient's chest level. If necessary, raise the bed slightly to increase the gravity flow. Remove kinks in the tubing. • Monitor the patient for decreased breath sounds, and percuss for dullness.
No drainage appearing in collection chamber	• If draining blood or other fluid, suspect a clot or obstruction in the tubing. Gently milk the tubing to expel the obstruction, if your facility's policy permits. • Monitor the patient for lung-tissue compression caused by accumulated pleural fluid.
Substantial increase in bloody drainage, indicating possible active bleeding or drainage of old blood	• Monitor the patient's vital signs. Look for an increased pulse rate, decreased blood pressure, and orthostatic changes that may indicate acute blood loss. • Measure drainage every 15 to 30 minutes to determine whether it's occurring continuously or if drainage increase occurred as a result of position change. Report drainage greater than 200 ml in 1 hour.
No bubbling in suction-control chamber	• Check for obstructions in the tubing. Make sure all connections are tight. • Check that the suction apparatus is turned on. Increase the suction slowly until you see gentle bubbling.
Loud, vigorous bubbling in suction-control chamber	• Turn down the suction source until bubbling is just visible.
Constant bubbling in water-seal chamber	• Assess the chest drainage unit and tubing for an air leak. • If an air leak isn't noted in the external system, notify the practitioner immediately. Leaking and trapping of air in the pleural space can result in a tension pneumothorax.

(continued)

Troubleshooting chest drains *(continued)*

Problem	Interventions
Evaporation causing water level in suction-control chamber to drop below desired -20 cm H_2O	• Using a syringe and needle, add water or normal saline solution through a resealable diaphragm on the back of the suction-control chamber.
Trouble breathing immediately after special procedure due to obstructed drainage resulting from improper chest drainage unit positioning	• Raise the head of the bed, and reposition the unit so that gravity promotes drainage. • Perform a quick respiratory assessment, and take the patient's vital signs. Make sure enough water is in the water-seal and suction-control chambers.
Disconnected, contaminated chest drainage unit	• Clamp the chest tube proximal to the latex connecting tubing. • Insert the distal end of the chest tube into a container of sterile water or saline until the end is 1″ to 1½″ (2 to 4 cm) below the top of the water. Unclamp the chest tube. • Obtain a new closed chest drainage system and set it up. • Attach the chest tube to the new unit. • To prevent a tension pneumothorax (which may occur when clamping stops air and fluid from escaping), never leave the chest tube clamped for more than 1 minute.

Removing a chest tube

After the patient's lung has reexpanded, you may assist the practitioner in removing the chest tube. First, obtain the patient's vital signs and perform a respiratory assessment. After explaining the procedure to the patient, administer an analgesic, as ordered, 30 minutes before tube removal. Then follow these steps.

• Place the patient in semi-Fowler's position or on his unaffected side.

• Place a linen-saver pad under the affected side to protect the bed linen from drainage and to provide a place to put the chest tube after removal.

• Put on clean gloves and remove the chest tube dressings, being careful not to dislodge the chest tube. Discard soiled dressings.

• The practitioner puts on sterile gloves, holds the chest tube in place with sterile forceps, and cuts the suture anchoring the tube.

• The chest tube is securely clamped, and the patient is instructed to perform Valsalva's maneuver by exhaling fully and bearing down. Valsalva's maneuver effectively increases intrathoracic pressure.

• The practitioner holds an airtight dressing, usually petroleum gauze, so that he can cover the insertion site with it immediately after removing the tube. After he removes the tube and covers the insertion site, secure the dressing with tape. Be sure to cover the dressing completely with tape to make it as airtight as possible.

• Dispose of the chest tube, soiled gloves, and equipment according to your facility's policy.

• Take the patient's vital signs, and assess the depth and quality of his respirations. Assess him carefully for signs and symptoms of pneumothorax, subcutaneous emphysema, or infection.

Removing contact lenses

Contact lens removal techniques depend largely on the type of lenses the patient wears and how readily they come off of the eye. For successful removal of soft and rigid lenses, follow the steps outlined below. If you have trouble removing lenses manually, try using a specially made suction cup.

Soft lenses

With the patient looking up and her upper lid raised, use your dominant index finger to slide the lens onto the lower cornea. Pinch the lens between your index finger and thumb to remove it (as shown).

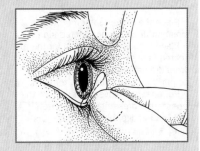

Rigid lenses

Place one thumb on each eyelid and move the lids toward each other, pressing gently against the eyeball. When the lids meet the lens edges, the suction breaks and the lens is released (as shown). Catch the lens in your lower hand, or remove it from the patient's lashes.

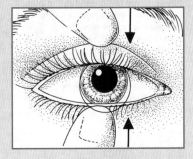

Using a suction cup

Separate the lids with your nondominant hand. Squeeze the suction cup with your dominant hand, and place it gently against the lens (as shown). Open your fingers slightly to create suction between the lens and the cup. Rock the lens gently to remove it.

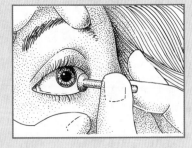

Fitting a patient for a crutch

Position the crutch so that it extends from a point 4″ to 6″ (10 to 15 cm) to the side and 4″ to 6″ in front of the patient's feet to 1½″ to 2″ (4 to 5 cm) below the axillae (about the width of two fingers). Then adjust the handgrips so that the patient's elbows are flexed at a 15-degree angle when he's standing with the crutches in the resting position.

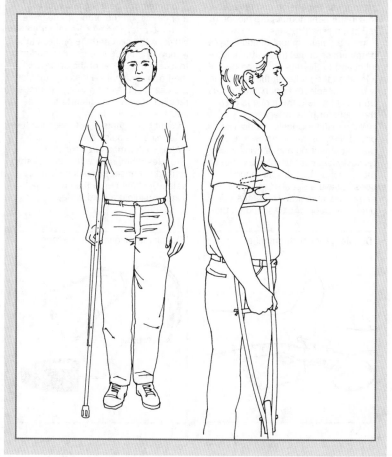

Using a Doppler device

More sensitive than palpation for determining pulse rate, the Doppler ultrasound blood flow detector is especially useful when a pulse is faint or weak. Unlike palpation, which detects arterial wall expansion and retraction, this instrument detects the motion of red blood cells (RBCs).

• Apply a small amount of coupling gel or transmission gel (not water-soluble lubricant) to the ultrasound probe.

• Position the probe on the skin directly over the selected artery. In the illustration below left, the probe is over the posterior tibial artery.

• When using a Doppler model like the one in the illustration below left, turn the instrument on and, moving counterclockwise, set the volume control to the lowest setting. If your model doesn't have a speaker, plug in the earphones and slowly raise the volume. The Doppler ultrasound stethoscope shown in the illustration below right is basically a stethoscope fitted with an audio unit, volume control, and transducer, which amplifies the movement of RBCs.

• To obtain the best signals with either device, tilt the probe 45 degrees from the artery, being sure to put gel between the skin and the probe. Slowly move the probe in a circular motion to locate the center of the artery and the Doppler signal—a hissing noise at the heartbeat. Avoid moving the probe rapidly because this distorts the signal.

• Count the signals for 60 seconds to determine the pulse rate.

• After you've measured the pulse rate, clean the probe with a soft cloth soaked in antiseptic solution or soapy water. Don't immerse the probe or bump it against a hard surface.

Doppler probe with amplifier

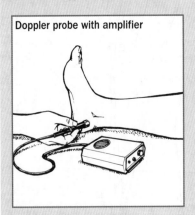

Doppler ultrasound stethoscope

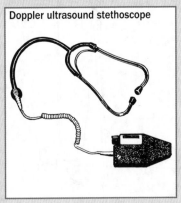

Changing a central venous dressing

Expect to change your patient's central venous dressing every 48 hours if it's gauze and at least every 7 days if it's transparent. Many facilities specify dressing changes whenever the dressing becomes soiled, moist, or loose. These illustrations show the key steps you'll perform.

First, put on clean gloves and remove the old dressing by pulling it toward the exit site of a long-term catheter or toward the insertion site of a short-term catheter. This technique helps you avoid pulling out the line. Remove and discard your gloves.

Next, put on sterile gloves and clean the skin around the site using an alcohol pad. Start at the center and move outward, using a circular motion.

Allow the skin to dry and clean the site with chlorhexidine swabs using a vigorous side-to-side motion.

After the solution has dried, cover the site with a dressing, such as the transparent semipermeable dressing shown here. Write the time and date on the dressing.

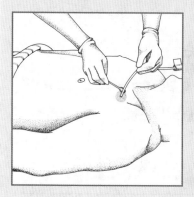
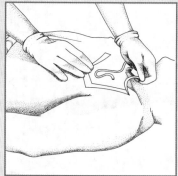

Applying a transparent semipermeable dressing

To secure the I.V. insertion site, you can apply a transparent semipermeable dressing as follows:

• Make sure the insertion site is clean and dry.
• Remove the dressing from the package and, using sterile technique, remove the protective seal. Avoid touching the sterile surface.
• Place the dressing directly over the insertion site and the hub, as shown below. Don't cover the tubing. Also, don't stretch the dressing because doing so may cause itching.
• Tuck the dressing around and under the cannula hub to make the site impervious to microorganisms.
• To remove the dressing, grasp one corner and then lift and stretch it. If removal is difficult, try loosening the edges with alcohol or water.

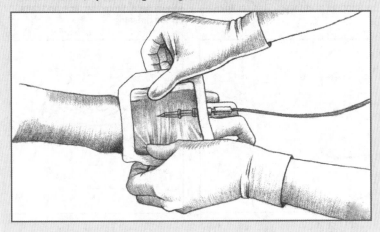

Securing an ET tube

Before taping an endotracheal (ET) tube in place, make sure the patient's face is clean, dry, and free from beard stubble. If possible, suction his mouth and dry the tube just before taping. Also, check the reference mark on the tube to ensure correct placement. After taping, always check for bilateral breath sounds to ensure that the tube hasn't been displaced by manipulation.

To tape the tube securely, use one of these three methods.

Method 1

Cut two 2" (5-cm) strips and two 15" (38-cm) strips of 1" cloth adhesive tape. Then cut a 13" (33-cm) slit in one end of each 15" strip (as shown).

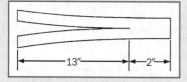

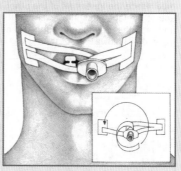

Apply skin adhesive to the patient's cheeks. Place the 2" strips on his cheeks, creating a new surface on which to anchor the tape securing the tube. When frequent retaping is necessary, this helps preserve the patient's skin integrity. If the patient's skin is excoriated or at risk, you can use a transparent semipermeable dressing to protect the skin.

Apply the adhesive to the tape on the patient's face and to the part of the tube where you'll be applying the tape. On the side of the mouth where the tube will be anchored, place the unslit end of the long tape on top of the tape on the patient's cheek.

Wrap the top half of the tape around the tube twice, pulling the tape tightly around the tube. Then, directing the tape over the patient's upper lip, place the end of the tape on his other cheek. Cut off excess tape. Use the lower half of the tape to secure an oral airway, if necessary (as shown above right).

Or, twist the lower half of the tape around the tube twice and attach it to the original cheek (as shown above right). Taping in opposite directions places equal traction on the tube.

If you've taped in an oral airway or are concerned about the tube's stability, apply the other 1" strip of tape in the same manner, starting on the other side of the patient's face. If the tape around the tube is too bulky, use only the upper part of the tape and cut off the lower part. If the patient has copious oral secretions, seal the tape by cutting a 1" (piece of paper tape, coating it with benzoin tincture, and placing the paper tape over the adhesive tape.

Method 2

Cut one piece of 1" cloth adhesive tape long enough to wrap around the patient's head and overlap in front. Then cut an 8" (20.3-cm) piece of tape, and center it on the longer piece, sticky sides together. Next, cut a 5" (12.7-cm) slit in each end of the longer tape (as shown below).

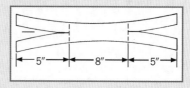

(continued)

Securing an ET tube *(continued)*

Apply skin adhesive to the patient's cheeks, under his nose, and under his lower lip.

Place the top half of one end of the tape under the patient's nose, and wrap the lower half around the ET tube. Place the lower half of the other end of the tape along his lower lip, and wrap the top half around the tube (as shown below).

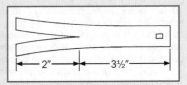

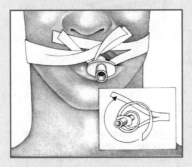

Apply skin adhesive to the part of the ET tube that will be taped. Wrap the split ends of each piece of tape around the tube, one piece on each side. Overlap the tape to secure it.

Apply the free ends of the tape to both sides of the patient's face. Then insert tracheostomy ties through the holes in the tape and knot the ties (as shown below).

Method 3

Cut a tracheostomy tie in two pieces, one a few inches longer than the other, and cut two 6″ (15.2-cm) pieces of 1″ cloth adhesive tape. Then cut a 2″ (5.1-cm) slit in one end of both pieces of tape. Fold back the other end of the tape ½″ (1.3 cm) so that the sticky sides are together, and cut a small hole in it (as shown above right).

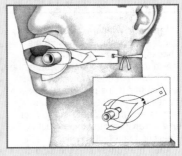

Bring the longer tie behind the patient's neck. Knotting the ties on the side prevents him from lying on the knot and developing a pressure ulcer.

Applying an eye patch

An eye patch may be applied for various reasons: to protect the eye after injury or surgery, to prevent accidental damage to an anesthetized eye, to promote healing, to absorb secretions, or to prevent the patient from touching or rubbing his eye.

A thicker patch, called a *pressure patch,* may be used to help corneal abrasions heal, compress postoperative edema, or control hemorrhage from traumatic injury. Application requires an ophthalmologist's prescription and supervision.

To apply a patch, choose a gauze pad of appropriate size for the patient's face, place it gently over the closed eye (as shown), and secure it with two or three strips of tape. Extend the tape from midforehead across the eye to below the earlobe.

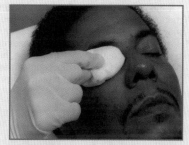

A pressure patch, which is markedly thicker than a single-thickness gauze patch, exerts extra tension against the closed eye. After placing the initial gauze pad, build it up with additional gauze pieces. Tape it firmly so that the patch exerts even pressure against the closed eye (as shown).

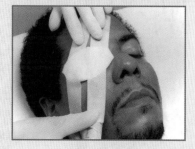

For increased protection of an injured eye, place a plastic or metal shield (as shown) on top of the gauze pads and apply tape over the shield.

Occasionally, you may use a head dressing to secure a pressure patch. The dressing applies additional pressure or, in burn patients, holds the patch in place without tape.

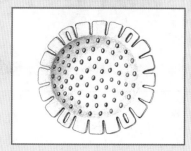

Locating the fundus

A full-term pregnancy stretches the ligaments supporting the uterus, placing the uterus at risk for inversion during palpation and massage. To guard against this, use your hands to support and fix the uterus in a safe position.

To do this, place one hand against the patient's abdomen at the symphysis pubis level. This steadies the fundus and prevents downward displacement. Place the other hand at the top of the fundus, cupping it.

· Gently compress the uterus between both hands to evaluate uterine firmness.
· Note the level of the fundus above or below the umbilicus in fingerbreadths or centimeters.
· If the uterus seems soft and boggy, gently massage the fundus with a circular motion until it becomes firm. Simply cupping the uterus between your hands may also stimulate contraction. Alternatively, massage the fundus with the side of the hand above the fundus. Without digging into the abdomen, gently compress and release, always supporting the lower uterine segment with the other hand. Observe for lochia flow during massage.
· Massage long enough to produce firmness. The sensitive fundus needs only gentle pressure.

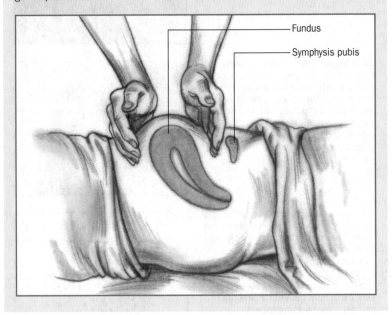

Fundus

Symphysis pubis

Administering gastric feeding

• Elevate the bed to semi-Fowler's or high Fowler's position.

• Remove the cap or plug from the feeding tube. Attach the catheter-tip or bulb syringe to aspirate stomach contents.

• Examine the aspirate, and place a small amount on the pH test strip. Probability of gastric placement is increased if the aspirate has a typical gastric fluid appearance (grassy green, clear and colorless with mucus shreds, or brown) and a pH lower than 5.0.

• To assess gastric emptying, aspirate and measure residual gastric contents. Hold feedings if residual volume is greater than the predetermined amount specified in the physician's order. Reinstill any aspirate obtained.

• Connect the gavage bag tubing to the feeding tube.

• If you're using a bulb or catheter-tip syringe, remove the bulb or plunger and attach the syringe to the pinched-off feeding tube.

• Fill the syringe with formula, and release the feeding tube. The height at which you hold the syringe will determine the flow rate. When the syringe is three-quarters empty, pour more formula into it.

• Never allow the syringe to empty completely.

• If you're using an infusion controller, thread the tube from the formula container through the controller according to the manufacturer's directions. Purge the tubing of air, and attach it to the feeding tube.

• Program the ordered flow rate and open the regulator clamp.

• After administering the appropriate amount of formula, flush the tubing by adding 60 ml of water to the gavage bag or bulb syringe or manually flush it using a barrel syringe.

• If you're administering a continuous feeding, flush the feeding tube every 4 hours. Monitor gastric emptying every 4 hours.

• To discontinue gastric feeding, close the regulator clamp on the gavage bag tubing, disconnect the syringe or tubing from the feeding tube, or turn off the infusion controller.

• Cover the end of the feeding tube with its plug or cap.

• Leave the patient in semi-Fowler's or high Fowler's position for at least 30 minutes.

• Change equipment every 24 hours or according to your facility's or manufacturer's policy.

Managing gastric feeding problems

Complication	Intervention
Aspiration of gastric secretions	• Discontinue feeding immediately. • Perform tracheal suction of aspirated contents, if possible. • Notify the physician. Prophylactic antibiotics and chest physiotherapy may be ordered. • Check tube placement before feeding to prevent complication.
Hyperglycemia	• Monitor blood glucose levels. • Notify the physician of elevated levels. • Administer insulin, if ordered. • Change the formula to one with a lower sugar content as ordered.
Tube obstruction	• Flush the tube with warm water. If necessary, replace the tube. • Flush the tube with 60 ml of water after each feeding to remove excess formula, which could occlude the tube.
Vomiting, bloating, diarrhea, or cramps	• Reduce the flow rate. • Warm the formula to prevent GI distress. • For 30 minutes after feeding, position the patient on his right side with his head elevated to facilitate gastric emptying. • Notify the physician. He may want to reduce the amount of formula being given during each feeding or order medication to increase GI motility.

Reinserting a gastrostomy feeding button

If your patient's gastrostomy feeding button pops out (with coughing, for example), it needs to be reinserted. Here are some steps to follow.

Prepare the equipment

Collect the feeding button, an obturator, and water-soluble lubricant. If the button is to be reinserted, wash it with soap and water and rinse thoroughly.

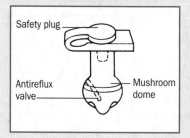

Insert the button

· Check the depth of the patient's stoma to make sure you have a feeding button of the correct size.
· Clean around the stoma.
· Lubricate the obturator with a water-soluble lubricant, and distend the button several times to ensure patency of the antireflux valve within the button.
· Lubricate the mushroom dome and the stoma.
· Gently push the button through the stoma into the stomach.

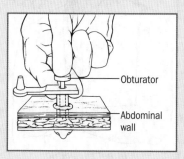

· Remove the obturator by gently rotating it as you withdraw it, to keep the antireflux valve from adhering to it.
· If the valve sticks nonetheless, gently push the obturator back into the button until the valve closes.
· After removing the obturator, make sure the valve is closed.
· Close the flexible safety plug, which should be relatively flush with the skin surface.

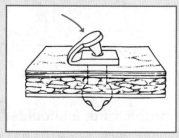

· If you need to administer a feeding right away, open the safety plug and attach the feeding adapter and feeding tube.
· Deliver the feeding as ordered.

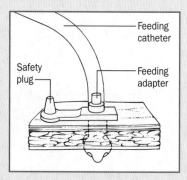

Using a hydraulic lift

After placing the patient supine in the center of the sling, position the hydraulic lift above him. Then attach the chains to the hooks on the sling.

Turn the lift handle clockwise to raise the patient to the sitting position. If he's positioned properly, continue to raise him until he's suspended just above the bed.

After positioning the patient above the wheelchair, turn the lift handle counterclockwise to lower him onto the seat. When the chains become slack, stop turning and unhook the sling from the lift.

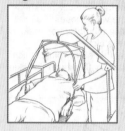

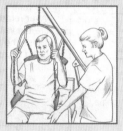

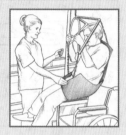

Immobilizing a shoulder dislocation

When a shoulder dislocation has been reduced, an external immobilization device, such as the elastic shoulder immobilizer or the stockinette Velpeau splint, can maintain the position until healing takes place. The device should remain on for about 3 weeks.

Elastic shoulder immobilizer

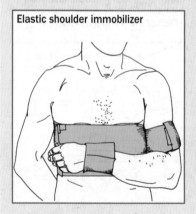

Stockinette Velpeau splint

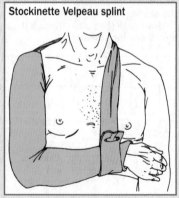

Setting up continuous bladder irrigation

With continuous bladder irrigation, a triple-lumen catheter allows irrigating solution to flow into the bladder through one lumen and flow out through another, as shown here. The third lumen is used to inflate the balloon that holds the catheter in place.

• Insert the spike of the tubing into the container of irrigating solution. (If you have a two-container system, insert one spike into each container.)
• Squeeze the drip chamber on the spike of the tubing.
• Open the flow clamp, and flush the tubing to remove air that could cause bladder distention. Then close the clamp.
• Clean the opening to the inflow lumen of the catheter with the alcohol or povidone-iodine pad.
• Insert the distal end of the tubing securely into the inflow lumen (third port) of the catheter.
• Make sure the catheter's outflow lumen is securely attached to the drainage bag tubing.
• Open the flow clamp under the container of irrigating solution, and set the drip rate as ordered.

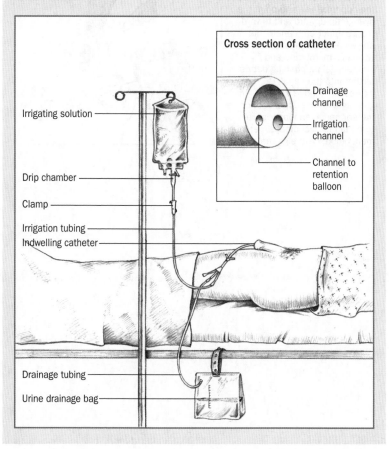

Cross section of catheter

Drainage channel

Irrigation channel

Channel to retention balloon

Irrigating solution

Drip chamber

Clamp

Irrigation tubing

Indwelling catheter

Drainage tubing

Urine drainage bag

Irrigating the ear canal

· Gently pull the auricle up and back to straighten the ear canal. (For a child, pull the ear down and back.)
· Have the patient hold an emesis basin beneath the ear to catch returning irrigant. Position the tip of the irrigating syringe at the meatus of the auditory canal. Don't block the meatus because you'll impede backflow and raise pressure in the canal.

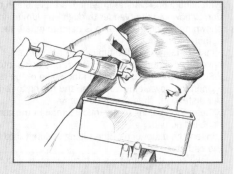

· Tilt the patient's head toward the opposite ear, and point the syringe tip upward and toward the posterior ear canal. This angle prevents damage to the tympanic membrane and guards against pushing debris farther into the canal.
· Direct a steady stream of irrigant against the upper wall of the ear canal, and inspect return fluid for cloudiness, cerumen, blood, or foreign matter.

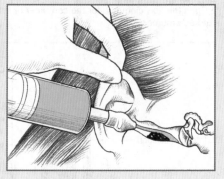

Irrigating the eye

Depending on the type and extent of injury, the patient's eye may need to be irrigated using different devices.

Squeeze bottle

For moderate-volume irrigation—to remove eye secretions, for example—apply sterile ophthalmic irrigant to the eye directly from the squeeze bottle container. Direct the stream at the inner canthus, and position the patient so the stream washes across the cornea and exits at the outer canthus.

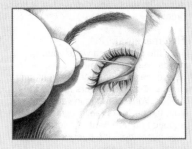

I.V. tube

For copious irrigation—to treat chemical burns, for example—set up an I.V. bag and tubing without a needle. Use the procedure described for moderate irrigation to flush the eye for at least 15 minutes. Alkali burns may require irrigation for several hours.

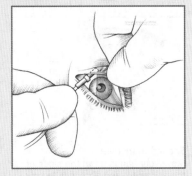

Morgan lens

Connected to irrigation tubing, a Morgan lens permits continuous lavage and delivers medication to the eye. Use an adapter to connect the lens to the I.V. tubing and the solution container. Begin the irrigation at the prescribed flow rate. To insert the device, ask the patient to look down as you insert the lens under the upper eyelid. Then have her look up as you retract and release the lower eyelid over the lens.

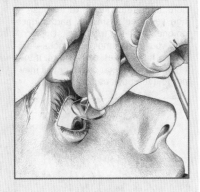

Performing Leopold's maneuvers

You can determine fetal position, presentation, and attitude by performing Leopold's maneuvers. Ask the patient to empty her bladder, assist her to a supine position, and expose her abdomen. Then perform the four maneuvers in order.

First maneuver

Face the patient and warm your hands. Place them on her abdomen to determine fetal position in the uterine fundus. Curl your fingers around the fundus. With the fetus in vertex position, the buttocks feel irregularly shaped and firm. With the fetus in breech position, the head feels hard, round, and movable.

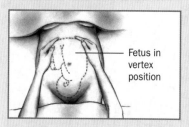

Fetus in vertex position

Second maneuver

Move your hands down the sides of the abdomen, and apply gentle pressure. If the fetus lies in vertex position, you'll feel a smooth, hard surface on one side—the fetal back. Opposite, you'll feel lumps and knobs—the knees, hands, feet, and elbows. If the fetus lies in breech position, you may not feel the back at all.

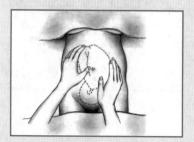

Third maneuver

Spread apart the thumb and fingers of one hand. Place them just above the patient's symphysis pubis. Bring your fingers together. If the fetus lies in vertex position and hasn't descended, you'll feel the head. If the fetus lies in vertex position and has descended, you'll feel a less distinct mass.

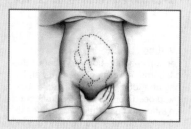

Fourth maneuver

Use this maneuver in late pregnancy when the fetus is in cephalic presentation. The purpose of the fourth maneuver is to determine flexion or extension of the fetal head and neck. Place your hands on both sides of the lower abdomen. Apply gentle pressure with your fingers as you slide your hands downward, toward the symphysis pubis. If the head and neck are flexed, your hands will meet obstruction—the cephalic prominence—on the side opposite the fetal back. If the head and neck are extended, the cephalic prominence will be palpated on the same side as the fetal back. Flexion of the fetal head and neck facilitates vaginal delivery.

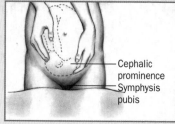

Cephalic prominence
Symphysis pubis

Measuring neonatal size

Besides weight, anthropometric measurements include head and chest circumferences and head-to-heel length. These measurements serve as a baseline and show whether the neonate's size is within normal ranges.

Measuring head circumference
· Slide the tape measure over the neonate's head. To arrive at the greatest circumference, draw the tape snugly across the center of the forehead and the most prominent portion of the posterior head (the occiput).

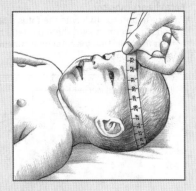

Measuring chest circumference
· Place the tape under the back, and wrap it snugly around the chest at the nipple line. To ensure accuracy, keep the back and front of the tape level.
· Take the measurement after the neonate inspires and before he begins to exhale.

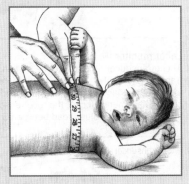

Measuring head-to-heal length
· Fully extend the neonate's legs with the toes pointing up. Measure the distance from the heel to the top of the head. If possible, have someone extend the legs by pressing down gently on the needs, or use a length board if available.

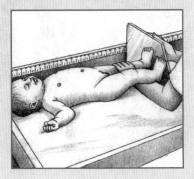

Applying external fetal monitoring devices

To ensure clear tracings that define fetal status and labor progress, be sure to precisely position external monitoring devices, such as an ultrasound transducer or a tocotransducer.

Fetal heart monitor

Palpate the uterus to locate the fetus's back. If possible, place the ultrasound transducer over this site where the fetal heartbeat sounds the loudest. Then tighten the belt. Use the fetal heart tracing on the monitor strip to confirm the transducer's position.

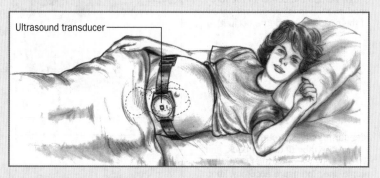

Ultrasound transducer

Labor monitor

A tocotransducer records uterine motion during contractions. Place the tocotransducer over the uterine fundus where it contracts, either midline or slightly to one side. Place your hand on the fundus, and palpate a contraction to verify proper placement. Secure the tocotransducer's belt; then adjust the pen set so that the baseline values read between 5 and 15 mm Hg on the monitor strip.

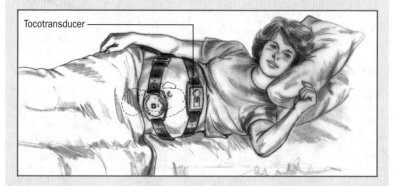

Tocotransducer

Applying an internal electronic fetal monitor

During internal electronic fetal monitoring, a spiral electrode monitors the fetal heart rate and an internal catheter monitors uterine contractions.

Inserting the spiral electrode

The spiral electrode is inserted after a vaginal examination that determines the position of the fetus. As shown, the electrode is attached to the presenting fetal part, usually the scalp or buttocks.

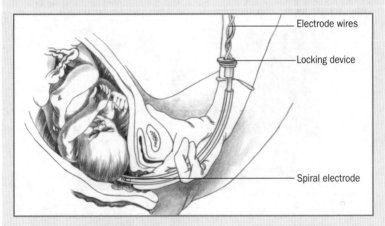

Inserting the intrauterine catheter

The intrauterine catheter is inserted up to a premarked level on the tubing and then connected to a monitor that interprets uterine contraction pressures.

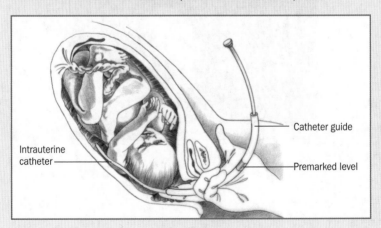

Using a bedside hemoglobin monitor

Monitoring hemoglobin levels at the patient's bedside is a straightforward procedure. A photometer, such as the HemoCue analyzer featured here, relies on capillary action to draw blood into a disposable microcuvette.

This method of obtaining blood minimizes a health care worker's exposure to the patient's blood and decreases the risk of cross-contamination. Follow these steps when using the HemoCue system.

After you pierce the skin, the microcuvette draws blood automatically.

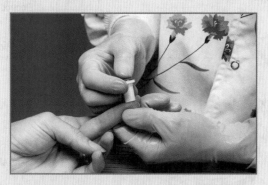

Next, place the microcuvette in the photometer. The photometer screen displays the hemoglobin levels.

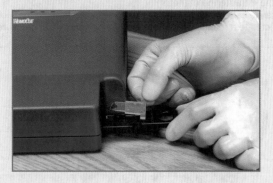

Setting up an ICP monitoring system

• Begin by opening a sterile towel. On the sterile field, place a 20-ml luer-lock syringe, an 18G needle, a 250-ml bag filled with normal saline solution (with outer wrapper removed), and a disposable transducer.

• Put on sterile gloves and gown according to your facility's policy, and fill the 20-ml syringe with normal saline solution from the I.V. bag.

• Remove the injection cap from the patient line, and attach the syringe. Turn the system stopcock off to the short end of the patient line, and flush through to the drip chamber (as shown below left). Allow a few drops to flow through the flow chamber (the manometer), the tubing, and the one-way valve into the drainage bag. (Fill the tubing and the manometer slowly to minimize air bubbles. If any air bubbles surface, be sure to force them from the system.) In some systems, the drainage system will prime itself with the patient's cerebrospinal fluid.

• Attach the manometer to the I.V. pole at the head of the bed.

• Slide the drip chamber onto the manometer, and align the chamber to the zero point, which should be at the inner canthus of the patient's eye.

• Next, connect the transducer to the monitor.

• Put on a clean pair of sterile gloves.

• Keeping one hand sterile, turn the patient stopcock off to the short end of the patient line.

• Align the zero point with the center line of the patient's head, level with the middle of the ear.

• Lower the flow chamber to zero, and turn the stopcock off to the dead-end cap. With a clean hand, balance the system according to monitor guidelines.

• Turn the system stopcock off to drainage, and raise the flow chamber to the ordered height (as shown below right).

• Return the stopcock to the ordered position, and observe the monitor for the return of intracranial pressure (ICP) patterns.

• The holder is raised and lowered to keep the patient's ICP at exact readings specified by the neurologist. If the neurologist orders cerebrospinal fluid to drain if ICP reaches 10, then the chamber is raised to 10.

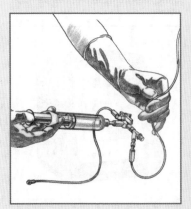

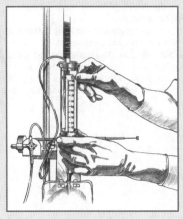

Using an electronic vital signs monitor

Preparing the device
· Make sure that the power switch is off. Then plug the monitor into a properly grounded wall outlet. Secure the dual air hose to the front of the monitor.
· Connect the pressure cuff's tubing into the other ends of the dual air hose, and tighten connections to prevent air leaks.
· Squeeze all air from the cuff, and wrap the cuff loosely around the patient's arm or leg, allowing two fingerbreadths between cuff and arm or leg. Never apply the cuff to a limb that has an I.V. line in place. Position the cuff's "artery" arrow over the palpated brachial artery. Then secure the cuff for a snug fit.

Selecting parameters
· When you turn on the monitor, it will default to a manual mode. (In this mode, you can obtain vital signs yourself before switching to the automatic mode.) Press the auto/manual button to select the automatic mode. The monitor will give you baseline data for the pulse rate, systolic and diastolic pressures, and mean arterial pressure.
· Compare your previous manual results with these baseline data. If they match, you're ready to set the alarm parameters. Press the select button to blank out all displays except systolic pressure.
· Use the high and low limit buttons to set the specific parameters for systolic pressure. You'll also do this three more times for mean arterial pressure, pulse rate, and diastolic pressure. After you've set the parameters

for diastolic pressure, press the select button again to display all current data. Even if you forget to do this last step, the monitor will automatically display current data 10 seconds after you set the last parameters.

Collecting data
· You need to tell the monitor how often to obtain data. Press the set button until you reach the desired time interval in minutes. If you've chosen the automatic mode, the monitor will display a default cycle time of 3 minutes. You can override the default cycle time to set the interval you prefer.
· You can obtain a set of vital signs at any time by pressing the start button. Also, pressing the cancel button will stop the interval and deflate the cuff. You can retrieve stored data by pressing the prior data button. The monitor will display the last data obtained along with the time elapsed since then. Scrolling backward, you can retrieve data from the previous 99 minutes.

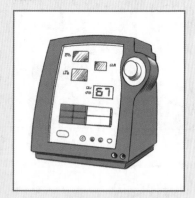

Inserting a nasogastric tube

· Help the patient into high Fowler's position unless contraindicated.

· Measure the tube by holding the end of the tube at the tip of the patient's nose, extending the tube to the patient's earlobe and then down to the xiphoid process.

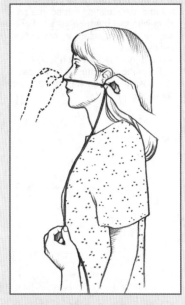

· Mark this distance on the tubing with tape.

· Assess airflow in both nostrils. Choose the nostril with the better airflow.

· Lubricate the first 3″ (7.6 cm) of the tube with a water-soluble gel.

· Instruct the patient to hold her head straight and upright.

· Grasp the tube with the end pointing downward, and carefully insert it into the more patent nostril.

· Aim the tube downward and toward the ear closer to the chosen nostril, and advance it slowly.

· When the tube reaches the nasopharynx, you'll feel resistance. Instruct the patient to lower her head slightly; rotate the tube 180 degrees toward the opposite nostril.

· Unless contraindicated, direct the patient to sip water through a straw and swallow as you slowly advance the tube.

· Watch for respiratory distress as you advance the tube.

· Stop advancing the tube when the tape mark reaches the patient's nostril.

· Attach a catheter-tip or bulb syringe to the tube and inject air while listening over the stomach (you should hear a "slooosh").

· Then aspirate stomach contents.

· Place a small amount of aspirate on the pH test strip. Probability of gastric placement is increased if the aspirate has a typical gastric fluid appearance (grassy green, clear and colorless with mucus shreds, or brown) and a pH lower than 5.0.

· If you don't obtain stomach contents, position the patient on her left side to move the contents into the stomach's greater curvature, and aspirate again.

· If you still can't aspirate stomach contents, advance the tube 1″ to 2″ (2.5 to 5 cm).

· After placement is confirmed, secure the tube to the patient's nose with hypoallergenic tape.

Clearing a nasoenteric-decompression tube obstruction

If your patient's nasoenteric-decompression tube appears to be obstructed, perform these measures to restore patency.

· First, disconnect the tube from suction and irrigate with normal saline solution. Use gravity flow to help clear the obstruction, unless ordered otherwise.

· If irrigation doesn't reestablish patency, tug slightly on the tube to free it from the gastric mucosa because it may be positioned against the intestinal wall.

· If gentle tugging doesn't restore patency, the tube may be kinked. Before manipulating the tube to try to clear the obstruction, take the following precautions:

– Never reposition or irrigate a nasoenteric-decompression tube (without a surgeon's order) in a patient who has had GI surgery.

– Avoid manipulating a tube in a patient who had the tube inserted during surgery because this may disturb new sutures.

– Don't try to reposition a tube in a patient who was difficult to intubate (because of an esophageal stricture, for example).

Taping a nephrostomy tube

To tape a nephrostomy tube directly to the skin, cut a wide piece of hypoallergenic adhesive tape twice lengthwise to its midpoint.

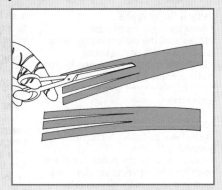

Apply the uncut end of the tape to the skin so that the midpoint meets the tube. Wrap the middle strip around the tube in a spiral fashion. Tape the other two strips to the patient's skin on both sides of the tube.

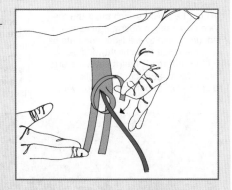

For greater security, repeat this step with a second piece of tape, applying it in the reverse direction. You may also apply two more strips of tape perpendicular to and over the first two pieces.

Always apply another strip of tape lower down on the tube in the direction of the drainage tube to further anchor the tube. Don't put tension on sutures that prevent tube distention.

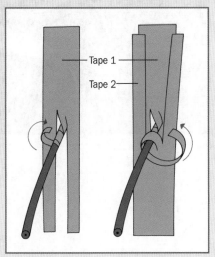

Using pulse oximetry

Using a finger probe

· Select a finger for the test.

· Make sure the patient isn't wearing false fingernails or nail polish.

· Place the transducer (photodetector) probe over the patient's finger so that the light beams and sensors oppose each other.

· If the patient has long fingernails, position the probe perpendicular to the finger, if possible, or clip the fingernail.

· Always position the patient's hand at heart level to eliminate venous pulsations and to promote an accurate reading.

· Turn the power switch on; if the device is working properly, a beep will sound, a display will light momentarily, and the pulse searchlight will flash.

· After four to six heartbeats, the arterial oxygen saturation and pulse rate displays will supply information with each beat and the pulse amplitude indicator will begin tracking the patient's pulse.

Using an ear probe

· Using an alcohol pad, massage the patient's earlobe for 10 to 20 seconds. Mild erythema indicates adequate vascularization.

· Following the manufacturer's instructions, attach the ear probe to the patient's earlobe or pinna.

· Be sure to establish good contact with the ear; an unstable probe may set off the low perfusion alarm.

· A saturation reading and pulse waveform will appear after a few seconds.

· Leave the ear probe in place for 3 or more minutes until readings stabilize at the highest point. An alternate method is to take three separate readings and average them.

· Make sure you revascularize the patient's earlobe each time.

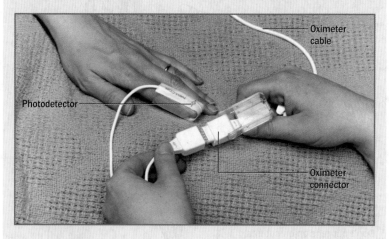

Photodetector

Oximeter cable

Oximeter connector

Troubleshooting pulse oximeter problems

To maintain a continuous display of arterial oxygen saturation (Spo_2) levels, you need to keep the monitoring site clean and dry. Make sure the skin doesn't become irritated from adhesives used to keep disposable probes in place. You may need to change the site if this happens. Disposable probes that irritate the skin can be replaced by nondisposable models that don't need tape.

A common problem with pulse oximeters is failure of the device to obtain a signal. If this happens, first check the patient's vital signs. If they're sufficient to produce a signal, check for the following problems.

Poor connection

Check that the sensors are properly aligned. Make sure that wires are intact and securely fastened and that the pulse oximeter is plugged into a power source.

Inadequate or intermittent blood flow to the site

Check the patient's pulse rate and capillary refill time, and take corrective action if blood flow to the site is decreased. This may require you to loosen restraints, remove tight-fitting clothes, take off a blood pressure cuff, or check arterial and I.V. lines. If none of these interventions works, you may need to find an alternate site. Finding a site with proper circulation may be a challenge when the patient is receiving vasoconstrictive drugs.

Equipment malfunction

Remove the pulse oximeter from the patient, and attempt to obtain an Spo_2 level on yourself or another healthy person. If you can obtain a normal value, the equipment is functioning properly.

Performing percussion and vibration

To perform percussion, instruct the patient to breathe slowly and deeply (using the diaphragm) to promote relaxation. Hold your hands in a cupped shape, with fingers flexed and thumbs pressed tightly against your index fingers. Percuss each segment for 1 to 2 minutes by alternating your hands against the patient in a rhythmic manner. Listen for a hollow sound on percussion to verify correct performance of the technique.

To perform vibration, ask the patient to inhale deeply and then exhale slowly through pursed lips. During exhalation, firmly press your fingers and the palms of your hands against the chest wall. Tense the muscles of your arms and shoulders in an isometric contraction to send fine vibrations through the chest wall. Vibrate during five exhalations over each chest segment.

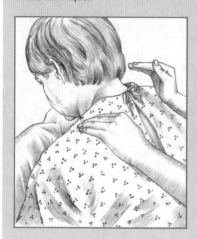
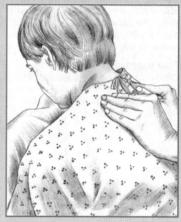

Caring for a PEG or PEJ site

The exit site of a percutaneous endoscopic gastrostomy (PEG) or percutaneous endoscopic jejunostomy (PEJ) tube requires routine observation and care. Follow these care guidelines:

· Change the dressing daily while the tube is in place.

· After removing the dressing, carefully slide the tube's outer bumper away from the skin (as shown top right) about ½" (1.5 cm).

· Examine the skin around the tube. Look for redness and other signs of infection or erosion.

· Gently depress the skin surrounding the tube, and inspect for drainage (as shown bottom right). Expect minimal wound drainage initially after implantation. This should subside in about 1 week.

· Inspect the tube for wear and tear. (A tube that wears out will need replacement.)

· Clean the site with the prescribed cleaning solution.

· Apply povidone-iodine ointment over the exit site according to your facility's guidelines.

· Rotate the outer bumper 90 degrees (to avoid repeating the same tension on the same skin area), and slide the outer bumper back over the exit site.

· If leakage appears at the PEG site, or if the patient risks dislodging the tube, apply a sterile gauze dressing over the site. Don't put sterile gauze underneath the outer bumper. Loosening the anchor this way allows the feeding tube free play, which could lead to wound abscess.

· Write the date and time of the dressing change on the tape.

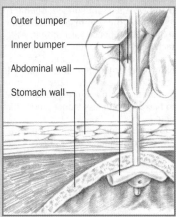

Outer bumper

Inner bumper

Abdominal wall

Stomach wall

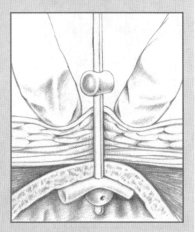

Applying a pneumatic antishock garment

After taking the patient's baseline vital signs and explaining the treatment, prepare to apply the antishock garment. On a smooth surface, open the garment with Velcro fasteners down.

Open all stopcock valves; then attach the foot pump tubing to the valve on the pressure control unit. Can the patient be turned from side to side? If not, slide the garment under him. If he can be turned, place the garment next to him and, with assistance, move him onto it.

Before closing the garment, remove any sharp objects, such as pieces of glass, stones, keys, or a buckle that could injure the patient or tear the garment. As appropriate, pad pressure points and apply lanolin to protect the patient's skin from irritation.

Place the upper edge of the garment just below the patient's lowest rib. Wrap the right leg compartment around the patient's right leg. Secure the compartment by fastening all the Velcro straps from ankle to thigh. Repeat this procedure for the left leg; then wrap the abdomen. Double-check that all valves are properly positioned.

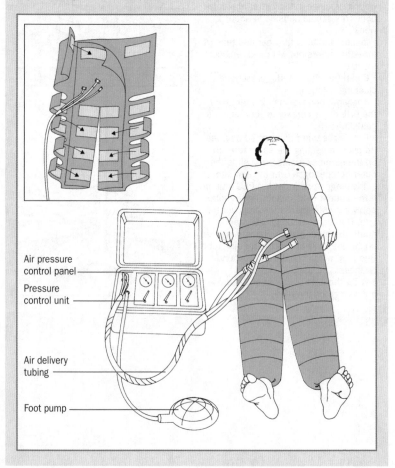

Air pressure control panel

Pressure control unit

Air delivery tubing

Foot pump

Positioning patients

This chart lists various positions in which patients may be placed. These positions may be used for patient comfort, but proper positioning also maintains functional body alignment and patient safety, promotes respiration and circulation, relieves pressure, and aids in administering treatment.

Position	Implementation	Rationale	Indications
Elevation of extremity	Use the bed controls to elevate the lower extremities, or use pillows to elevate the upper and lower extremities.	• Promotes circulation and comfort • Enables examinations and procedures	• Thrombophlebitis • After cast application • Edema • After surgery on extremity
Dorsal recumbent (supine)	Place the patient on his back with the knees slightly flexed. Place a pillow beneath the head for comfort.	• Immobilizes the spine	• Spinal cord injury • Urinary catheter insertion • Vaginal examination
Fowler's	Elevate the head of the bed to 45 degrees, and raise the bed section under the patient's knees, flexing the knees slightly.	• Enables examination • Immobilizes the spine • Promotes drainage, cardiac output, and ventilation • Prevents aspiration of food and secretions	• Head injury, cranial surgery, increased intracranial pressure (ICP) • After abdominal surgery • Dyspnea • Vomiting • After thyroidectomy • After eye surgery
High Fowler's	Elevate the head of the bed to 90 degrees, and raise the bed section under the patient's knees, flexing the knees slightly.	• Promotes drainage, cardiac output, and ventilation • Prevents aspiration of food and secretions	• Head injury, cranial surgery, increased ICP • Dyspnea, respiratory distress • Feeding (during and after meals) • Hiatal hernia
Lateral (side-lying)	Place the patient on his side, with weight being mostly supported by the lateral aspect of the lower scapula and the lower ileum. Support with pillows.	• Promotes safety • Prevents atelectasis, pressure ulcers, and aspiration of food and secretions	• After abdominal surgery • Coma • Pressure ulcer • Enema or rectal irrigation

(continued)

Positioning patients (continued)

Position	Implementation	Rationale	Indications
Lithotomy	Place the patient on his back (either flat or with the head slightly elevated). Knees should be flexed at right angles and feet placed in stirrups.	• Enables examination of the pelvis	• Perineal or rectal procedure
Prone	Place the patient on his stomach with the head turned to one side. Position the arms at the side or above the head. Make sure that the legs are extended.	• Enables examination of the back and spine • Promotes gas exchange	• Immobilization • Acute respiratory distress syndrome • After lumbar puncture or myelogram
Reverse Trendelenburg's	Elevate the head of the bed and lower the feet.	• Provides counterbalance for traction • Promotes blood flow to the lower extremities	• Cervical traction • After lower extremity vessel surgery
Semi-Fowler's	Elevate the head of the bed to 30 degrees, and raise the bed section under the patient's knees, flexing the knees slightly.	• Promotes drainage, cardiac output, and ventilation • Prevents aspiration of food and secretions	• Head injury, cranial surgery, increased ICP • After abdominal surgery • Dyspnea • Vomiting • After thyroidectomy • After eye surgery
Sims'	Position the patient on his side with a small pillow beneath the head. Flex one knee toward the abdomen, with the other knee only slightly flexed. Place one arm behind the body and the other in a comfortable position. Support with pillows.	• Enables examination of the back and rectum • Prevents pressure ulcers and atelectasis	• Coma • Rectal injuries

Positioning patients (continued)

Position	Implementation	Rationale	Indications
Trendelenburg's	Position the patient in a supine position with the feet elevated 30 to 40 degrees higher than the head.	• Promotes postural drainage and venous return	• Shock • Cystic fibrosis

Using sequential compression therapy

· Measure the circumference of the upper thigh while the patient rests in bed. Do this by placing the measuring tape under the thigh at the gluteal furrow.

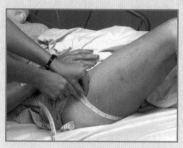

· Find the patient's thigh measurement on the sizing chart, and locate the corresponding size of the compression sleeve.
· Lay the unfolded sleeves on a flat surface with the cotton lining facing up (as shown below).

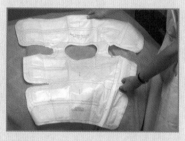

· Notice the markings on the lining denoting the ankle and the area behind the knee at the popliteal pulse point. Use these markings to position the sleeve at the appropriate landmarks.

· Place the patient's leg on the sleeve lining. Position the back of the knee over the popliteal opening.
· Make sure the back of the ankle is over the ankle marking.
· Starting at the side opposite the clear plastic tubing, wrap the sleeve snugly around the patient's leg.
· Fasten the sleeve securely with the Velcro fasteners. For the best fit, first secure the ankle and calf sections and then the thigh.
· The sleeve should fit snugly but not tightly. Check the fit by inserting two fingers between the sleeve and the patient's leg at the knee opening. Loosen or tighten the sleeve by readjusting the Velcro fastener.

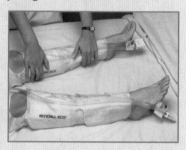

· Connect each sleeve to the tubing leading to the controller.
· Plug the compression controller into the proper wall outlet. Turn on the power.
· The controller automatically sets the compression sleeve pressure at 45 mm Hg, which is the midpoint of the normal range (35 to 55 mm Hg).

Making a sling

Place the apex of a triangular bandage behind the patient's elbow on the injured side. Hold one end of the bandage so it extends up toward the patient's neck on the uninjured side, and let the other end hang straight down. The bandage's long side should parallel the midline of the patient's body.

Adjust the bandage so that the forearm and upper arm form an angle of slightly less than 90 degrees to increase venous return from the hand and forearm and to facilitate drainage from swelling. Then tie the two bandage ends at the side of the patient's neck, rather than at the back, to prevent neck flexion and avoid irritation and pressure over a cervical vertebra.

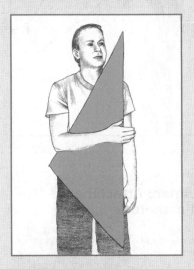

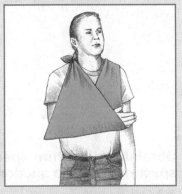

Loop the top corner of the bandage over the shoulder on the uninjured side and around the back of the patient's neck. Then bring the lower end of the bandage over the flexed forearm and up to the shoulder on the injured side.

Carefully secure the sling with a safety pin above and behind the elbow. For a child younger than age 7, use tape instead of a pin to prevent the chance of an injury.

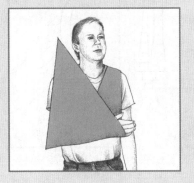

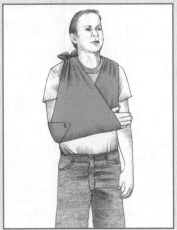

Obtaining a nasopharyngeal specimen

Pass the swab into the nasopharynx about 3″ to 4″ (7.5 to 10 cm). Quickly but gently rotate the swab to collect the specimen. Then remove the swab, taking care not to injure the nasal mucous membrane. Insert the swab into the culture tube and label it.

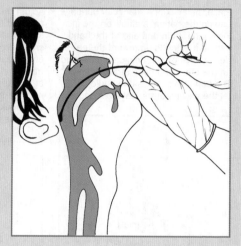

Obtaining a sputum specimen: Attaching specimen trap to suction catheter

Wearing gloves, push the suction tubing onto the male adapter of the in-line trap.

Insert the suction catheter into the rubber tubing of the trap.

After suctioning, disconnect the in-line trap from the suction tubing and catheter. To seal the container, connect the rubber tubing to the male adapter of the trap.

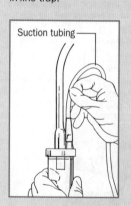

Suction tubing

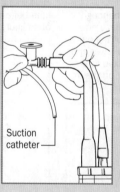

Suction catheter

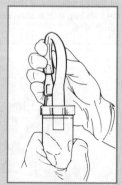

Aspirating a urine specimen

Clamp the indwelling urinary catheter distal to the aspiration port for about 30 minutes. Wipe the port with an alcohol pad, and insert a needle and a 10-ml or 20-ml syringe into the port perpendicular to the tube. Aspirate the required amount of urine, and expel it into the specimen container. Remove the clamp on the drainage tube.

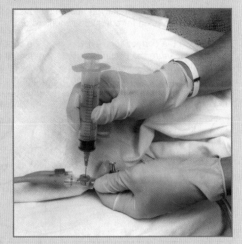

Using an air splint

In an emergency, an air splint can be applied to immobilize a fracture or control bleeding, especially from a forearm or lower leg. This compact, comfortable splint is made of double-walled plastic and provides gentle, diffuse pressure over an injured area. The appropriate splint is chosen, wrapped around the affected extremity, secured with Velcro or other strips, and then inflated. The fit should be snug enough to immobilize the extremity without impairing circulation.

An air splint may actually control bleeding better than a local pressure bandage. The device's clear plastic construction simplifies inspection of the affected site for bleeding, pallor, or cyanosis. An air splint also allows the patient to be moved without further damage to the injured limb.

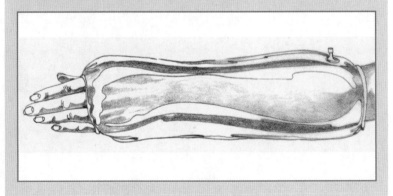

Measuring for antiembolism stockings

Measure the patient carefully to ensure that his antiembolism stockings provide enough compression for adequate venous return.

To choose the correct *knee-length* stocking, measure the circumference of the calf at its widest point (below left) and the leg length from the bottom of the heel to the back of the knee (bottom left).

To choose a *thigh-length* stocking, measure the calf as for a knee-length stocking and the thigh at its widest point (below right). Then measure leg length from the bottom of the heel to the gluteal fold (bottom right).

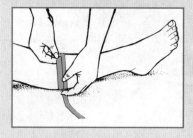

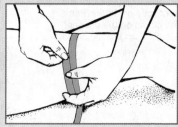

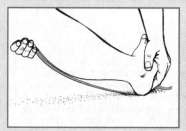

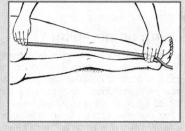

Applying an antiembolism stocking

Gather the loose part of the stocking at the toes, and pull this portion toward the heel.

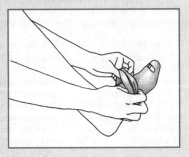

Then gather the loose part of the stocking and bring it over the heel with short, alternating front and back pulls.

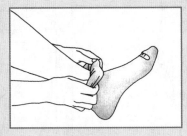

Insert the index and middle fingers into the gathered part of the stocking at the ankle, and ease it upward by rocking it slightly up and down.

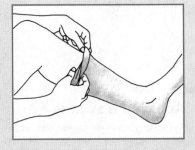

Wrapping a stump

Proper stump care protects the limb, reduces swelling, and prepares the limb for a prosthesis. As you perform the procedure, teach the patient.

Start by obtaining two 4″ elastic bandages. Center the end of the first 4″ bandage at the top of the patient's thigh. Unroll the bandage downward over the stump and to the back of the leg.

Make three figure-eight turns to adequately cover the ends of the stump. As you wrap, include the roll of flesh in the groin area. Use enough pressure to ensure that the stump narrows toward the end so that it fits comfortably into the prosthesis.

Use the second 4″ bandage to anchor the first bandage around the waist. For a below-the-knee amputation, use the knee to anchor the bandage in place. Secure the bandage with clips, safety pins, or adhesive tape. Check the stump bandage regularly, and rewrap it if it bunches at the end.

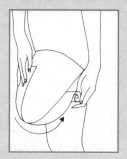
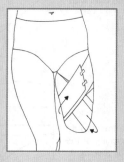
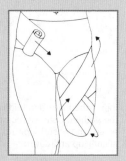

Applying a swathe

To further immobilize an arm after applying a sling, wrap a folded triangular bandage or wide elastic bandage around the patient's upper torso and the upper arm on the injured side. Don't cover the patient's uninjured arm. Make the swathe just tight enough to secure the injured arm to the body. Tie or pin the ends of the bandage just in front of the axilla on the uninjured side.

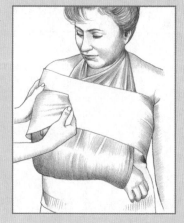

Measuring tracheal cuff pressure

• Attach the cuff pressure manometer to the pilot balloon port.
• Place the diaphragm of the stethoscope over the trachea, and listen for an air leak (a loud, gargling sound).

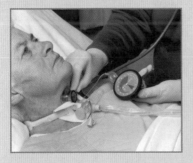

• As soon as you hear an air leak, release the red button and gently squeeze the handle of the cuff pressure manometer to inflate the cuff (as shown below). Continue to add air to the cuff until you no longer hear an air leak.

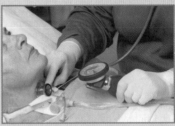

• If you don't hear an air leak, press the red button under the dial of the cuff pressure manometer to slowly release air from the balloon on the tracheal tube (as shown below). Auscultate for an air leak.

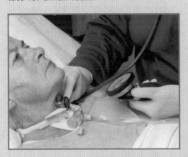

• When the air leak ceases, read the dial on the cuff pressure manometer (as shown below). This is the minimal pressure required to effectively occlude the trachea around the tracheal tube. In many cases, this pressure will fall within the green area (16 to 24 cm H_2O) on the manometer dial.

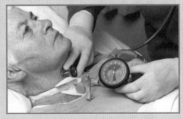

Performing open tracheal suctioning

• Remove the top from the normal saline solution or water bottle.

• Open the package containing the sterile solution container.

• Using strict sterile technique, open the suction catheter kit and put on the gloves. If using individual supplies, open the suction catheter and the gloves, placing the nonsterile glove on your nondominant hand and then the sterile glove on your dominant hand.

• Using your nondominant (nonsterile) hand, pour the normal saline solution or sterile water into the solution container.

• Place a small amount of water-soluble lubricant on the sterile area. Lubricant may be used to facilitate passage of the catheter during naso-tracheal suctioning.

• Using your dominant (sterile) hand, remove the catheter from its wrapper. Keep it coiled so it can't touch a non-sterile object. Using your other hand to manipulate the connecting tubing, attach the catheter to the tubing.

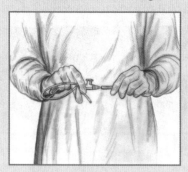

• Using your nondominant hand, set the suction pressure according to facility policy. Typically, pressure may be set between 80 and 120 mm Hg. Higher pressures don't enhance secretion removal and may cause traumatic injury. Occlude the suction port to assess suction pressure (as shown here).

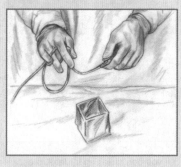

• Dip the catheter tip in the saline solution to lubricate the outside of the catheter and reduce tissue trauma during insertion.

• With the catheter tip in the sterile solution, occlude the control valve with the thumb of your nondominant hand. Then suction a small amount of solution through the catheter to lubricate the inside of the catheter, thus facilitating passage of secretions through it.

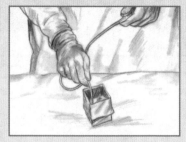

• For nasal insertion of the catheter, lubricate the tip of the catheter with the sterile, water-soluble lubricant to reduce tissue trauma during insertion.
• Insert the catheter into the patient's nostril while gently rolling it between your fingers to help it advance through the turbinates.
• As the patient inhales, quickly advance the catheter as far as possible. To avoid oxygen loss and tissue trauma, don't apply suction during insertion.
• If the patient coughs as the catheter passes through the larynx, briefly hold the catheter still and then resume advancement when the patient inhales.
• If the patient isn't intubated or is intubated but isn't receiving supplemental oxygen or aerosol, instruct him to take three to six deep breaths to help minimize or prevent hypoxia during suctioning.
• If the patient is being mechanically ventilated, preoxygenate him using either a handheld resuscitation bag or the sigh mode on the ventilator.

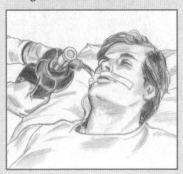

• Using your sterile hand, gently insert the suction catheter into the artificial airway (as shown below). Advance the catheter, without applying suction, until you meet resistance. If the patient coughs, pause briefly and then resume advancement.

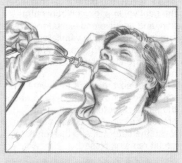

• Using your nonsterile hand, disconnect the patient from the ventilator.
• After inserting the catheter, apply suction intermittently by removing and replacing the thumb of your nondominant hand over the control valve. Simultaneously use your dominant hand to withdraw the catheter as you roll it between your thumb and forefinger. This rotating motion prevents the catheter from pulling tissue into the tube as it exits, thus avoiding tissue trauma. Never suction more than 10 seconds at a time, to prevent hypoxia.

Performing closed tracheal suctioning

The closed tracheal suction system can ease removal of secretions and reduce patient complications. Consisting of a sterile suction catheter in a clear plastic sleeve, the system permits the patient to remain connected to the ventilator during suctioning.

As a result, the patient can maintain the tidal volume, oxygen concentration, and positive end-expiratory pressure delivered by the ventilator while being suctioned. In turn, this reduces the occurrence of suction-induced hypoxemia.

Another advantage of this system is a reduced risk of infection, even when the same catheter is used many times. The caregiver doesn't need to touch the catheter, and the ventilator circuit remains closed.

Implementation

To perform the procedure, gather a closed suction control valve, a T-piece to connect the artificial airway to the ventilator breathing circuit, and a catheter sleeve that encloses the catheter and has connections at each end for the control valve and the T-piece. Then follow these steps:

· Remove the closed suction system from its wrapping. Attach the control valve to the connecting tubing.

· Depress the thumb suction control valve, and keep it depressed while setting the suction pressure to the desired level.

· Connect the T-piece to the ventilator breathing circuit, making sure that the irrigation port is closed; then connect the T-piece to the patient's endotracheal or tracheostomy tube (as shown below).

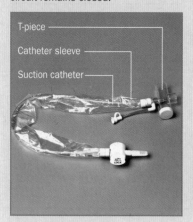

T-piece
Catheter sleeve
Suction catheter

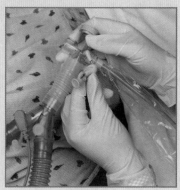

• With one hand keeping the T-piece parallel to the patient's chin, use the thumb and index finger of the other hand to advance the catheter through the tube and into the patient's tracheobronchial tree (as shown below).

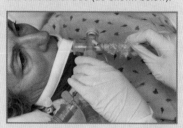

• It may be necessary to gently retract the catheter sleeve as you advance the catheter.
• While continuing to hold the T-piece and control valve, apply intermittent suction and withdraw the catheter until it reaches its fully extended length in the sleeve. Repeat the procedure as necessary.
• After you've finished suctioning, flush the catheter by maintaining suction while slowly introducing normal saline solution or sterile water into the irrigation port.
• Place the thumb control valve in the off position.
• Dispose of and replace the suction equipment and supplies according to your facility's policy.
• Change the closed suction system per manufacturer and facility policy.

Assisting with a bedside tracheotomy

To perform a tracheotomy, the surgeon will first clean the area from the chin to the nipples with povidone-iodine solution. Next, he'll place sterile drapes on the patient and locate the area for the incision—usually 1 to 2 cm below the cricoid cartilage. Then he'll inject a local anesthetic.

He'll make a horizontal or vertical incision in the skin. (A vertical incision helps avoid arteries, veins, and nerves on the lateral borders of the trachea.) Then he'll dissect subcutaneous fat and muscle and move the muscle aside with vein retractors to locate the tracheal rings. He'll make an incision between the second and third tracheal rings (as shown below) and use hemostats to control bleeding.

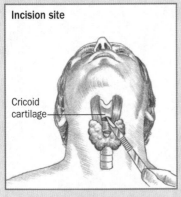

Incision site

Cricoid cartilage

He'll inject a local anesthetic into the tracheal lumen to suppress the cough reflex, and then he'll create a stoma in the trachea. When this is done, carefully apply suction to remove blood and secretions that may obstruct the airway or be aspirated into the lungs. The surgeon then will insert the tracheostomy tube and obturator into the stoma (as shown top of next column). After inserting the tube, he'll remove the obturator.

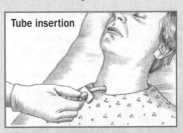

Tube insertion

Apply a sterile tracheostomy dressing, and anchor the tube with tracheostomy ties (as shown below). Check for air movement through the tube and auscultate the lungs to ensure proper placement.

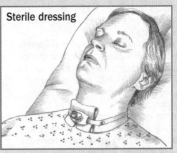

Sterile dressing

An alternative approach

In another approach, the surgeon inserts the tracheostomy tube percutaneously. Using either a series of dilators or a pair of forceps, he creates a stoma for tube insertion. Unlike the surgical technique, this method dilates rather than cuts the tissue structures.

After the skin is prepared and anesthetized, the surgeon makes a 1-cm midline incision. When the stoma reaches the desired size, the surgeon inserts the tracheostomy tube. When the tube is in place, inflate the cuff, secure the tube, and check the patient's breath sounds. Next, obtain a portable chest X-ray.

Deflating and inflating a tracheostomy cuff

As part of tracheostomy care, you may be required to deflate and inflate a tracheostomy cuff. If so, gather a 5-ml or 10-ml syringe, padded hemostat, and stethoscope, and follow these steps.

· Read the cuff manufacturer's instruction because cuff types and procedures vary.

· Assess the patient's condition, explain the procedure to him, and reassure him. Wash your hands thoroughly.

· Help the patient into semi-Fowler's position, if possible, or place him in a supine position so secretions above the cuff site will be pushed up into his mouth if he's receiving positive-pressure ventilation.

· Suction the oropharyngeal cavity to prevent pooled secretions from descending into the trachea after cuff deflation.

· Release the padded hemostat clamping the cuff inflation tubing, if a hemostat is present.

· Insert a 5-ml or 10-ml syringe into the cuff pilot balloon, and very slowly withdraw all air from the cuff. Leave the syringe attached to the tubing for later reinflation of the cuff.

· Remove the ventilation device. Suction the lower airway through the existing tube to remove all secretions, and then reconnect the patient to the ventilation device.

· Maintain cuff deflation for the prescribed time. Observe the patient for adequate ventilation, and suction as necessary. If the patient has difficulty breathing, reinflate the cuff immediately by depressing the syringe plunger very slowly. Use a stethoscope to listen over the trachea for the air leak, and then inject the least amount of air needed to achieve an adequate tracheal seal.

· When inflating the cuff, you may use the minimal-leak technique or the minimal occlusive-volume technique to help gauge the proper inflation point.

· If you're inflating the cuff using cuff pressure measurement, be careful not to exceed 25 mm Hg.

· After you've inflated the cuff, if the tubing doesn't have a one-way valve at the end, clamp the inflation line with a padded hemostat (to protect the tubing) and remove the syringe.

· Check for a minimal-leak cuff seal. You shouldn't feel air coming from the patient's mouth, nose, or tracheostomy site, and a conscious patient shouldn't be able to speak. Be alert for air leaks from the cuff itself.

· Note the exact amount of air used to inflate the cuff to detect tracheal malacia if more air is consistently needed.

· Make sure the patient is comfortable and can easily reach the call button and communication aids.

· Properly clean or dispose of all equipment, supplies, and trash according to your facility's policy. Replenish used supplies, and make sure all necessary emergency supplies are at the bedside.

Positioning TENS electrodes

In transcutaneous electrical nerve stimulation (TENS), electrodes placed around peripheral nerves (or an incisional site) transmit mild electrical pulses to the brain. The current is thought to block pain impulses. The patient can influence the level and frequency of his pain relief by adjusting the controls on the device.

Typically, electrode placement varies even though patients may have similar complaints. Electrodes can be placed in several ways:
• to cover the painful area or surround it, as with muscle tenderness or spasm or painful joints

• to "capture" the painful area between electrodes, as with incisional pain.

In peripheral nerve injury, electrodes should be placed proximal to the injury (between the brain and the injury site) to avoid increasing pain. Placing electrodes in a hypersensitive area also increases pain. In an area lacking sensation, electrodes should be placed on adjacent dermatomes.

These illustrations show combinations of electrode placement (solid squares) and areas of nerve stimulation (shaded areas) for low back and leg pain.

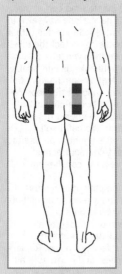 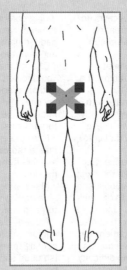 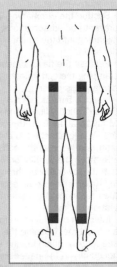

Using a transfer board

For the patient who can't stand, a transfer board allows safe transfer from bed to wheelchair. To perform this transfer, follow these steps.
· First, explain and demonstrate the procedure. Eventually, the patient may become proficient enough to transfer himself independently or with supervision.
· Help the patient put on pajama bottoms or a robe and shoes or slippers.
· Lock the bed wheels.
· Place the wheelchair angled slightly and facing the foot of the bed. Lock the wheels, and remove the armrest closest to the patient. Make sure that the bed is flat, and adjust its height so that the bed is level with the wheelchair seat.
· Help the patient to a sitting position on the edge of the bed, with his feet resting on the floor. Make sure that the front edge of the wheelchair seat is aligned with the back of the patient's knees (as shown below left). Although it's important that the patient have an even surface on which to transfer, he may find it easier to transfer to a slightly lower surface.

· Ask the patient to lean away from the wheelchair while you slide one end of the transfer board under him.
· Now place the other end of the transfer board on the wheelchair seat, and help the patient return to the upright position.
· Stand in front of the patient to prevent him from sliding forward. Tell him to push down with both arms, lifting the buttocks up and onto the transfer board. The patient then repeats this maneuver, edging along the board, until he's seated in the wheelchair. If the patient can't use his arms to assist with the transfer, stand in front of him, put your arms around him and, if he's able, have him put his arms around you. Gradually slide him across the board until he's safely in the chair (as shown below right).
· When the patient is in the chair, fasten the seat belt, if necessary, to prevent falls.
· Then remove the transfer board, replace the wheelchair armrest and footrest, and reposition the patient in the chair.

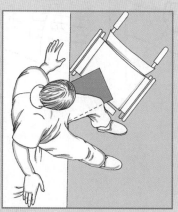
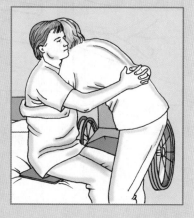

Taping a venous access site

If you'll be using tape to secure the access device to the insertion site, use one of the basic methods described below. Use sterile tape if you'll be placing a transparent dressing over the tape.

Chevron method

• Cut a long strip of ½″ tape, and place it sticky side up under the cannula and parallel to the short strip of tape.

• Cross the ends of the tape over the cannula so that the tape sticks to the patient's skin.

• Apply a piece of 1″ tape across the two wings of the chevron.

• Loop the tubing and secure it with another piece of 1″ tape. When the dressing is secured, apply a label. On the label, write the date and time of insertion, type and gauge of the needle, and your initials.

U method

• Cut a 2″ (5.1-cm) strip of ½″ tape. With the sticky side up, place it under the hub of the cannula.

• Bring each side of the tape up, folding it over the wings of the cannula in a U shape. Press it down parallel to the hub.

• Apply tape to stabilize the catheter.

• When a dressing is secured, apply a label. On the label, write the date and time of insertion, type and gauge of the needle or cannula, and your initials.

H method

• Cut three strips of 1″ tape.

• Place one strip of tape over each wing, keeping the tape parallel to the cannula.

• Now place the other strip of tape perpendicular to the first two. Put it either directly on top of the wings or just below the wings, directly on top of the tubing.

• Make sure the cannula is secure; then apply a dressing and a label. On the label, write the date and time of insertion, type and gauge of needle or cannula, and your initials.

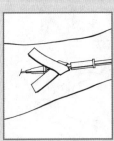

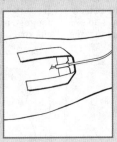

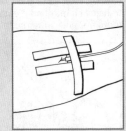

Using a walker

Sitting down

• First, tell the patient to stand with the back of his stronger leg against the front of the chair, his weaker leg slightly off the floor, and the walker directly in front of him.

• Tell him to grasp the armrests on the chair one arm at a time while supporting most of his weight on the stronger leg. (In these illustrations, the patient has left leg weakness.)

• Tell the patient to lower himself into the chair and slide backward. After he's seated, he should place the walker beside the chair.

Getting up

• After bringing the walker to the front of his chair, tell the patient to slide forward in the chair. Placing the back of his stronger leg against the seat, he should then advance the weaker leg.

• Next, with both hands on the armrests, the patient can push himself to a standing position. Supporting himself with the stronger leg and the opposite hand, the patient should grasp the walker's handgrip with his free hand.

• Then the patient should grasp the free handgrip with his other hand.

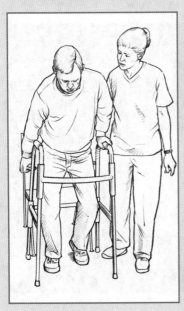

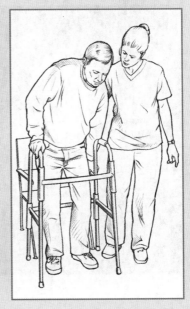

Using a warming system

Shivering, the compensatory response to falling body temperature, may use more oxygen than the body can supply—especially in a surgical patient. In the past, patients were covered with blankets to warm their bodies. Now, health care facilities may supply a warming system, such as the Bair Hugger patient-warming system (shown below).

This system helps to gradually increase body temperature by drawing air through a filter, warming the air to the desired temperature, and circulating it through a hose to a warming blanket placed over the patient.

When using the warming system, follow these guidelines:

· Place the warming blanket directly over the patient with the paper side facing down and the clear tubular side facing up.

· Use a bath blanket in a single layer over the warming blanket to minimize heat loss.

· Make sure the connection hose is at the foot of the bed.

· Take the patient's temperature during the first 15 to 30 minutes and at least every 30 minutes while the warming blanket is in use.

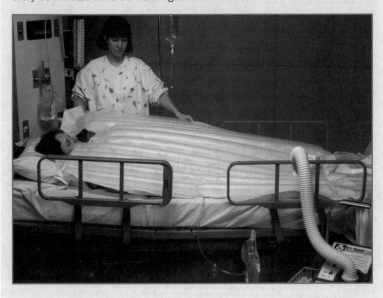

Specialized aspects of care

CDC isolation precautions

The Centers for Disease Control and Prevention (CDC) and the Hospital Infection Control Practices Advisory Committee developed the CDC Guidelines for Isolation Precautions in Hospitals to help hospitals maintain up-to-date isolation practices. CDC guidelines contain two tiers of precautions: standard precautions and transmission-based precautions.

Standard precautions

Standard precautions are to be used when caring for all hospital patients, regardless of their diagnoses or presumed infections. Standard precautions are the primary strategy for preventing nosocomial infection and replace the earlier, universal precautions. Standard precautions refer to protection from:
• blood
• all body fluids, secretions, and excretions except sweat, regardless of whether they contain visible blood
• skin that isn't intact
• mucous membranes.

Transmission-based precautions

Transmission-based precautions are instituted when caring for patients with known or suspected highly transmissible infections that necessitate more stringent precautions than those described in the standard precautions. There are three types of transmission-based precautions: contact, airborne, and droplet.

Contact precautions

Contact precautions reduce the risk of transmitting infectious agents by direct or indirect contact. Direct-contact transmission can occur through patient care activities that require physical contact. Indirect-contact transmission involves a susceptible host coming in contact with a contaminated object, usually inanimate, in the patient's environment. Contact precautions include the use of gloves, a mask, and a gown—in addition to standard precautions—to avoid contact with the infectious agent. Stringent hand washing is also necessary after removing the protective items.

Airborne precautions

Airborne precautions reduce the risk of airborne transmission of infectious agents. Microorganisms carried through the air can be dispersed widely by air currents, making them available for inhalation or deposit on a susceptible host in the same room or a longer distance away from the infected patient.

Airborne precautions include special air-handling and ventilation procedures to prevent the spread of infection. They require the use of respiratory protection, such as a mask—in addition to standard precautions—when entering an infected patient's room.

Droplet precautions

Droplet precautions reduce the risk of transmitting infectious agents in large-particle (exceeding 5 micrometers) droplets. Such transmission involves the contact of infectious agents with the conjunctivae or nasal or oral mucous membranes of a susceptible person. Large-particle droplets don't remain in the air and generally travel short distances of 3′ (0.9 m) or less. They require the use of a mask—in addition to standard precautions—to protect the mucous membranes.

Indications for contact precautions

Disease	Precautionary period
Acute viral (acute hemorrhagic) conjunctivitis	Duration of illness
Clostridium difficile enteric infection	Duration of illness
Diphtheria (cutaneous)	Duration of illness
Enteroviral infection, in diapered or incontinent patient	Duration of illness
Escherichia coli disease, in diapered or incontinent patient	Duration of illness
Hepatitis A, in diapered or incontinent patient	Duration of illness
Herpes simplex virus infection (neonatal or mucocutaneous)	Duration of illness
Impetigo	Until 24 hours after initiation of effective therapy
Infection or colonization with multidrug-resistant bacteria	Until off antibiotics and culture is negative
Major abscesses, cellulitis, or pressure ulcer	Until 24 hours after initiation of effective therapy
Parainfluenza virus infection, in diapered or incontinent patient	Duration of illness
Pediculosis (lice)	Until 24 hours after initiation of effective therapy
Respiratory syncytial virus infection, in an infant or a young child	Duration of illness
Rotavirus infection, in diapered or incontinent patient	Duration of illness
Rubella, congenital syndrome	Precautions during any admission until infant is 1 year old, unless nasopharyngeal and urine cultures negative for virus after age 3 months
Scabies	Until 24 hours after initiation of effective therapy
Shigellosis, in diapered or incontinent patient	Duration of illness
Smallpox	Duration of illness; requires airborne precautions

Indications for contact precautions *(continued)*

Disease	Precautionary period
Staphylococcal furunculosis, in an infant or a young child	Duration of illness
Viral hemorrhagic infections (Ebola, Lassa, Marburg)	Duration of illness
Zoster (chickenpox, disseminated zoster, or localized zoster in immunodeficient patient)	Until all lesions are crusted; requires airborne precautions

Indications for airborne precautions

Disease	Precautionary period
Chickenpox (varicella)	Until lesions are crusted and no new lesions appear
Herpes zoster (disseminated)	Duration of illness
Herpes zoster (localized in immunocompromised patient)	Duration of illness
Measles (rubeola)	Duration of illness
Smallpox (variola major)	Duration of illness, until all scabs fall off
Tuberculosis (TB)—pulmonary or laryngeal, confirmed or suspected	Depends on clinical response; patient must be on effective therapy, be improving clinically (decreased cough and fever and improved findings on chest X-ray), and have three consecutive negative sputum smears collected on different days, or TB must be ruled out

Indications for droplet precautions

Disease	Precautionary period
Adenovirus infection in an infant or a young child	Duration of illness
Diphtheria (pharyngeal)	Until off antibiotics and two cultures taken at least 24 hours apart are negative
Influenza	Duration of illness
Invasive *Haemophilus influenzae* type B disease, including meningitis, pneumonia, and sepsis	Until 24 hours after initiation of effective therapy
Invasive *Neisseria meningitidis* disease, including meningitis, pneumonia, epiglottiditis, and sepsis	Until 24 hours after initiation of effective therapy
Mumps	For 9 days after onset of swelling
Mycoplasma pneumoniae infection	Duration of illness
Parvovirus B19	Duration of hospitalization when chronic disease occurs in an immunodeficient patient; for patient with transient aplastic crisis or red cell crisis, maintain precautions for 7 days
Pertussis	Until 5 days after initiation of effective therapy
Pneumonic plague	Until 72 hours after initiation of effective therapy
Rubella (German measles)	Until 7 days after onset of rash
Streptococcal pharyngitis, pneumonia, or scarlet fever in an infant or a young child	Until 24 hours after initiation of effective therapy

Recommended barriers to infection

This list presents the minimum requirements for using gloves, gowns, masks, and eye protection to avoid coming in contact with and spreading pathogens. In addition to washing your hands thoroughly in all cases, refer to your facility's guidelines and use your judgment when assessing the need for barrier protection in specific situations.

Key

Gloves

Gown

Mask

Eyewear

Bathing, for patient with open lesions

if soiling likely

Bedding, changing visibly soiled

if soiling likely

Bleeding or pressure application to control it if soiling likely

if soiling likely

if splattering likely

if splattering likely

Blood glucose (capillary) testing

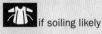

Cardiopulmonary resuscitation

if splattering likely

if splattering likely

if splattering likely

Central venous line insertion and venesection

Chest drainage system change

if splattering likely

if splattering likely

if splattering likely

Chest tube insertion or removal

if splattering likely

if splattering likely

if splattering likely

(continued)

Recommended barriers to infection *(continued)*

Cleaning (stools, spilled blood or body substances, or surface contaminated by blood or body fluids)

 if soiling likely

Colonoscopy, flexible sigmoidoscope

Coughing, frequent and forceful by patient; direct contact with secretions

Dialysis, peritoneal (initiating acute treatment, performing an exchange, terminating acute treatment, dismantling tubing from cycler, discarding peritoneal drainage, irrigating peritoneal catheter, changing tubing, or assisting with insertion of acute peritoneal catheter outside sterile field)

 if splattering likely

 if splattering likely

Dressing change for burns

Dressing removal or change for wounds with little or no drainage

Dressing removal or change for wounds with large amounts of drainage

 if soiling likely

Emptying drainage receptacles, including suction containers, urine receptacles, bedpans, emesis basins

 if soiling likely

 if splattering likely

 if splattering likely

Enema

 if soiling likely

Fecal impaction, removal of

Fecal incontinence, placement of indwelling catheter for, and emptying bag of

 if soiling likely

I.V. or intra-arterial line (insertion, removal, tubing change at catheter hub)

Recommended barriers to infection *(continued)*

Intubation or extubation

if splattering likely

if splattering likely

if splattering likely

Invasive procedures (lumbar puncture, bone marrow aspiration, paracentesis, liver biopsy) outside the sterile field

Irrigation, wound

if soiling likely

if splattering likely

if splattering likely

Nasogastric (NG) tube, insertion or irrigation

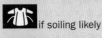if soiling likely

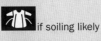if splattering likely

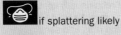if splattering likely

Ostomy care, irrigation, and teaching

if soiling likely

Pelvic examination and Papanicolaou test

Postmortem care

if soiling likely

Pressure ulcer care

Specimen collection (blood, stools, urine, sputum, wound)

Suctioning, nasotracheal or endotracheal

if soiling likely

if splattering likely

if splattering likely

Suctioning, oral or nasal

(continued)

Recommended barriers to infection *(continued)*

Tracheostomy suctioning and cannula cleaning

 if soiling likely

 if splattering likely

 if splattering likely

Tracheostomy tube change

 if splattering likely

Tracheostomy tube change *(continued)*

 if splattering likely

Urine and stool testing

Wound packing

 if soiling likely

Hand hygiene and hand rubs

The Centers for Disease Control and Prevention (CDC) defines *hand hygiene* as "any method that removes or destroys microorganisms on hands." It's a general term that refers to hand washing, antiseptic hand washing, antiseptic hand rubs, and surgical hand antisepsis.

Hand washing
Redefined by the CDC guideline, hand washing refers to washing hands with plain (such as nonantimicrobial) soap and water. Use of an antiseptic agent (such as chlorhexidine, triclosan, or iodophor) to wash hands is an antiseptic hand wash. Hand washing is appropriate whenever the hands are soiled or contaminated with infectious material, after using or cleaning the toilet, or before preparing food. Surgical personnel preoperatively perform surgical hand antisepsis to eliminate transient bacteria and reduce resident hand flora. Whether it involves a plain or antiseptic agent, hand washing is still the single most effective method of preventing the spread of infection.

Hand rubs
Hand hygiene also includes the use of rubs or hand sanitizers. An antiseptic hand rub involves applying an antiseptic, alcohol-containing product designed to reduce the number of viable microorganisms on the skin to all surfaces of the hands and rubbing until the product has dried (usually within 30 seconds). These products are also referred to as waterless antiseptic agents because no water is required. Alcohol hand rubs usually contain emollients to prevent skin drying and chapping. Hand rubs and sanitizers are appropriate for decontaminating the hands after minimal contamination.

Reportable diseases and infections

The Centers for Disease Control and Prevention (CDC), the Occupational Safety and Health Administration, The Joint Commission, and the American Hospital Association all require health care facilities to document and report certain diseases acquired in the community or in hospitals and other health care facilities.

Generally, the health care facility reports diseases to the appropriate local authorities. These authorities notify the state health department, which in turn reports the diseases to the appropriate federal agency or national organization.

The list of diseases that appears here is the CDC's list of nationally notifiable infectious diseases for 2006. Each state also keeps a list of reportable diseases appropriate to its region.

- Acquired immunodeficiency syndrome
- Anthrax
- Arboviral neuroinvasive and nonneuroinvasive diseases (California serogroup virus, eastern equine encephalitis virus, Powassan virus, St. Louis encephalitis virus, western equine encephalitis virus, West Nile virus)
- Botulism (food-borne, infant, other [wound and unspecified])
- Brucellosis
- Chancroid
- *Chlamydia trachomatis,* genital infections
- Cholera
- Coccidioidomycosis
- Cryptosporidiosis
- Cyclosporiasis
- Diphtheria
- Ehrlichiosis (human granulocytic, human monocytic, human [other or unspecified agent])
- Giardiasis
- Gonorrhea
- *Haemophilus influenzae,* invasive disease
- Hansen's disease (leprosy)
- Hantavirus pulmonary syndrome
- Hemolytic uremic syndrome, postdiarrheal
- Hepatitis, viral, acute (hepatitis A acute, hepatitis B acute, hepatitis B virus perinatal infection, hepatitis C acute)
- Hepatitis, viral, chronic (chronic hepatitis B, hepatitis C virus infection [past or present])
- Human immunodeficiency virus (adult 13 years or older], pediatric [younger than 13 years])
- Influenza-associated pediatric mortality
- Legionellosis
- Listeriosis
- Lyme disease
- Malaria
- Measles
- Meningococcal disease
- Mumps
- Pertussis
- Plague
- Poliomyelitis (paralytic)
- Psittacosis (ornithosis)
- Q fever
- Rabies (animal, human)
- Rocky Mountain spotted fever
- Rubella (German measles) and congenital syndrome
- Salmonellosis
- Severe acute respiratory syndrome-associated coronavirus disease
- Shiga toxin-producing *Escherichia coli*
- Shigellosis
- Streptococcal disease, invasive, group A
- Streptococcal toxic shock syndrome
- *Streptococcus pneumoniae,* drug-resistant, invasive disease
- *Streptococcus pneumoniae,* invasive, in children younger than 5 years
- Syphilis (primary; secondary; latent; early latent; late latent; latent unknown duration; neurosyphilis; late nonneurologic)
- Syphilis, congenital (syphilitic stillbirth)
- Tetanus
- Toxic shock syndrome
- Trichinellosis (trichinosis)
- TB
- Tularemia
- Typhoid fever
- Vancomycin-intermediate *Staphylococcus aureus*
- Vancomycin-resistant *Staphylococcus aureus*
- Varicella (morbidity)
- Varicella (deaths only)
- Yellow fever

Preoperative care

Preoperative care begins when surgery is planned and ends with the administration of anesthesia. This phase of care includes a preoperative interview and assessment to collect baseline subjective and objective data from the patient and his family; diagnostic tests, such as urinalysis, electrocardiogram, and chest radiography; preoperative teaching; securing informed consent from the patient; and physical preparation.

During the preoperative phase, the nurse performs a thorough assessment of the patient's emotional and physical status to determine teaching needs and to identify patients at risk for surgery, and documents baseline data for future comparisons.

Anxiety can interfere with the effectiveness of anesthesia and the patient's ability to actively participate in his care. Providing information about what will occur during surgery and sensations the patient can expect to feel helps to decrease anxiety.

Many interventions and activities contribute to patient safety. According to the Patient Care Partnership, the patient has the right to be informed by physicians and other direct caregivers of relevant, current, and understandable information concerning diagnosis, treatment, and progress.

Informed consent is required by law to help protect the patient's rights, autonomy, and privacy. Failure to obtain informed consent can result in assault and battery or negligence charges against the health care providers. The surgeon should provide the patient with information regarding the extent and type of surgery, alternative therapies, and usual risks and benefits. A consent form that includes all of this information must be signed by the patient and a witness, verifying that the patient has received the required information.

The nurse is responsible for making sure that the consent form is signed and that the patient understands the information before receiving preoperative medications. The nurse promotes patient safety by restricting activity after administration of sedatives and by completing a preoperative checklist to make sure that all procedures are carried out.

The patient shouldn't have ingested food or fluids for 8 hours before surgery. Just before the patient is moved to the surgical area, make sure that he's wearing a hospital gown, his identification band is in place, and his vital signs have been recorded. Check to see that hairpins, nail polish, and jewelry have been removed. Note whether dentures, contact lenses, or prosthetic devices have been removed or left in place. Preoperative medications should be administered as ordered.

Obtaining informed consent

Informed consent means that the patient is given a full explanation of the procedure, its risks and complications, and the risk if the procedure isn't performed at this time. Although obtaining informed consent is the physician's responsibility, the nurse is responsible for verifying that this step has been completed.

You may be asked to witness the patient's signature. However, if you didn't hear the physician's explanation to the patient, you must sign that you are witnessing only the patient's signature.

Consent forms must be signed before the patient receives his preoperative medication because forms signed after sedatives are given are legally invalid. Adults and emancipated minors can sign their own consent forms. Children's consent forms and those of adults with impaired mental status must be signed by a parent or legal guardian.

Surgical verifications

Wrong-site, wrong-procedure, and wrong-person surgery are errors that may occur in the operating room or in other settings, such as during ambulatory care or interventional radiology.

Several factors may contribute to an increased risk of wrong-site, wrong-procedure, or wrong-person surgery, including inadequate assessment of the patient, inadequate review of the medical records, inaccurate communication among members of the health care team, the involvement of multiple surgeons in the procedure, failure to include the patient in the site-identification process, and the practice of relying solely on the surgeon for site identification. Consistent use of a universal protocol by all members of the surgical team is essential.

These steps make up the universal protocol established by The Joint Commission:

- preoperative verification of information gathering and verification of procedure
- marking the site so that the mark is visible after the patient is prepped and draped
- calling a "time out" before beginning the procedure to conduct a final verification of patient, procedure, and site, and to answer any questions or concerns that the patient or surgical or procedure team may have.

Postoperative care

Postoperative care begins when the patient arrives in the postanesthesia care unit and continues as he moves on to the short procedure unit, medical-surgical unit, or intensive care area. Postoperative care aims to minimize complications by early detection and prompt treatment of the condition, such as postoperative pain, inadequate oxygenation, or other adverse physiologic effects.

Recovery from general anesthesia takes longer than induction because the anesthetic is retained in fat and muscle. Fat has a meager blood supply; thus, it releases the anesthetic slowly, providing enough anesthesia to maintain adequate blood and brain levels during surgery. The patient's recovery time varies with his amount of body fat, his overall condition, his premedication regimen, and the type, dosage, and duration of anesthesia. The effects of anesthesia and surgery can place the patient at risk for many physiologic disorders.

During the postoperative phase, the nurse is initially responsible for assessing the patient's physical status and monitoring changes that occur during the recovery process. When the patient's condition stabilizes, nursing care focuses on returning him to a functional level of wellness as soon as possible within the limitations created by surgery. The speed of a patient's recovery depends on how effectively the nurse can anticipate potential complications, begin the necessary preventive and supportive measures, and involve the patient's family in the recovery process. Facilitating communication among the patient, his family, and members of the health care team is also the nurse's responsibility.

If the patient is discharged home after surgery, it's the nurse's responsibility to help the patient and his family translate instructions on the discharge sheet into useful ways to deal with practical matters at home. Areas to be discussed include diet, bowel movements, resumption of sexual activity, wound care, driving, activity restriction, return to work, and medications. Each patient's care plan should be individualized to improve wellness and to maximize independence.

PQRST: The alphabet of pain assessment

Use the PQRST mnemonic device to obtain more information about the patient's pain. Asking the patient these questions elicits important details about his pain.

P *rovocative or palliative*
- What provokes or worsens your pain?
- What relieves the pain or causes it to subside?

Q *uality or quantity*
- What does the pain feel like? Is it aching, intense, knifelike, burning, or cramping?
- Are you having pain right now? If so, is it more or less severe than usual?
- To what degree does the pain affect your normal activities?
- Do you have other symptoms along with the pain, such as nausea or vomiting?

R *egion and radiation*
- Where's your pain?
- Does the pain radiate to other parts of your body?

S *everity*
- How severe is your pain? How would you rate it on a 0-to-10 scale, with 0 being no pain and 10 being the worst pain imaginable?
- How would you describe the intensity of your pain at its best? At its worst? Right now?

T *iming*
- When did your pain begin?
- At what time of day is your pain best? At what time is it worst?
- Is the onset sudden or gradual?
- Is the pain constant or intermittent?

Pain responses

Behavioral responses
Behavioral responses include altered body position, moaning, sighing, grimacing, withdrawal, crying, restlessness, muscle twitching, and immobility.

Sympathetic responses
Sympathetic responses are commonly associated with mild to moderate pain and include pallor, elevated blood pressure, dilated pupils, skeletal muscle tension, dyspnea, tachycardia, and diaphoresis.

Parasympathetic responses
Parasympathetic responses are commonly associated with severe, deep pain and include pallor, decreased blood pressure, bradycardia, nausea and vomiting, weakness, dizziness, and loss of consciousness.

Assess pain at least every 2 hours and during rest, during activity, and through the night when pain is commonly heightened. Ability to sleep doesn't indicate absence of pain.

Visual pain rating scale

You can evaluate pain in a nonverbal manner for pediatric patients age 3 and older and for adults with language difficulties. One instrument is the Wong-Baker FACES pain rating scale; another, two simple faces such as the ones shown here. Ask the patient to choose the face that describes how he's feeling—either happy because he has no pain, or sad because he has some or a lot of pain. Alternatively, to pinpoint varying levels of pain, you can ask the patient to draw a face.

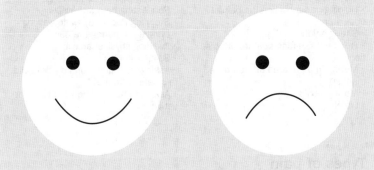

Differentiating acute and chronic pain

Acute pain may cause certain physiologic and behavioral changes that you won't observe in a patient with chronic pain.

Type of pain	Physiologic evidence	Behavioral evidence
Acute	• Increased respirations • Increased pulse • Increased blood pressure • Dilated pupils • Diaphoresis	• Restlessness • Distraction • Worry • Distress
Chronic	• Normal respirations, pulse, blood pressure, and pupil size • No diaphoresis	• Reduced or absent physical activity • Despair, depression • Hopelessness

Pain behavior checklist

A pain behavior is something a patient uses to communicate pain, distress, or suffering. Note if your patient displays any of these behaviors during assessment.

- Grimacing
- Moaning
- Sighing
- Clenching teeth
- Holding or supporting the painful body area
- Sitting rigidly
- Frequently shifting posture or position
- Moving in a guarded or protective manner
- Moving very slowly
- Limping

- Taking medication
- Using a cane, a cervical collar, or another prosthetic device
- Walking with an abnormal gait
- Requesting help with walking
- Stopping frequently while walking
- Lying down during the day
- Avoiding physical activity
- Being irritable
- Asking such questions as "Why did this happen to me?"
- Asking to be relieved from tasks or activities

Types of pain

- Nociceptive pain—ongoing activation of pain receptors; classified as somatic or visceral
  – Somatic pain—caused by injury to skin, bone, joint, connective tissue, and muscle; described as dull, aching, prickly, or burning
  – Visceral pain—caused by ongoing injury to internal organ or supporting tissues; described as cramping, pressurelike, or stabbing
- Neuropathic pain—caused by injury to the nervous system; pain may be sustained even after injury is healed; described as burning, tingling, or shooting pain, like electricity; can be caused by injury or disease
- Psychogenic pain—caused by psychological factors; may occur with or without disease or injury

Treating pain

Give medications
• If the patient is allowed oral intake, begin with a nonopioid analgesic, such as acetaminophen or aspirin, every 4 to 6 hours as ordered.
• If the patient needs more relief than a nonopioid analgesic provides, you may give a mild opioid as ordered.
• If the patient needs still more pain relief, you may administer a strong opioid as prescribed.
• If ordered, teach the patient how to use a patient controlled analgesia device. This device can help the patient manage his pain and decrease his anxiety.

Provide emotional support
• Show your concern by spending time talking with the patient. Because of his pain and his inability to manage it, he may be anxious and frustrated. Such feelings can worsen his pain.

Perform comfort measures
• Periodically reposition the patient to reduce muscle spasms and tension and to relieve pressure on bony prominences. Increasing the angle of the bed can reduce pull on an abdominal incision, diminishing pain. If appropriate, elevate a limb to reduce swelling, inflammation, and pain.
• Give the patient a back massage to help reduce tense muscles.
• Perform passive range-of-motion exercises to prevent stiffness and further loss of mobility, relax tense muscles, and provide comfort.
• Provide oral hygiene. Keep a fresh water glass or cup at the bedside because many pain medications tend to dry the mouth.
• Wash the patient's face and hands to soothe him, which may reduce his perception of pain.

Use cognitive therapy
• Help the patient enhance the effect of analgesics by using such techniques as distraction, guided imagery, deep breathing, and relaxation.
• For distraction, have the patient recall a pleasant experience or focus his attention on an enjoyable activity. For instance, have him use music as a distraction by turning on the radio when the pain begins. Tell him to close his eyes and concentrate on listening; raise or lower the volume as his pain increases or subsides. Note, however, that distraction is usually effective only against episodes of pain lasting less than 5 minutes.
• For guided imagery, help the patient concentrate on a peaceful, pleasant image such as walking on the beach. Encourage him to concentrate on the details of the image he has selected by asking about its sight, sound, smell, taste, and touch. The positive emotions evoked by this exercise minimize pain.
• For deep breathing, have the patient stare at an object, then slowly inhale and exhale as he counts aloud to maintain a comfortable rate and rhythm. Tell him to concentrate on the rise and fall of his abdomen. Encourage him to feel more and more weightless with each breath while he concentrates on the rhythm of his breathing or on any restful image.
• For muscle relaxation, have the patient focus on a particular muscle group. Ask him to tense the muscles and note the sensation. After 5 to 7 seconds, tell him to relax the muscles and concentrate on the relaxed state. Tell him to note the difference between the tense and relaxed states. After he tenses and relaxes one muscle group, have him proceed to another and another until he has covered his entire body.

Guide to making wound care decisions

Ask yourself these questions to help you determine what kind of care your patient's wound needs and how you should proceed. Be sure to assess the wound and document it according to facility policy and procedure.

How should I clean the wound?
☐ Water ☐ Saline ☐ Commercial wound cleaner

Is the wound clean or necrotic?
☐ Clean ☐ Necrotic

Is gangrene present?
☐ Yes ☐ No

Is there blood flow to the area?
☐ Yes ☐ No

Is the wound infected?
☐ Yes ☐ No

Does the wound need debridement?
☐ Yes ☐ No

What kind of debridement is appropriate?
☐ Sharp ☐ Chemical ☐ Mechanical ☐ Autolytic

Is the wound partial thickness or full thickness?
☐ Partial thickness ☐ Full thickness

How much drainage is present?
☐ None ☐ Minimal ☐ Moderate ☐ Heavy

How does the surrounding skin appear?
☐ Intact ☐ Irritated ☐ Denuded

What cover or dressing is appropriate?
☐ Transparent film ☐ Hydrogel ☐ Hydrocolloid
☐ Alginate ☐ Foam ☐ Gauze ☐ Other

Wound age

When determining wound age, you need to first determine if the wound is acute or chronic. Be careful—you can't base your determination solely on time because there isn't a set time frame before an acute wound becomes a chronic wound.

Wound type	Characteristics
Acute	• A new or relatively new wound • Occurs suddenly • Healing progresses in a timely, predictable manner • Typically heals by primary intention • Examples: surgical and traumatic wounds
Chronic	• May develop over time • Healing has slowed or stopped • Typically heals by secondary intention • Examples: pressure, vascular, and diabetic ulcers

Assessing the wound bed

Assess these characteristics:

• size and depth (in centimeters); use photography, a disposable tape measure, or a wound tracing
• tunneling (extensions of the wound bed into adjacent tissue) and undermining (extensions of the wound bed under the skin); measure in centimeters as you would for wound depth
• texture (healthy granulation tissue has a soft, bumpy appearance)
• moisture (the wound bed should be moist enough so that cells and chemicals needed for healing can move on the wound surface but it shouldn't be overly moist or dry)
• odor (a clean, uninfected wound produces little, if any, odor)
• condition of the wound margins and surrounding skin
  – the skin should appear smooth, not rolled, and tightly adhered to the wound bed
  – white, or macerated, skin indicates too much moisture
  – induration (hardened) tissue indicates infection.

Assessing drainage

A thorough wound assessment includes assessing drainage, the wound bed, and pain. Begin by removing the dressing. Then consider these questions:
· Is the dressing saturated or dry?
· Is the drainage well contained, or does it ooze from the edges of the wound? (If the wound is oozing, consider using a more absorbent dressing.)

· If the patient has an occlusive dressing, were the edges well sealed?
· Do you note a scant, moderate, or large amount of drainage?
· What color, consistency, and texture is the drainage?
· Does the drainage have an odor?

Drainage descriptors

The terminology in this chart can help you describe the color and consistency of wound drainage.

Description	Color and consistency
Serous	· Clear or light yellow · Thin and watery
Sanguineous	· Red (with fresh blood) · Thin
Serosanguineous	· Pink to light red · Thin · Watery
Purulent	· Creamy yellow, green, white, or tan · Thick and opaque

Measuring a wound

When measuring a wound, you must determine its length, width, and depth. You must also assess and measure the surrounding areas.

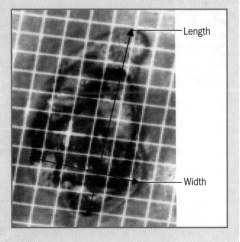

Length
· First, determine the longest distance across the open area of the wound, regardless of orientation.
· In this photo, note the line used to illustrate length.

Width
· Next, determine the longest distance across the wound at a right angle to the length.
· In this photo, note the relationship between length and width.

Depth
· If the wound is like the full-thickness ischial pressure ulcer in this photo, you'll need to record its depth—determined by measurements taken when inserting a swab into the deepest part of the wound.
· Also measure areas of tunneling or undermining.

Surrounding areas
· Note areas of reddened, intact skin and white skin.
· These areas are measured and recorded as surrounding erythema and maceration, not as part of the wound itself.

Wound depth

A wound is classified as partial thickness or full thickness according to its depth. Partial-thickness wounds involve only the epidermis or extend into the dermis but not through it. Full-thickness wounds extend through the dermis into tissues beneath and may expose adipose tissue, muscle, or bone.

Partial-thickness wound

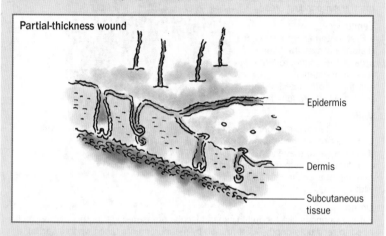

Epidermis

Dermis

Subcutaneous tissue

Full-thickness wound

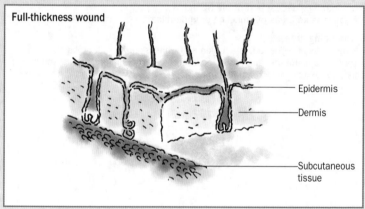

Epidermis

Dermis

Subcutaneous tissue

Measuring wound depth

To measure the depth of a wound, you'll need gloves, a cotton-tipped swab, and a disposable measuring device. You can also use this method to measure wound tunneling or undermining.

Put on gloves, and then gently insert the swab into the deepest portion of the wound.

Grasp the swab with your fingers at the point that corresponds to the wound's margin. You can carefully mark the swab where it meets the edge of the skin.

Remove the swab and measure the distance from your fingers or from the mark on the swab to the end of the swab to determine the depth.

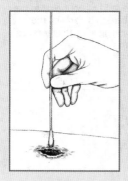
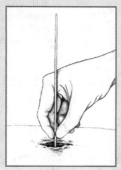
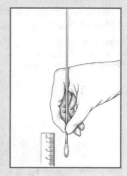

Measuring wound tunneling

Tunneling is tissue destruction that occurs around the wound perimeter underlying intact skin, causing the wound edges to pull away from the wound's base. Measuring and documenting the location and depth of tunneling is important because tunneling may be more extensive in one part of a wound than another.

What you'll need
- Sterile gloves
- Sterile cotton-tipped applicators
- Measuring guide

How you do it
- Wash your hands.
- Put on sterile gloves.

- Gently probe the wound bed and edges with your finger or a sterile cotton-tipped applicator to assess for wound tunneling.
- Gently insert the applicator into the wound in the direction where the deepest tunneling occurs, as shown bottom left.
- Grasp the applicator where it meets the wound edge.
- Remove the applicator, keeping your hand in place, and place it next to the measuring guide to determine the length of tunneling in centimeters, as shown bottom right.

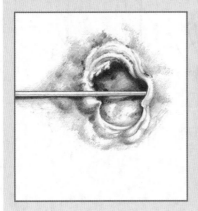

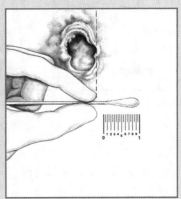

Recognizing wound failure to heal

Sign	Causes	Interventions
Wound bed		
Too dry	• Exposure of tissue and cells normally in a moist environment to air • Inadequate hydration	• Add moisture regularly. • Use a dressing that maintains moisture, such as a hydrocolloid or hydrogel dressing.
No change in size or depth for 2 weeks	• Pressure or trauma to the area • Poor nutrition, poor circulation, or inadequate hydration • Poor control of disease processes such as diabetes • Inadequate pain control • Infection	• Reassess the patient for local or systemic problems that impair wound healing, and intervene as necessary.
Increase in size or depth	• Debridement • Ischemia due to excess pressure or poor circulation • Infection	• If caused by debridement, no intervention is necessary. • Poor circulation may not be resolvable, but consider adding warmth to the area and administering a vasodilator or antiplatelet medication.
Necrosis	• Ischemia	• Perform debridement if the remaining living tissue has adequate circulation.
Increase in drainage or change in drainage from clear to purulent	• Infection • Autolytic or enzymatic debridement	• If caused by autolytic or enzymatic debridement, no intervention is necessary; an increase or change of color in drainage is expected because of the breakdown of dead tissue. • If debridement isn't the cause, assess the wound for infection.
Tunneling	• Pressure over bony prominences • Presence of foreign body • Deep infection	• Protect the area from pressure. • Irrigate and inspect tunneling as carefully as possible for a hidden suture or leftover bit of dressing material. • If tunneling doesn't shorten in length each week, thoroughly clean and obtain a tissue biopsy for infection and, with a chronic wound, for possible malignancy.

(continued)

Recognizing wound failure to heal *(continued)*

Sign	Causes	Interventions
Wound edges		
Red, hot skin; tenderness; and induration	• Inflammation due to excess pressure or infection	• Protect the area from pressure. • If pressure relief doesn't resolve the inflammation within 24 hours, topical antimicrobial therapy may be indicated.
Maceration (white skin)	• Excess moisture	• Protect the skin with petroleum jelly or barrier wipe. • If practical, obtain an order for a more absorptive dressing.
Rolled skin edges	• Too-dry wound bed	• Obtain an order for moisture-retentive dressings. • If rolling isn't resolved in 1 week, debridement of the edges may be necessary.
Undermining or ecchymosis of surrounding skin (loose or bruised skin edges)	• Excess shearing force to the area	• Initiate measures to protect the area, especially during patient transfers.

Complications of wound healing

Hemorrhage

Internal hemorrhage can result in the formation of a hematoma, which typically occurs around bruises.

External hemorrhage (visible bleeding from the wound) results from the rupture of newly developed blood vessels. Each time new blood vessels suffer damage, the body must repair the vessels, delaying healing. The fragility of new blood vessels is one reason to protect the wound with a dressing.

Infection

Infection requires prompt attention because, if left untreated, cellulitis or a bacterial infection could develop and spread to surrounding tissue. Signs and symptoms of infection include:
• redness and warmth at the wound margins and surrounding tissue
• fever
• edema
• pain at the wound site or a sudden increase in existing pain
• pus
• an increase in exudate or a change in its color
• odor
• discolored granulation tissue

• further wound breakdown or a lack of progress toward healing.

Fistula formation

A fistula is an abnormal passage between two organs or between an organ and the skin. In a wound, it may appear as undermining or a sinus tract (also known as *tunneling*). If a sinus tract is present, its extent and direction must be determined.

Dehiscence and evisceration

Dehiscence is a separation of skin and tissue layers. It usually occurs 3 to 11 days after the injury and may follow surgery. Dehiscence is most likely to occur when collagen fibers aren't mature enough to hold the incision closed without sutures. Similar to dehiscence, evisceration involves the protrusion of underlying visceral organs.

Dehiscence and evisceration may require emergency surgery, especially if they involve an abdominal wound. If a wound opens without evisceration, it may need to heal by secondary intention. Poor nutrition and advanced age increase a patient's risk of dehiscence and evisceration.

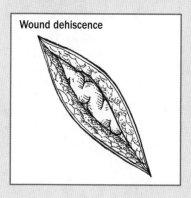

Wound dehiscence

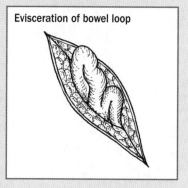

Evisceration of bowel loop

Tailoring wound care to wound color

Wound color	Management technique
Red	• Cover the wound, keep it moist and clean, and protect it from trauma. • Use a transparent dressing, such as Tegaderm or OpSite, over a gauze dressing moistened with normal saline solution, or use a hydrogel, foam, or hydrocolloid dressing to insulate and protect the wound.
Yellow	• Clean the wound and remove the yellow layer. • Cover the wound with a moisture-retentive dressing, such as a hydrogel or foam dressing or a moist gauze dressing with or without a debriding enzyme. • Consider hydrotherapy with whirlpool or pulsatile lavage.
Black	• Debride the wound as ordered. Use an enzyme product (such as Accuzyme or Panafil), conservative sharp debridement, or hydrotherapy with whirlpool or pulsatile lavage. • For wounds with inadequate blood supply and uninfected heel ulcers, don't debride. Keep them clean and dry.

Caring for a traumatic wound

When treating a patient with a traumatic wound, always begin by assessing the ABCs: airway, breathing, and circulation. Move on to the wound itself only after ABCs are stable. Here are the basic steps to follow in caring for each type of traumatic wound.

Abrasion

• Flush the area of the abrasion with normal saline solution or wound cleaning solution.
• Use a sterile 4″ × 4″ gauze pad moistened with normal saline solution to remove dirt or gravel, and gently rub toward the entry point to work contaminants back out the way they entered.
• If the wound is extremely dirty, you may need to scrub it with a surgical brush. Be as gentle as possible because this is a painful process for the patient.
• Allow a small wound to dry and form a scab. Cover larger wounds with a nonadherent pad or petroleum gauze and a light dressing. Apply antibacterial ointment if ordered.

Laceration

• Moisten a sterile 4″ × 4″ gauze pad with normal saline solution or wound cleaning solution. Gently clean the wound, beginning at the center and working out to approximately 2″ (5 cm) beyond the edge of the wound. Whenever the pad becomes soiled, discard it and use a new one. Continue until the wound appears clean.
• If necessary, irrigate the wound using a 50 ml catheter-tip syringe and normal saline solution.
• Assist the practitioner in suturing the wound if necessary; apply sterile strips of porous tape if suturing isn't needed.

• Apply antibacterial ointment, as ordered, to prevent infection.
• Apply a dry sterile dressing over the wound to absorb drainage and help prevent bacterial contamination.

Bite

• Immediately irrigate the wound with copious amounts of normal saline solution. Don't immerse and soak the wound; this may allow bacteria to float back into the tissue.
• Clean the wound with sterile 4″ × 4″ gauze pads and an antiseptic solution such as povidone-iodine.
• Assist with debridement if ordered.
• Apply a loose dressing. If the bite is on an extremity, elevate it to reduce swelling.
• Ask the patient about the animal that bit him to determine whether there's a risk of rabies. Administer rabies and tetanus shots as needed.

Penetrating wound

• If the wound is minor, allow it to bleed for a few minutes before cleaning it. A larger puncture wound may require irrigation.
• Cover the wound with a dry dressing.
• If the wound contains an embedded foreign object, such as a shard of glass or metal, stabilize the object until the practitioner can remove it. When the object is removed and bleeding is under control, clean the wound as you would a laceration.

Management of pressure ulcers algorithm

1 Pressure ulcer identification

2 Initial assessment

3 Education and development of treatment plan

| **4** Nutritional assessment and support | **5** Management of tissue loads | **6** Ulcer care; managing bacterial colonization and infection |

7 Is ulcer healing?

YES

8 Monitor

NO

9 Reassessment of treatment plan and evaluation of adherence

Return to **3**

Key

Yes-no decision

Interventions

Education and counseling

Refer to previous node

Source: "Treatment of Pressure Ulcers." *Clinical Practice Guideline Number 15,* AHCPR Publication Number 95-0652: December 1994.

Treatment of venous ulcers algorithm

Establish etiology. Review patient history and wound management. Perform leg examination.

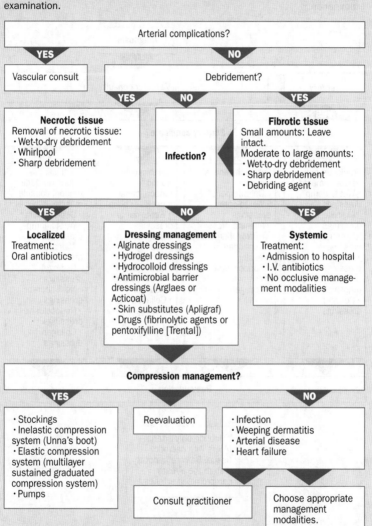

Adapted with permission from "Arterial vs. Venous Ulcers: Diagnosis and Treatment," *Advances in Skin and Wound Care* 14(3):147, May-June 2001.

Treatment of arterial ulcers algorithm

Establish etiology. Review patient history and wound management. Perform leg examination.

	Diagnosis	

Surgery	**Vascular consult**

YES

Surgery candidate?

NO — **NO** — **NO** — **NO**

Preulceration:	Partial-thickness wound:	Full-thickness wound (involving tendon, capsule, muscle, or bone):	Full-thickness wound (excluding tendon, capsule, muscle, or bone):
• Debridement* • Wet-to-damp dressings • Alginate dressings • Hydrogel dressings • Nonadherent dressings • Nonocclusive dressings • Collagen dressings	• Debridement* • Wet-to-damp dressings • Alginate dressings • Hydrogel dressings • Nonadherent dressings • Nonocclusive dressings • Collagen dressings	• Wet-to-damp dressings • Hydrogel dressings • Nonadherent dressings • Nonocclusive dressings • Collagen dressings	• Debridement* • Wet-to-damp dressings • Alginate dressings • Hydrogel dressings • Nonadherent dressings • Nonocclusive dressings • Collagen dressings

Reevaluation

*Debride only arterial ulcers with necrotic tissue. Be careful not to disturb the already compromised arteries.

Adapted with permission from "Arterial vs. Venous Ulcers: Diagnosis and Treatment," *Advances in Skin & Wound Care* 14(3):147, May-June 2001.

Treatment of diabetic ulcers algorithm

> Establish etiology.
> Review past medical treatments.
> Review medication history.
> Perform noninvasive vascular assessment.
> Evaluate the patient's footwear.

Ischemic: Ankle-brachial index < 0.8
Vascular consult (if indicated)

Neuropathic: Ankle-brachial index > 0.9
Assess degree of neuropathy.

Debridement

Ischemic
Remove eschar:
• Enzymatic debridement
• Nonaggressive dressing treatment

Nonischemic, neuropathic
• Debride hyperkeratotic rim
• Perform aggressive sharp debridement

Infection?

YES   **NO**   **YES**

Localized soft tissue
• Broad-spectrum oral antibiotics
• Reevaluation in 1 week
• Non-weight-bearing activity (if possible)
• Control of diabetes

Wound care

Localized bone; systemic
• Admission to hospital
• Appropriate cultures
• I.V. antibiotics
• Possibly, surgical intervention
• Antiseptic soaks

Adapted with permission from *Advances in Skin & Wound Care* 13(1):35, January-February 2000.

Wound dressings

Before selecting a dressing, consider its basic purpose: to provide an optimal environment for the body to heal itself. Some dressings absorb moisture from a wound bed, whereas others add moisture to it. Always remember the cardinal rule: Keep moist tissue moist and dry tissue dry.

Ideally, a dressing should conform to the wound and adhere to surrounding skin while still remaining easily removable.

Functions of a wound dressing
· To protect the wound from contamination and trauma
· To provide compression if bleeding or swelling is likely to occur
· To apply medications
· To absorb drainage or debrided necrotic tissue
· To fill or pack the wound
· To protect the skin surrounding the wound

Moisture scale
Use this chart to quickly determine the category of dressing that's appropriate for your patient.

Absorb moisture		Neutral (maintain existing moisture level)		Add moisture	
· Alginates · Specialty absorptives · Vacuum-assisted closure (VAC) device · Gauze	· Foams · Hydrocolloids · Compression dressings	· Composites · MiniVAC device	· Transparent films · Biological dressings · Collagen dressings · Contact layers · Warm-Up Therapy System	· Sheet hydrogels	· Amorphous hydrogel · Debriding agents

Alginate dressings

Alginate dressings are nonwoven, absorbent dressings made from seaweed. They're available as soft, white, sterile pads or ropes.

Safe to use on infected wounds, these dressings absorb excessive exudate. As they absorb exudate, the dressings turn into a gel that keeps the wound bed moist and promotes healing.

These nonadhesive, nonocclusive dressings also promote autolysis.

Indications for use
Use alginate dressings on:
• wounds with moderate to heavy drainage
• wounds with tunneling.

Advantages
• Hold up to 20 times their own weight in fluid
• May be cut to fit wound dimensions
• May be layered for more absorption
• Come in ropes for deep wound packing

Disadvantages
• May require the use of irrigation to remove the dressing from the wound
• Require secondary dressings
• Can't be used on dry eschar or wounds with light drainage
• May dehydrate the wound bed of a dryer wound

Antimicrobial dressings

Antimicrobial dressings protect against bacteria and provide a moist environment for wound healing—an improvement on topical antibiotic therapy. Active ingredients, such as silver, iodine, and polyhexethylene, provide the antimicrobial effects.

Antimicrobial dressings come in many forms, including transparent dressings, gauze, island dressings, foams, and absorptive fillers.

Indications for use
Use antimicrobial dressings as primary or secondary dressings on:
• infected wounds
• draining wounds
• nonhealing wounds.
You can also use them to manage minimal to heavy drainage.

Advantages
• Reduce and prevent infection
• Work against a broad spectrum of microorganisms

Disadvantages
• May produce a hypersensitivity reaction in patients sensitive to such product ingredients as silver or iodine
• May sting when applied

Biological dressings

Biological dressings are temporary dressings that function like skin grafts. They may be made from amnionic or chorionic membranes, woven from manmade fibers, or harvested from animals (usually pigs) or cadavers.

Eventually, the body rejects a biological dressing; if that occurs before the underlying wound heals, the dressing must be replaced with a skin graft.

Indications for use
Use biological dressings on:
• ulcers of varying thickness (depending on the product)
• skin grafting donor sites
• burns.

Advantages
• Shorten healing times
• Prevent infection and fluid loss
• Ease patient discomfort

Disadvantages
• May cause allergic reactions
• May require secondary dressings

Collagen dressings

Collagen dressings accelerate wound healing by encouraging the organization of new collagen fibers and granulation tissue. They're made with bovine or avian collagen.

Indications for use
Use collagen dressings on:
• chronic, nonhealing, granulated wound beds
• wounds with tunneling.

Advantages
• Come in gel, granule, and sheet forms (some also contain alginate)
• Work well on chronic, clean wounds
• Can be used on wounds with minimal to heavy drainage (depending on the product selected)

Disadvantages
• May cause an allergic reaction in patients sensitive to collagen, bovine, or avian products
• Require secondary dressings
• Aren't appropriate for third-degree burns or wounds with dry beds

Composite dressings

Composite dressings are hybrid dressings that combine two or more types of dressings into one. For example, a three-layer composite dressing can include a bacterial barrier; an absorbent foam, hydrocolloid, or hydrogel layer; an adherent or nonadherent layer; and an adhesive border.

Indications for use

Use composite dressings as primary or secondary dressings on wounds with minimal to heavy drainage.

They can also be used to protect peripheral and central I.V. lines.

Advantages

- Available in various combinations to suit each patient's wound care needs
- Come in multiple sizes and shapes

Disadvantages

- May not provide a moist wound environment (depending on the product selected) and may dry the wound bed
- Can't be cut to fit without losing some dressing integrity
- Can't be used on third-degree burns

Contact layer dressings

Contact layer dressings are single-layer dressings made of woven or perforated material that lie directly on the wound's surface. The nonadherent contact layer prevents other dressings from sticking to this surface.

Indications for use

Use contact layer dressings to let drainage flow to a secondary dressing while preventing that secondary dressing from adhering to the wound.

Advantages

- Decrease the pain experienced during dressing changes
- May be used with topical medications, fillers, or gauze dressings
- Can be cut to fit or overlap the wound's edges

Disadvantages

- Require a secondary dressing
- Contraindicated for use on third-degree burns, infected wounds, and wounds with tunneling

Foam dressings

Foam dressings are nonadherent, somewhat absorbent, spongelike polymer dressings that may include an adhesive border. They provide a moist healing environment and thermal insulation.

Indications for use

Use foam dressings as primary or secondary dressings on wounds with minimal to moderate drainage (including around tubes) when you need a nonadherent surface.

Advantages

· Nonadherent
· With an adhesive border, don't require a secondary dressing
· Can be used on infected wounds if changed daily
· May be used in combination with other products
· Can manage heavier drainage because they wick moisture from the wound and allow evaporation (hydropolymer foam dressings)

Disadvantages

· Without an adhesive border, may require a secondary dressing, tape, wrap, or net
· Not recommended for nondraining wounds
· May cause maceration if not changed regularly

Hydrocolloid dressings

Hydrocolloid dressings are adhesive, moldable wafers made of a carbohydrate-based material. Most have a waterproof backing. They're impermeable to oxygen, water, and water vapor, and most provide some degree of absorption. These dressings turn to gel as they absorb moisture, help maintain a moist wound bed, and promote autolytic debridement.

Indications for use

Use hydrocolloid dressings on wounds with minimal to moderate drainage, including wounds with necrosis or slough.

Hydrocolloid sheet dressings can also serve as secondary dressings.

Advantages

· Don't stick to a moist wound base
· Maintain moisture by becoming gelatinous as they absorb drainage
· May require changing only two to three times each week
· Can easily be removed from the wound base
· Come in contoured forms for use on specific sites
· Come in several varieties (sheets, powder, or gel) in thin and traditional thickness

Disadvantages

· Can't be used on burns or dry wounds
· Can cause skin stripping when removed
· Can cause maceration or hypergranulation

Hydrogel dressings

Hydrogel dressings are water- or glycerin-based polymer dressings that don't adhere to wounds. They provide limited absorption (some are 96% water themselves) and come as tubes of gel or in flexible sheets. Hydrogel dressings add moisture and promote autolytic debridement.

Indications for use
Use hydrogel dressings on:
- dry wounds
- wounds with minimal drainage
- wounds with necrosis or slough.

Advantages
- Come in sheet and amorphous gel form
- Can cool a wound, soothing and easing pain

Disadvantages
- Require a secondary dressing (gel form)
- Can macerate surrounding skin
- May necessitate daily dressing changes
- Vary in viscosity among brands and according to the product's base (water or glycerin)

Specialty absorptive dressings

Specialty absorptive dressings have multiple layers of a highly absorbent material, such as cotton or rayon, and may have adhesive borders. Types include gels, pads, gauze, and pillows.

Indications for use
Use specialty absorptive dressings on infected or noninfected wounds with heavy drainage.

Advantages
- Highly absorbent
- Typically require less frequent changes
- Come in several forms

Disadvantages
- Can't be used on burns or wounds with little or no drainage

Transparent film dressings

Clear, adherent, and nonabsorbent, transparent film dressings are semipermeable to oxygen and water vapor, but not to water itself. Transparency allows visual inspection of the wound with the dressing in place. These polyurethane dressings maintain a moist wound environment and promote autolysis.

Indications for use
Use transparent film dressings on:
• partial-thickness wounds with minimal exudate
• wounds with eschar (dry, leathery, black necrotic tissue) to promote autolysis.

Advantages
• May require less-frequent changes
• Allow you to see the wound
• Adherent but don't stick to the wound
• Not bulky

Disadvantages
• Don't absorb drainage, making them appropriate only for partial-thickness wounds with minimal exudate
• Can strip skin when the adhesive pulls at the skin around the wound during dressing removal

Wound fillers

Wound fillers are specialized dressings used to fill deeper wounds. They're made of various materials and come in many forms, including pastes, granules, powders, beads, and gels. Wound fillers can add moisture to the wound bed or absorb drainage, depending on the product.

Indications for use
Use wound fillers as primary dressings on infected or noninfected wounds with minimal to moderate drainage that require packing.

Advantages
• Come in several forms with different absorption capabilities

Disadvantages
• Can't be used on third-degree burns, dry wounds, or wounds with tunnels and sinus tracts
• Can alarm sensitive patients because of the wormlike appearance of some products

Debriding agents

When applied directly to necrotic or devitalized tissue, debriding agents, which are chemical or enzyme preparations, remove the dead tissue in the wound. If the wound contains eschar, the eschar is crosshatched before application so the debriding agent can penetrate the tissue.

Indications for use

Use debriding agents to debride wounds with moderate to large amounts of necrotic tissue, especially in cases where surgical debridement isn't an option.

Advantages

· May contain chlorophyll, which helps to control odor
· Debride effectively even when used in small amounts

Disadvantages

· May contain known allergens
· May require secondary dressings
· May cause irritation if they come in contact with surrounding skin
· May cause a burning sensation in the wound during application that can last for several hours
· May turn drainage green and be wrongly interpreted as infection if the product contains chlorophyll

Provant Wound Closure System

The Provant Wound Closure System is a noninvasive treatment that stimulates healing by directing a treatment signal $2\frac{3}{4}''$ to $3\frac{1}{4}''$ (7 to 8 cm) into the tissues around the wound. This signal induces the proliferation of fibroblasts and epithelial cells as well as the secretion of multiple growth factors, resulting in faster healing.

Treatment doesn't require removal of existing dressings. Clinical studies indicate that the Provant Wound Closure System effectively promotes healing, even in cases of chronic, severe pressure ulcers.

Indications for use

Use the Provant Wound Closure System on wounds in the inflammatory phase of healing.

Advantages

· Requires no special training
· Requires only two 30-minute treatments per day
· May be used over existing dressings

Disadvantages

· Can't be used for pregnant patients or those with cardiac pacemakers
· Won't help heal bone or deep internal organs

Vacuum-assisted closure device

Vacuum-assisted closure (VAC), also called *negative pressure wound therapy,* can be used when a wound fails to heal in a timely manner. VAC therapy encourages healing by applying localized subatmospheric pressure at the site of the wound. This reduces edema and bacterial colonization and stimulates the formation of granulation tissue.

The large-capacity VAC device is cumbersome to move. An alternative is the MiniVAC device, a smaller, portable version that runs on batteries and has a 50-ml drainage capacity.

Two VAC devices are the VAC Freedom (a portable, lightweight device with a 300-ml drainage capacity) and the VAC-ATS (a device with touch-screen operations and a 500-ml drainage capacity), which is ideal for use on patients in acute care settings with heavily draining wounds.

Indications

VAC therapy helps manage slow-healing acute, subacute, or chronic exudative wounds with cavities. It's ideal for pressure ulcers or surgical wounds with depths greater than ⅜" (1 cm).

Advantages

· Cleans deeply and can manage moderate to large amounts of drainage
· Can manage multiple wounds when dressings are cut to bridge two or more wounds
· Has rechargeable batteries and is small enough to fit in a pouch worn at the waist or over the shoulder (Mini-VAC and VAC Freedom)

Disadvantages

· Contraindicated for untreated osteomyelitis, malignancies, and wounds with necrotic tissue or fistulas
· The 5' to 6' (1.5 to 2 m) vacuum tube requires the patient to remain in one place or carry the unit along
· Either requires electricity (the VAC and VAC-ATS) or has batteries that must be recharged (the MiniVAC and VAC Freedom)
· Can result in bruising at the wound base if used incorrectly (for example, if the pressure is improperly set)

Warm-Up Therapy System

The Warm-Up Therapy System, also called *noncontact normothermic wound therapy*, is a temporary therapy that increases the temperature of the wound bed, thereby promoting increased blood flow in the area of the wound.

The dressing in this system contains a special electronic warming card. When in place, the card heats to 100.4° F (38° C), bathing the wound in radiant heat. The closely sealed wound covering promotes a moist environment in the wound bed. This system is designed to remain in place for 72 hours.

Indications for use

As ordered, use the Warm-Up Therapy System for acute or chronic, full- or partial-thickness wounds, regardless of etiology, that have failed to heal with traditional therapies, including wounds with compromised blood flow, such as arterial or diabetic foot ulcers.

Advantages
· May absorb a small to moderate amount of drainage in the wound covering

Disadvantages
· Contraindicated for third-degree burns
· Requires specific dressings and thorough patient teaching related to dressing changes and heat management

Evaluating nutritional disorders

This chart shows implications for nutritional assessment findings.

Body system or region	Sign or symptom
General	• Weakness and fatigue • Weight loss
Skin, hair, and nails	• Dry, flaky skin • Rough, scaly skin with bumps • Petechiae or ecchymoses • Sore that won't heal • Thinning, dry hair • Spoon-shaped, brittle, or ridged nails
Eyes	• Night blindness; corneal swelling, softening, or dryness; Bitot's spots • Red conjunctiva
Throat and mouth	• Cracks at corner of mouth • Magenta tongue • Beefy, red tongue • Soft, spongy, bleeding gums • Swollen neck (goiter)
Cardiovascular	• Edema • Tachycardia, hypotension
GI	• Ascites
Musculoskeletal	• Bone pain and bowleg • Muscle wasting
Neurologic	• Altered mental status • Paresthesia

Implications

• Anemia, electrolyte imbalance
• Decreased calorie intake, increased calorie use, or inadequate nutrient intake or absorption

---

• Vitamin A, vitamin B complex, or linoleic acid deficiency
• Vitamin A deficiency
• Vitamin C or K deficiency
• Protein, vitamin C, or zinc deficiency
• Protein deficiency
• Iron deficiency

• Vitamin A deficiency

• Riboflavin deficiency

• Riboflavin or niacin deficiency
• Riboflavin deficiency
• Vitamin B_{12} deficiency
• Vitamin C deficiency
• Iodine deficiency

• Protein deficiency
• Fluid volume deficit

• Protein deficiency

• Vitamin D or calcium deficiency
• Protein, carbohydrate, and fat deficiency

• Dehydration and thiamine or vitamin B_{12} deficiency
• Vitamin B_{12}, pyridoxine, or thiamine deficiency

How to take anthropometric arm measurements

Follow this procedure when measuring midarm circumference, triceps skin-fold thickness, and midarm muscle circumference.

1. Locate the midpoint on the patient's upper arm using a nonstretching tape measure, and mark it with a felt-tip pen.

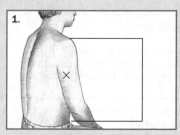

2. Determine the triceps skin-fold thickness by grasping the patient's skin between your thumb and forefinger approximately ⅜" (1 cm) above the midpoint. Place the calipers at the midpoint and squeeze the calipers for about 3 seconds. Record the measurement registered on the handle gauge to the nearest 0.5 mm. Take two more readings, and then average all three to compensate for possible error.

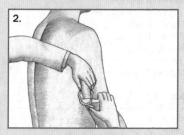

3. From the midpoint, measure the midarm circumference. Calculate midarm muscle circumference by multiplying the triceps skin-fold thickness (in centimeters) by 3.143 and subtracting the result from the midarm circumference.

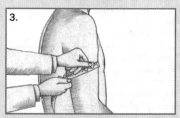

4. Record all three measurements as percentages of the standard measurements by using the following formula:

$$\frac{\text{actual measurement} \times 100}{\text{standard measurement}}$$

Compare the patient's percentage measurement with the standard. A measurement of less than 90% of the standard indicates calorie deprivation; a measurement of over 90% indicates adequate or more than adequate energy reserves.

Measurement	Standard	90%
Midarm circumference	Men: 29.3 cm Women: 28.5 cm	Men: 26.4 cm Women: 25.7 cm
Triceps skin-fold thickness	Men: 12.5 mm Women: 16.5 mm	Men: 11.3 mm Women: 14.9 mm
Midarm muscle circumference	Men: 25.3 cm Women: 23.2 cm	Men: 22.8 cm Women: 20.9 cm

Adapted from Blackburn GL, Bistrian BR, Maini BS, Schlamm HT, Smith MF. Nutritional and metabolic assessment of the hospital patient. *JPEN J Parenter Enteral Nutr.* 1977;1:11–22, with permission from the American Society for Parenteral and Enteral Nutrition (A.S.P.E.N.). A.S.P.E.N. does not endorse the use of this material in any form other than its entirety.

Tips for detecting nutritional problems

Nutritional problems may stem from physical conditions, drugs, diet, or lifestyle factors. This list can help you identify risk factors that make your patient particularly susceptible to nutritional problems.

Physical conditions
· Chronic illnesses, such as diabetes and neurologic, cardiac, or thyroid problems
· Family history of diabetes or heart disease
· Draining wounds or fistulas
· Weight issues—weight loss of 5% of normal body weight; weight less than 90% of ideal body weight; weight gain or loss of 10 lb (4.5 kg) or more in past 6 months; obesity; or weight gain of 20% above normal body weight
· History of GI disturbances
· Anorexia or bulimia
· Depression or anxiety
· Severe trauma
· Recent chemotherapy or radiation therapy
· Physical limitations, such as paresis or paralysis
· Recent major surgery
· Pregnancy, especially teen or multiple-birth pregnancy

Drugs and diet
· Fad diets
· Steroid, diuretic, or antacid use
· Mouth, tooth, or denture problems
· Excessive alcohol intake
· Strict vegetarian diet
· Liquid diet or nothing by mouth for more than 3 days

Lifestyle factors
· Lack of support from family or friends
· Financial problems

Mineral requirements, deficiencies, and toxicities

This table lists the daily requirements of common minerals as well as the signs and symptoms of deficiency and toxicity for each.

Minerals and adult requirements	Signs and symptoms of deficiencies	Signs and symptoms of toxicities
Major minerals		
Calcium 1,000 mg (ages 19 to 50) 1,200 mg (> age 50)	• Arm and leg numbness, brittle fingernails, heart palpitations, insomnia, muscle cramps, osteoporosis	• Renal calculi, impaired iron absorption
Chloride 750 mg	• Disturbance in acid-base balance	• None
Magnesium Men: 400 mg (ages 19 to 30) 420 mg (> age 30) Women: 310 mg (ages 19 to 30) 320 mg (> age 30)	• Confusion, disorientation, nervousness, irritability, rapid pulse, tremors, muscle control loss, neuromuscular dysfunction	• Cardiac rhythm disturbances, hypotension, respiratory failure
Phosphorus 700 mg	• Appetite loss, fatigue, irregular breathing, nervous disorders, muscle weakness	• None
Potassium 2,000 mg	• Muscular weakness, paralysis, anorexia, confusion, slow irregular heartbeat, weak reflexes	• Cardiac disturbances, paralysis
Sodium 500 mg	• Appetite loss, intestinal gas, muscular atrophy, vomiting, weight loss	• Edema and elevated blood pressure
Sulfur No recommended intake	• None	• None
Trace minerals		
Chromium 50 to 200 mcg	• Glucose intolerance (in diabetes patients)	• None
Cobalt Unknown	• Indigestion, diarrhea or constipation, weight loss, fatigue, poor memory	• None
Copper 1.5 to 3 mg	• General weakness, impaired respiration, skin sores, bone disease	• Vomiting, diarrhea

Mineral requirements, deficiencies, and toxicities *(continued)*

Minerals and adult requirements	Signs and symptoms of deficiencies	Signs and symptoms of toxicities
Fluoride Men: 3.8 mg Women: 3.1 mg	• Dental caries	• Mottling and pitting of permanent teeth, increased bone density and calcification
Iodine 150 mcg	• Cold hands and feet, dry hair, irritability, nervousness, obesity, simple goiter	• Enlarged thyroid gland
Iron Men: 10 mg Women: 15 mg (ages 19 to 50) 10 mg (> age 50)	• Brittle nails, constipation, respiratory problems, tongue soreness or inflammation, anemia, pallor, weakness, cold sensitivity, fatigue	• Abdominal cramps and pains, nausea, vomiting, hemosiderosis, hemochromatosis
Manganese 2 to 5 mg	• Ataxia, dizziness, hearing disturbance or loss	• Severe neuromuscular disturbances
Molybdenum 45 mcg	• None	• Headache, dizziness, heartburn, weakness, nausea, vomiting, diarrhea
Selenium 55 mcg	• None	• Nausea, vomiting, abdominal pain, hair and nail changes, nerve damage, fatigue
Zinc Men: 11 mg Women: 8 mg	• Delayed sexual maturity, fatigue, smell and taste loss, poor appetite, prolonged wound healing, slowed growth, skin disorders	• Anemia, impaired calcium absorption, fever, muscle pain, dizziness, reproductive failure

Vitamin requirements, deficiencies, and toxicities

This table lists the daily requirements of common vitamins as well as the signs and symptoms of deficiency and toxicity for each.

Vitamins and adult requirements	Signs and symptoms of deficiencies	Signs and symptoms of toxicities
Water-soluble vitamins		
Vitamin B₁ (thiamine) *Men:* 1.2 mg *Women:* 1.1 mg	• Beriberi (fatigue, muscle weakness, confusion, edema, enlarged heart, heart failure)	• None
Vitamin B₂ (riboflavin) *Men:* 1.3 mg *Women:* 1.1 mg	• Ariboflavinosis (dermatitis, glossitis, photophobia)	• None
Vitamin B₃ (niacin) *Men:* 16 mg *Women:* 14 mg	• Pellagra (dermatitis, diarrhea, dementia, death)	• Flushing, gastric ulcers, low blood pressure, nausea, vomiting, diarrhea, liver damage
Vitamin B₆ (pyridoxine) *Men:* 1.3 mg (< age 50) 1.7 mg (> age 50) *Women:* 1.3 mg (< age 50) 1.5 mg (> age 50)	• Dermatitis, glossitis, seizures, anemia	• Depression, irritability, headaches, fatigue
Vitamin B₁₂ (cobalamin) 2.4 mcg	• Indigestion, diarrhea or constipation, weight loss, macrocytic anemia, fatigue, poor memory, irritability, paresthesia of hands and feet	• None
Vitamin C (ascorbic acid) *Men:* 90 mg *Women:* 75 mg	• Scurvy (bleeding gums, delayed wound healing, hemorrhaging, softening of the bones, easy fractures)	• Diarrhea, nausea, headaches, fatigue, hot flushes, insomnia
Biotin 30 mcg	• Anorexia, fatigue, depression, dry skin, heart abnormalities	• None
Folate (folic acid) 400 mcg	• Diarrhea, macrocytic anemia, confusion, depression, fatigue	• Masks vitamin B₁₂ deficiency
Pantothenic acid 5 mg	• General failure of all body systems	• None

Vitamin requirements, deficiencies, and toxicities *(continued)*

Vitamins and adult requirements	Signs and symptoms of deficiencies	Signs and symptoms of toxicities
Fat-soluble vitamins		
Vitamin A (retinol) *Men:* 1,000 mcg retinol equivalents *Women:* 800 mcg retinol equivalents	• Night blindness, bone growth cessation, dry skin, decreased saliva, diarrhea	• Headaches, vomiting, double vision, hair loss, liver damage
Vitamin D (calciferol) 5 mcg (≤ age 50) 10 mcg (ages 51 to 70) 15 mcg (≥ age 70)	• Rickets (retarded bone growth, bone malformations, decreased serum calcium, abdominal protrusion); osteomalacia (softening of bones, decreased serum calcium, muscle twitching)	• Renal calculi, kidney damage, muscle and bone weakness, excessive bleeding, headaches, excessive thirst
Vitamin E (tocopherol) 15 mg	• Red blood cell hemolysis, edema, skin lesions	• None
Vitamin K (menadione) *Men:* 80 mcg *Women:* 65 mcg	• Hemorrhaging	• None

Fat: Good, bad, and worst

Fats (fatty acids) come in many varieties—some good, some bad, and some really bad. To help your patient plan a heart-healthy diet, make sure that you understand the various types of fat.

Good

Monounsaturated fats

Monounsaturated fats are found mainly in canola oil, olive oil, peanut oil, and avocados. These fats are liquid at room temperature.

Polyunsaturated fats

Polyunsaturated fats are found in soybean, sesame, sunflower, and safflower seeds and their oils. They're also the main fats found in seafood. These fats are liquid or soft at room temperature. Specific polyunsaturated fatty acids, such as linoleic acid and alpha-linoleic acid, are called essential fatty acids because they're necessary for cell structure and making hormones. Essential fatty acids must be obtained from foods.

Bad

Saturated fats

Saturated fats are found chiefly in animal sources, such as meat, poultry, whole or reduced-fat milk, and butter. Some vegetable oils, such as coconut, palm kernel oil, and palm oil, are saturated. Saturated fats are usually solid at room temperature.

Dietary cholesterol

Dietary cholesterol is found in foods of animal origin, such as meat, pork, poultry, fish, eggs, and full-fat dairy products.

Worst

Trans fatty acids

Trans fatty acids (trans-fats, for short) form when vegetable oils are processed into margarine or shortening. Sources of trans-fats in the diet include snack foods and baked goods made with partially hydrogenated vegetable oil or vegetable shortening. Trans fatty acids also occur naturally in some animal products such as dairy products.

Potassium-rich foods

These foods are high in potassium content. They should be ingested by patients who have experienced potassium loss, such as that which occurs from taking diuretics. Other patients, such as ones with renal failure, should avoid potassium-rich foods.

Fruits
- Avocados
- Bananas
- Cantaloupe
- Dried fruit
- Fresh peaches
- Grapefruit juice
- Honeydew melon
- Orange juice
- Oranges

Beans
- Baked beans
- Black beans
- Black-eyed peas
- Butter beans
- Chickpeas
- Crowder peas
- Great Northern beans
- Kidney beans
- Lentils
- Lima beans
- Navy beans
- Pinto beans
- Split peas

Vegetables
- Broccoli
- Greens
- Spinach
- Tomatoes
- Tomato juice
- Tomato soup

Potatoes
- Baked sweet potato
- Baked white potato
- French fries
- Home fries

- Instant potato mixes
- Potato chips
- Yams

Miscellaneous foods
- Molasses
- Nuts
- Salt substitutes

Tips to reduce sodium intake

Only a small amount of sodium occurs naturally in foods; most sodium is added to them during processing. To help your patient cut down on sodium intake, provide these suggestions.

Read labels
- Read food labels for sodium content.
- Use food products with reduced sodium or no added salt.
- Be aware that soy sauce, broth, and foods that are pickled or cured have high sodium contents.

Cook wisely
- Instead of cooking with salt, use herbs, spices, cooking wines, lemon, lime, or vinegar to enhance food flavors.
- Cook pasta and rice without salt.
- Rinse canned foods, such as tuna, to remove some sodium.
- Avoid adding salt to foods, especially at the table.
- Avoid condiments, such as soy and teriyaki sauces, and monosodium glu-

tamate (MSG), or use lower-sodium versions.

Watch your diet
- Eat fresh poultry, fish, and lean meat rather than canned, smoked, or processed versions (which typically contain a lot of sodium).
- Whenever possible, eat fresh foods rather than canned or convenience foods.
- Limit intake of cured foods (bacon and ham), foods packed in brine (pickles, olives, and sauerkraut) and condiments (mustard, ketchup, horseradish, and Worcestershire sauce).
- When dining out, ask how food is prepared. Ask that your food be prepared without added salt or MSG.

Transcultural communication

Communication styles vary among cultures. Qualities viewed as desirable in one culture (such as maintaining eye contact, having a certain degree of openness, offering insight, and portraying emotional expression) may not be considered appropriate in another culture. For example:

• Direct eye contact is considered inappropriate and disrespectful in some Asian American, African American, Native American, and Appalachian cultures.

• Some Middle Eastern cultures focus solely on the present; they usually view the future as something to be accepted as it occurs, rather than planned.

• Some Asians strongly value harmonious interpersonal relationships. As a result, they may nod, smile, and provide answers they feel are expected to maintain harmony rather than expressing their true feelings and concerns.

Avoid making assumptions about a patient's behavior or communication style. An individual's cultural background may explain a communication style you would otherwise deem "inappropriate" or "abnormal."

Cultural considerations in patient care

As a health care professional, you'll interact with a diverse, multicultural patient population. Each culture has its own set of beliefs about health and illness, dietary practices, and other matters that you need to be familiar with when providing care.

Health and illness philosophy	Dietary practices	Other considerations
African Americans		
• May believe illness is related to supernatural causes, such as punishment from God or an evil spell • Believe health is a feeling of well-being • May seek advice and remedies from faith or folk healers	• May have food restrictions based on religious beliefs, such as not eating pork if Muslim • May view cooked greens as good for health	• Tend to be affectionate, as shown by touching and hugging friends and loved ones • If Muslim, must have head covered at all times • Respect elders, especially for their wisdom • Primary religions: Baptist, other Protestant denominations, Muslim
Arab Americans		
• Believe health is a gift from God and that one should care for oneself by eating right and minimizing stressors • May believe illness is caused by the evil eye, bad luck, stress, or an imbalance between hot and cold or moist and dry	• May not mix milk and fish, sweet and sour, or hot and cold • May not use ice in drinks; may believe hot soup can help recovery	• Respect elders and professionals • Traditional women may avoid eye contact with male strangers • Use same-sex family members as interpreters

Cultural considerations in patient care *(continued)*

Health and illness philosophy	Dietary practices	Other considerations
Arab Americans *(continued)*		
• May use amulets to ward off evil eye during illness • May assume passive role as patient • Believe in complete rest and ridding self of all responsibilities during illness • May have low pain threshold and express pain vocally	• If Muslim, prohibited from drinking alcohol and eating pork or ham	• Primary religions: Muslim, Christian (Greek Orthodox, Protestant)
Chinese Americans		
• Believe health is a balance of the principles of *yin* and *yang* and that illness stems from an imbalance of these elements; believe good health requires harmony among body, mind, and spirit • May use herbalists or acupuncturists before seeking medical help; ginseng root is a common home remedy • May use good luck objects, such as jade or rope tied around waist • Family expected to take care of patient, who assumes a passive role • Tend not to readily express pain; stoic by nature	• Rice, noodles, and vegetables are staples; tend to use chopsticks • Choose foods to help balance the *yin* (cold) and *yang* (hot) • Drink hot liquids, especially when sick	• Health care providers should keep a comfortable distance when approaching patient • Elders shouldn't be addressed by first name (a sign of disrespect) • Lack of eye contact may be a sign of respect • Tend to be very modest; best to use same-sex clinicians • Primary religions: Buddhist, Catholic, Protestant
Japanese Americans		
• Believe that health is a balance of oneself, society, and the universe • May believe illness is related to karma, resulting from behavior in present or past life • May believe certain food combinations cause illness • May use prayer beads if Buddhist • May use tea to treat GI ailments and constipation • May not complain of symptoms until severe	• Eat rice with most meals; may use chopsticks • Diet high in salt; low in sugar, fat, protein, and cholesterol	• Usually quiet and polite; may ask few questions about care, deferring to health care providers • Elderly may nod but not necessarily understand • Very modest; tend to avoid touching; best to use same-sex clinicians • Primary religions: Buddhist, Shinto, Christian

(continued)

Cultural considerations in patient care *(continued)*

Health and illness philosophy	Dietary practices	Other considerations

Hispanic Americans

Health and illness philosophy	Dietary practices	Other considerations
• Believe that health is influenced by environment, fate, and God's will • May believe in Galen's theory that the body's four humors—blood, phlegm, yellow bile, and black bile—must be kept in balance • May use herbal teas and soup to aid in recuperation • May self-medicate • May express pain by nonverbal cues • May have family that wants to keep seriousness of illness from patient	• Beans and tortillas are staples • Eat lots of fresh fruits and vegetables	• Modest, especially women • Use same-sex family members as interpreters • Primary religion: Roman Catholic

Native Americans

Health and illness philosophy	Dietary practices	Other considerations
• Use herbs and roots; each tribe has its own unique medicinal practices • Typically use modern medicine where available • Use ancient symbol of Medicine Wheel • May consider number 4 sacred (associated with four primary laws of creation: life, unity, equality, and eternity) • Use tobacco for important religious, ceremonial, and medicinal purposes; may sprinkle it around patient's bed to protect and heal him	• Have balanced diet of seafood, fruits, greens, corn, rice, and garden vegetables; low in salt • Specific dietary practices based on location: Urban dwellers commonly eat meat, while rural residents may consume only lamb and goat	• Clan and tribe considered extended family • Elders respected • May be uncomfortable sharing their belief systems • Use "talking circle" to share information and support and to solve problems

Childbearing practices of selected cultures

A patient's cultural beliefs can affect her attitudes toward illness and traditional medicine. By trying to accommodate these beliefs and practices in your care plan, you can increase the patient's willingness to learn and comply with treatment regimens. Because cultural beliefs may vary within particular groups, individual practices may differ from those described here.

African Americans
- View pregnancy as a state of well-being
- May delay prenatal care
- Believe that taking pictures during pregnancy may cause stillbirth
- Believe that reaching up during pregnancy may cause the umbilical cord to strangle the baby
- May use self-treatment for discomfort
- May cry out during labor or may be stoic
- May receive emotional support during birth from mother or another woman
- May view vaginal bleeding during postpartum period as sickness
- May prohibit tub baths and shampooing hair in the postpartum period
- May view breast-feeding as embarrassing and therefore bottle-feed
- Consider infant who eats well "good"
- May introduce solid food early
- May oil the baby's skin
- May place a bellyband on the neonate to prevent umbilical hernia

Arab Americans
- May not seek prenatal care
- Seek medical assistance when medical resources at home fail
- Fast during pregnancy to produce a son
- May labor in silence to be in control
- Limit male involvement during childbirth

Asian Americans
- View pregnancy as a natural process
- Believe mother has "happiness in her body"
- Omit milk from diet because it causes stomach distress
- Believe inactivity and sleeping late can result in difficult birth
- Believe childbirth causes a sudden loss of "yang forces," resulting in an imbalance in the body
- Believe hot foods, hot water, and warm air restore the yang forces
- Are attended to during labor by other women (usually patient's mother)—not the father of the baby
- Have stoic response to labor pain
- May prefer herbal medicine
- Restrict activity for 40 to 60 days postpartum
- Believe that colostrum is harmful (old, stale, dirty, poisonous, or contaminated) to baby so may delay breast-feeding until milk comes in

Hispanic Americans
- View pregnancy as normal, healthy state
- May delay prenatal care
- Prefer a *patera* or midwife
- Bring together mother's legs after childbirth to prevent air from entering uterus
- Are strongly influenced by the mother-in-law and mother during labor and birth and may listen to them rather than the husband
- View crying or shouting out during labor as unacceptable
- May wear a religious necklace that's placed around the neonate's neck after birth
- Believe in hot and cold theory of disease and health
- Restricted to boiled milk and toasted tortillas for first 2 days after birth
- Must remain on bed rest for 3 days after birth
- Delay bathing for 14 days after childbirth
- Delay breast-feeding because colostrum is considered dirty and spoiled
- Don't circumcise male infants
- May place a bellyband on the neonate to prevent umbilical hernia

(continued)

Childbearing practices of selected cultures *(continued)*

Native Americans
• View pregnancy as a normal, natural process
• May start prenatal care late
• Prefer a female birth attendant or midwife
• May be assisted in birth by mother, father, or husband
• View birth as a family affair and may want entire family present
• May use herbs to promote uterine contractions, stop bleeding, or increase flow of breast milk
• Use cradle boards to carry baby and don't handle baby much
• May delay breast-feeding because colostrum is considered harmful and dirty
• May plan on taking the placenta home for burial

How certain cultures handle labor pain

Cultural and familial influences play a role in how a woman expresses or re-presses pain. These influences also determine whether she uses pharmacologic methods of pain relief. If her family views childbirth as a natural process or function for the female in the family unit, the woman is less likely to outwardly react to labor pains or require pharmacologic methods of pain relief.

Culture	Actions during pain
Middle-Eastern women	• Verbally expressive during labor • Commonly cry out and scream loudly • May refuse pain medication
Samoan women	• Believe they shouldn't express pain verbally • Believe the pain must simply be endured • May refuse pain medication
Filipino women	• Lie quietly during labor
Vietnamese, Laotian, and other women of Southeast Asian descent	• Believe that crying out during labor is shameful • Believe that pain during labor must be endured
Hispanic women	• Are taught by their *pateras* (midwives) to endure pain and to keep their mouths closed during labor • Believe that to cry out would cause the uterus to rise and retard labor

Beliefs and practices of selected religions

A patient's religious beliefs can affect his attitudes toward illness and traditional medicine. By trying to accommodate the patient's religious beliefs and practices in your care plan, you can increase his willingness to learn and comply with treatment regimens. Because religious beliefs may vary within particular sects, individual practices may differ from those described here.

Religion	Birth and death rituals
Adventist	None (baptism of adults only)
Baptist	At birth, none (baptism of believers only); before death, counseling by clergy member and prayer
Christian Science	At birth, none; before death, counseling by a Christian Science practitioner
Church of Christ	None (baptism at age 8 or older)
Eastern Orthodox	At birth, baptism and confirmation; before death, last rites (For members of the Russian Orthodox Church, arms are crossed after death, fingers set in cross, and unembalmed body clothed in natural fiber.)
Episcopal	At birth, baptism; before death, occasional last rites
Jehovah's Witnesses	None

Dietary restrictions	Practices in health crisis
Alcohol, coffee, tea, opioids, stimulants; in many groups, meat prohibited also	Communion and baptism performed. Some members believe in divine healing, anointing with oil, and prayer. Some regard Saturday as the Sabbath.
Alcohol; in some groups, coffee and tea prohibited also	Some believe in healing by laying on of hands. Resistance to medical therapy occasionally approved.
Alcohol, coffee, and tobacco prohibited	Many members refuse all treatment, including drugs, biopsies, physical examination, and blood transfusions and permit vaccination only when required by law. Alteration of thoughts is believed to cure illness. Hypnotism and psychotherapy are prohibited. (Christian Scientist nurses and nursing homes honor these beliefs.)
Alcohol discouraged	Communion, anointing with oil, laying on of hands, and counseling are performed by a minister.
For members of the Russian Orthodox Church and usually the Greek Orthodox Church, no meat or dairy products on Wednesday, Friday, and during Lent	Anointing of the sick. For members of the Russian Orthodox Church, cross necklace is replaced immediately after surgery and shaving of male patients is prohibited except in preparation for surgery. For members of the Greek Orthodox Church, communion and Sacrament of Holy Unction are performed.
For some members, abstention from meat on Friday, fasting before communion (which may be daily)	Communion, prayer, and counseling are performed by a minister.
Abstention from foods to which blood has been added	Typically, no blood transfusions are permitted; a court order may be required for emergency transfusion.

(continued)

Beliefs and practices of selected religions *(continued)*

Religion	Birth and death rituals
Judaism	Ritual circumcision on 8th day after birth; burial of dead fetus; ritual washing of dead; burial (including organs and other body tissues) occurs as soon as possible; no autopsy or embalming
Lutheran	Baptism usually performed 6 to 8 weeks after birth
Jesus Christ of Latter Day Saints (Mormon)	At birth, none (baptism at age 8 or older); before death, baptism and gospel preaching
Islam	If spontaneous abortion occurs before 130 days, fetus treated as discarded tissue; after 130 days, as a human being; before death, confession of sins with family present; after death, only relatives or friends may touch the body
Orthodox Presbyterian	Infant baptism; scripture reading and prayer before death
Pentecostal Assembly of God, Foursquare Church	None (baptism only after age of accountability)
Roman Catholicism	Infant baptism, including baptism of aborted fetus without sign of clinical death (tissue necrosis); before death, anointing of the sick
United Methodist	Baptism of children and adults

Dietary restrictions	Practices in health crisis
For Orthodox and Conservative Jews, kosher dietary laws (for example, pork and shellfish prohibited); for Reform Jews, usually no restrictions	Donation or transplantation of organs requires rabbinical consultation. For Orthodox and Conservative Jews, medical procedures may be prohibited on the Sabbath—from sundown Friday to sundown Saturday—and specific holidays.
None	Communion, prayer, and counseling are performed by a minister.
Alcohol, tobacco, tea, and coffee prohibited; meat intake limited	Believe in divine healing through the laying on of hands; communion on Sunday; some members may refuse medical treatment. Many wear a special undergarment.
Pork prohibited; daylight fasting during 9th month of Islamic calendar	Faith healing is for the patient's morale only; conservative members reject medical therapy.
None	Communion, prayer, and counseling are performed by a minister.
Abstention from alcohol, tobacco, meat slaughtered by strangling, any food to which blood has been added, and sometimes pork	Divine healing through prayer, anointing with oil, and laying on of hands are performed.
Fasting or abstention from meat on Ash Wednesday and on Fridays during Lent; this practice usually waived for the hospitalized and elderly	Burial of major amputated limb (sometimes) in consecrated ground; donation or transplantation of organs is allowed if the benefit to the recipient outweighs the donor's potential harm. Sacrament of the Sick is also performed when patients are ill, not just before death and sometimes performed shortly after admission.
None	Communion is performed before surgery or similar crisis; donation of body parts is encouraged

7 Maternal-neonatal care

Taking an obstetric history

When taking the pregnant patient's obstetric history, ask her about:
- genital tract anomalies
- medications used during this pregnancy
- history of hepatitis, pelvic inflammatory disease, acquired immunodeficiency syndrome, blood transfusions, and herpes or other sexually transmitted diseases (STDs)
- partner's history of STDs
- previous abortions
- history of infertility.

Pregnancy particulars

Ask the patient about past pregnancies. Note the number of past full-term and preterm pregnancies and obtain the following information about each of the patient's past pregnancies, if applicable:
- Was the pregnancy planned?
- Did any complications—such as spotting, swelling of the hands and feet, surgery, or falls—occur?
- Did the patient receive prenatal care? If so, when did she start?
- Did she take any medications? If so, what were they? How long did she take them? Why?
- What was the duration of the pregnancy?
- How was the pregnancy overall for the patient?

Birth and baby specifics

Obtain information about the birth and postpartum condition in all previous pregnancies:
- What was the duration of labor?
- What type of birth was it?
- What type of anesthesia did the patient have, if any?
- Did the patient experience complications during pregnancy or labor?
- What were the birthplace, condition, sex, weight, and Rh factor of the neonate?
- Was the labor as she had expected it? Better? Worse?
- Did she have stitches after birth?
- What was the condition of the neonate after birth?
- What was the neonate's Apgar score?
- Was special care needed for the neonate? If so, what?
- Did the neonate experience problems during the first several days after birth?
- What's the child's present state of health?
- Was the neonate discharged from the health care facility with the mother?
- Did the patient experience postpartum problems?

Summarizing pregnancy information

Typically, an abbreviation system is used to summarize a woman's pregnancy information. Although many variations exist, a common abbreviation system consists of five digits—GTPAL.

Gravida = the number of pregnancies, including the present one.
Term = the total number of infants born at term or 37 or more weeks.
Preterm = the total number of infants born before 37 weeks.
Abortions = the total number of spontaneous or induced abortions.
Living = the total number of children currently living.

For example, if a woman pregnant once with twins delivers at 35 weeks' gestation and the neonates survive, the abbreviation that represents this information is "10202." During her next pregnancy, the abbreviation would be "20202."

An abbreviated but less informative version reflects only the gravida and para (the number of pregnancies that reached the age of viability—generally accepted to be 24 weeks, regardless of whether the babies were born alive or not).

In some cases, the number of abortions also may be included. For example, "G3, P2, Ab1" represents a woman who has been pregnant three times, who has had two deliveries after 24 weeks' gestation, and who has had one abortion. "G2, P1" represents a woman who has been pregnant two times and has delivered once after 24 weeks' gestation.

Formidable findings

When performing the health history and assessment, look for these findings to determine if a pregnant patient is at risk for complications.

Demographic factors
· Maternal age younger than 16 years or older than 35 years
· Fewer than 11 years of education

Lifestyle
· Smoking (more than 10 cigarettes per day)
· Substance abuse
· Long commute to work
· Refusal to use seatbelts
· Alcohol consumption
· Heavy lifting or long periods of standing
· Lack of smoke detectors in home
· Unusual stress

Obstetric history
· Infertility
· Grand multiparity
· Incompetent cervix
· Uterine or cervical anomaly
· Previous preterm labor or birth
· Previous cesarean birth
· Previous infant with macrosomia
· Two or more spontaneous or elective abortions
· Previous hydatidiform mole or choriocarcinoma
· Previous ectopic pregnancy
· Previous stillborn neonate or neonatal death
· Previous multiple gestation
· Previous prolonged labor
· Previous low-birth-weight infant
· Previous midforceps delivery
· Diethylstilbestrol exposure in utero
· Previous infant with neurologic deficit, birth injury, or congenital anomaly
· Less than 1 year since last pregnancy

Medical history
· Cardiac disease
· Metabolic disease
· Renal disease
· Recent urinary tract infection or bacteriuria
· GI disorders *(continued)*

Formidable findings *(continued)*

- Seizure disorders
- Family history of severe inherited disorders
- Surgery during pregnancy
- Emotional disorders or mental retardation
- Previous surgeries, particularly involving reproductive organs
- Pulmonary disease
- Endocrine disorders
- Hemoglobinopathies
- Sexually transmitted disease (STD)
- Chronic hypertension
- History of abnormal Papanicolaou smear
- Malignancy
- Reproductive tract anomalies

Current obstetric status

- Inadequate prenatal care
- Intrauterine growth–restricted fetus
- Large-for-gestational-age fetus
- Gestational hypertension
- Abnormal fetal surveillance tests
- Polyhydramnios
- Placenta previa
- Abnormal presentation
- Maternal anemia
- Weight gain of less than 10 lb (4.5 kg)
- Weight loss of more than 5 lb (2.3 kg)

- Overweight or underweight status
- Fetal or placental malformation
- Rh sensitization
- Preterm labor
- Multiple gestation
- Premature rupture of membranes
- Abruptio placentae
- Postdate pregnancy
- Fibroid tumors
- Fetal manipulation
- Cervical cerclage
- Maternal infection
- Poor immunization status
- STD

Psychosocial factors

- Inadequate finances
- Social problems
- Adolescent
- Poor nutrition, poor housing
- More than two children at home with no additional support
- Lack of acceptance of pregnancy
- Attempt at or ideation of suicide
- No involvement of baby's father
- Minority status
- Parental occupation
- Inadequate support systems
- Dysfunctional grieving
- Psychiatric history

Making sense out of pregnancy signs

This chart organizes signs of pregnancy into three categories: presumptive, probable, and positive.

Sign	Time from implantation (in weeks)	Other possible causes
Presumptive		
Breast changes, including feelings of tenderness, fullness, or tingling; and enlargement or darkening of areola	2	• Hyperprolactinemia induced by tranquilizers • Infection • Prolactin-secreting pituitary tumor • Pseudocyesis • Premenstrual syndrome
Nausea or vomiting upon arising	2	• Gastric disorders • Infections • Psychological disorders, such as pseudocyesis and anorexia nervosa
Amenorrhea	2	• Anovulation • Blocked endometrial cavity • Endocrine changes • Medications (phenothiazines) • Metabolic changes
Frequent urination	3	• Emotional stress • Pelvic tumor • Renal disease • Urinary tract infection
Fatigue	12	• Anemia • Chronic illness
Uterine enlargement in which the uterus can be palpated over the symphysis pubis	12	• Ascites • Obesity • Uterine or pelvic tumor
Quickening (fetal movement felt by the woman)	18	• Excessive flatus • Increased peristalsis
Linea nigra (line of dark pigment on the abdomen)	24	• Cardiopulmonary disorders • Estrogen-progestin hormonal contraceptives • Obesity • Pelvic tumor

(continued)

Making sense out of pregnancy signs *(continued)*

Sign	Time from implantation (in weeks)	Other possible causes
Presumptive *(continued)*		
Melasma (dark pigment on the face)	24	• Cardiopulmonary disorders • Estrogen-progestin hormonal contraceptives • Obesity • Pelvic tumor
Striae gravidarum (red streaks on the abdomen)	24	• Cardiopulmonary disorders • Estrogen-progestin hormonal contraceptives • Obesity • Pelvic tumor
Probable		
Serum laboratory tests revealing the presence of human chorionic gonadotropin (hCG) hormone	1	• Possible cross-reaction of luteinizing hormone (similar to hCG) in some pregnancy tests
Chadwick's sign (vagina changes color from pink to violet)	6	• Hyperemia of cervix, vagina, or vulva
Goodell's sign (cervix softens)	6	• Estrogen-progestin hormonal contraceptives
Hegar's sign (lower uterine segment softens)	6	• Excessively soft uterine walls
Sonographic evidence of gestational sac in which characteristic ring is evident	6	• None
Ballottement (fetus can be felt to rise against abdominal wall when lower uterine segment is tapped during bimanual examination)	16	• Ascites • Uterine tumor or polyps
Braxton Hicks contractions (periodic uterine tightening)	20	• Hematometra • Uterine tumor
Palpation of fetal outline through abdomen	20	• Subserous uterine myoma

Making sense out of pregnancy signs *(continued)*

Sign	Time from implantation (in weeks)	Other possible causes
Positive		
Sonographic evidence of fetal outline	8	• None
Fetal heart audible by Doppler ultra-sound	10 to 12	• None
Palpation of fetal movement through abdomen	20	• None

Physiologic adaptations to pregnancy

Cardiovascular system
· Cardiac hypertrophy
· Displacement of the heart
· Increased blood volume and heart rate
· Supine hypotension
· Increased fibrinogen and hemoglobin levels
· Decreased hematocrit

GI system
· Gum swelling
· Lateral and posterior displacement of the intestines
· Superior and lateral displacement of the stomach
· Delayed intestinal motility and gastric and gallbladder emptying time
· Constipation
· Displacement of the appendix from McBurney point
· Increased tendency of gallstone formation

Endocrine system
· Increased basal metabolic rate (up 25% at term)
· Increased iodine metabolism
· Slight parathyroidism
· Increased plasma parathyroid hormone level
· Slightly enlarged pituitary gland
· Increased prolactin production

· Increased cortisol level
· Decreased maternal blood glucose level
· Decreased insulin production in early pregnancy
· Increased production of estrogen, progesterone, and human chorionic somatomammotropin

Respiratory system
· Increased vascularization of the respiratory tract
· Shortening of the lungs
· Upward displacement of the diaphragm
· Increased tidal volume, causing slight hyperventilation
· Increased chest circumference (by about $2\frac{3}{8}''$ [6 cm])
· Altered breathing, with abdominal breathing replacing thoracic breathing as pregnancy progresses
· Slight increase (two breaths per minute) in respiratory rate
· Increased pH, leading to mild respiratory alkalosis

Metabolic system
· Increased water retention
· Decreased serum protein level
· Increased intracapillary pressure and permeability

• Increased serum lipid, lipoprotein, and cholesterol levels
• Increased iron requirements and carbohydrate needs
• Increased protein retention
• Weight gain of 25 to 30 lb (11.5 to 13.5 kg)

Integumentary system
• Hyperactive sweat and sebaceous glands
• Hyperpigmentation
• Darkening of nipples, areolae, cervix, vagina, and vulva
• Pigmentary changes in nose, cheeks, and forehead (facial chloasma)
• Striae gravidarum and linea nigra
• Breast changes (such as leaking of colostrum)
• Palmar erythema and increased angiomas
• Faster hair and nail growth with thinning and softening

Genitourinary system
• Dilated ureters and renal pelvis
• Increased glomerular filtration rate and renal plasma flow early in pregnancy
• Increased urea and creatinine clearance

• Decreased blood urea and nonprotein nitrogen levels
• Glycosuria
• Decreased bladder tone
• Increased sodium retention from hormonal influences
• Increased uterine dimension
• Hypertrophied uterine muscle cells (5 to 10 times normal size)
• Increased vascularity, edema, hypertrophy, and hyperplasia of the cervical glands
• Increased vaginal secretions with a pH of 3.5 to 6.0
• Discontinued ovulation and maturation of new follicles
• Thickening of vaginal mucosa, loosening of vaginal connective tissue, and hypertrophy of small-muscle cells
• Changes in sexual desire

Musculoskeletal system
• Increase in lumbosacral curve accompanied by a compensatory curvature in the cervicodorsal region
• Stoop-shouldered stance due to enlarged breasts pulling the shoulders forward
• Separation of the rectus abdominis muscles in the third trimester, allowing protrusion of abdominal contents at the midline

Nägele's rule

Nägele's rule is considered the standard method for determining the estimated date of delivery. The procedure is as follows:
· Ask the patient to state the first day of her last menses.
· Subtract 3 months from that first day of her last menses.
· Add 7 days.

Example:

First day of last menstrual period = October 5

Subtract 3 months = July 5

Add 7 days = July 12

Estimated date of delivery = July 12

Fundal height throughout pregnancy

This illustration shows approximate fundal heights at various times during pregnancy. The times indicated are in weeks. Note that between weeks 38 and 40, the fetus begins to descend into the pelvis.

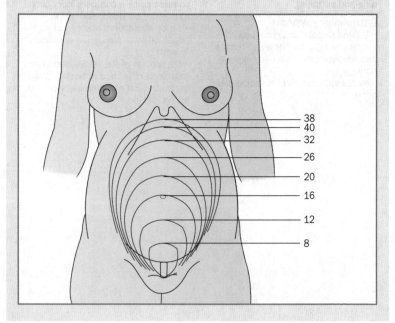

Dealing with pregnancy discomforts

This table lists common discomforts associated with pregnancy and suggestions for the patient on how to prevent and manage them.

Discomfort	Patient teaching
Urinary frequency	• Void as necessary. • Avoid caffeine. • Perform Kegel exercises.
Fatigue	• Try to get a full night's sleep. • Schedule a daily rest time. • Maintain good nutrition.
Breast tenderness	• Wear a supportive bra.
Vaginal discharge	• Wear cotton underwear. • Avoid tight-fitting pantyhose. • Bathe daily.
Backache	• Avoid standing for long periods. • Apply local heat, such as a heating pad (set on low) or a hot water bottle. Be sure to place a towel between the heat source and the skin to prevent burning. • Stoop to lift objects—don't bend.
Round ligament pain	• Slowly rise from a sitting position. • Bend forward to relieve pain. • Avoid twisting motions.
Constipation	• Increase fiber intake in the diet. • Set a regular time for bowel movements. • Drink more fluids, including water and fruit juices (unless contraindicated). Avoid caffeinated drinks.
Hemorrhoids	• Rest on the left side with the hips and lower extremities elevated to provide better oxygenation to the placenta and fetus. • Avoid constipation. • Apply witch hazel pads to the hemorrhoids. • Keep hemorrhoids reduced by using a well-lubricated gloved finger to push them gently inside the rectum; then tighten the rectal sphincter to support the hemorrhoids and contain them within the rectum. • Take sitz baths with warm water as often as needed to relieve discomfort. • Apply ice packs for reduction of swelling, if preferred over heat.
Varicosities	• Walk regularly. • Rest with the feet elevated daily. • Avoid standing for long periods. • Avoid crossing the legs. • Avoid wearing constrictive knee-high stockings; wear support stockings instead.

(continued)

Dealing with pregnancy discomforts *(continued)*

Discomfort	Patient teaching
Ankle edema	• Avoid standing for long periods. • Rest with the feet elevated. • Avoid wearing garments that constrict the lower extremities.
Headache	• Avoid eyestrain. • Rest with a cold cloth on the forehead.
Leg cramps	• Straighten the leg and dorsiflex the ankle. • Avoid pointing the toes.

Assessing pregnancy by weeks

Here are some assessment findings you can expect as pregnancy progresses in your patient.

Weeks 1 to 4
• Amenorrhea occurs.
• Breasts begin to change.
• Immunologic pregnancy tests become positive: Radioimmunoassay test results are positive a few days after implantation; urine human chorionic gonadotropin test results are positive 10 to 14 days after amenorrhea occurs.
• Nausea and vomiting begin between the fourth and sixth weeks.

Weeks 5 to 8
• Goodell's sign occurs (softening of the cervix and vagina).
• Ladin's sign occurs (softening of the uterine isthmus).
• Hegar's sign occurs (softening of the lower uterine segment).
• Chadwick's sign appears (purple-blue coloration of the vagina, cervix, and vulva).
• McDonald's sign appears (easy flexion of the fundus toward the cervix).
• Braun von Fernwald's sign occurs (irregular softening and enlargement of the uterine fundus at the site of implantation).

• Piskacek's sign may occur (asymmetrical softening and enlargement of the uterus).
• The cervical mucus plug forms.
• The uterus changes from pear-shaped to globular.
• Urinary frequency and urgency occur.

Weeks 9 to 12
• A fetal heartbeat is detected using ultrasonic stethoscope.
• Nausea, vomiting, and urinary frequency and urgency lessen.
• By the 12th week, the uterus is palpable just above the symphysis pubis.

Weeks 13 to 17
• The mother gains 10 to 12 lb (4.5 to 5.5 kg) during the second trimester.
• Uterine souffle is heard on auscultation.
• Mother's heartbeat increases by about 10 beats/minute between 14 and 30 weeks' gestation. Rate is maintained until 40 weeks' gestation.
• By the 16th week, the mother's thyroid gland enlarges by about 25%, and the uterine fundus is palpable halfway between the symphysis pubis and the umbilicus.

· Maternal recognition of fetal movements, or quickening, occurs between 16 and 20 weeks' gestation.

Weeks 18 to 22
· The uterine fundus is palpable just below the umbilicus.
· Fetal heartbeats are heard with the fetoscope at 20 weeks' gestation.
· Fetal rebound or ballottement is possible.

Weeks 23 to 27
· The umbilicus appears to be level with abdominal skin.
· Striae gravidarum are usually apparent.
· Uterine fundus is palpable at the umbilicus.
· The shape of the uterus changes from globular to ovoid.
· Braxton Hicks contractions start.

Weeks 28 to 31
· The mother gains 8 to 10 lb (3.5 to 4.5 kg) in the third trimester.
· The uterine wall feels soft and yielding.

· The uterine fundus is halfway between the umbilicus and xiphoid process.
· The fetal outline is palpable.
· The fetus is mobile and may be found in any position.

Weeks 32 to 35
· The mother may experience heartburn.
· Striae gravidarum become more evident.
· The uterine fundus is palpable just below the xiphoid process.
· Braxton Hicks contractions increase in frequency and intensity.
· The mother may experience shortness of breath.

Weeks 36 to 40
· The umbilicus protrudes.
· Varicosities, if present, become very pronounced.
· Ankle edema is evident.
· Urinary frequency recurs.
· Engagement, or lightening, occurs.
· The mucus plug is expelled.
· Cervical effacement and dilation begin.

Fetal developmental milestones

By the end of 4 weeks' gestation, the fetus begins to show noticeable signs of growth in all areas assessed. The fetus typically achieves specific developmental milestones by the end of certain gestational weeks.

By 4 weeks
• Head becomes prominent, accounting for about one-third of the entire embryo.
• Head is bent to such a degree that it appears as if it's touching the tail; embryo appears in a C shape.
• Heart appears in a rudimentary form as a bulge on the anterior surface.
• Eyes, ears, and nose appear in a rudimentary form.
• Nervous system begins to form.
• Extremities appear as buds.

By 8 weeks
• Organ formation is complete.
• Head accounts for about one-half of the total mass.
• Heart is beating and has a septum and valves.
• Arms and legs are developed.
• Abdomen is large, with evidence of fetal intestines.
• Facial features are readily visible; eye folds are developed.
• Gestational sac is visible on ultrasound.

By 12 weeks
• Nail beds are beginning to form on extremities; arms appear in normal proportions.
• Heartbeat can be heard using a Doppler ultrasound stethoscope.
• Kidney function is beginning; fetal urine may be present in amniotic fluid.
• Tooth buds are present.
• Placenta formation is complete with presence of fetal circulation.
• Gender is distinguishable with external genitalia's outward appearance.

By 16 weeks
• Fetal heart sounds are audible with stethoscope.

• Lanugo is present and well formed.
• Fetus demonstrates active swallowing of amniotic fluid.
• Fetal urine is present in amniotic fluid.
• The skeleton begins ossification.
• Intestines assume normal position in the abdomen.

By 20 weeks
• Mother can feel spontaneous movements by the fetus.
• Hair begins to form, including eyebrows and scalp hair.
• Fetus demonstrates definite sleep and wake patterns.
• Brown fat begins to form.
• Sebum is produced by the sebaceous glands.
• Meconium is evident in the upper portion of the intestines.
• Lower extremities are fully formed.
• Vernix caseosa covers the skin.

By 24 weeks
• Well-defined eyelashes and eyebrows are visible.
• Eyelids are open and pupils can react to light.
• Meconium may be present down to the rectum.
• Hearing is developing, with the fetus being able to respond to a sudden sound.
• Lungs are producing surfactant.
• Passive antibody transfer from the mother begins (possibly as early as 20 weeks' gestation).

By 28 weeks
• Surfactant appears in amniotic fluid.
• Alveoli in the lungs begin to mature.
• In the male, the testes start to move from the lower abdomen into the scrotal sac.

- Eyelids can open and close.
- Skin appears red.

By 32 weeks
- Fetus begins to appear more rounded as more subcutaneous fat is deposited.
- Moro reflex is active.
- Fetus may assume a vertex or breech position in preparation for birth.
- Iron stores are beginning to develop.
- Fingernails increase in length, reaching the tips of the fingers.
- Vernix caseosa thickens.

By 36 weeks
- Subcutaneous fat continues to be deposited.
- Soles of feet have one or two creases.
- Lanugo begins to decrease in amount.
- Fetus is storing additional glycogen, iron, carbohydrate, and calcium.
- Skin on the face and body begins to smooth.

By 40 weeks
- Fetus begins to kick actively and forcefully, causing maternal discomfort.
- Vernix caseosa is fully formed.
- Soles of the feet demonstrate creases covering at least two-thirds of the surface.
- Conversion of fetal hemoglobin to adult hemoglobin begins.
- In the male, testes descend fully into the scrotal sac.

Understanding chorionic villus sampling

Procedure

To collect a specimen for chorionic villus sampling, place the patient in the lithotomy position. The practitioner checks the placement of the uterus bimanually, inserts a Graves' speculum, and swabs the cervix with an antiseptic solution. If necessary, he may use a tenaculum to straighten an acutely flexed uterus, permitting cannula insertion.

Guided by ultrasound and possibly endoscopy, he directs the catheter through the cannula to the villi. He applies suction to the catheter to remove about 30 mg of tissue from the villi. He then withdraws the specimen, places it in a Petri dish, and examines it with a microscope. Part of the specimen is then cultured for further testing.

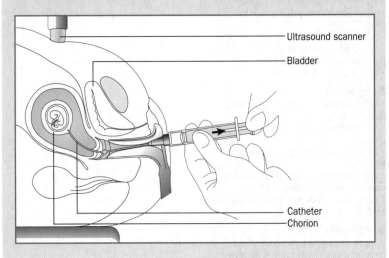

Ultrasound scanner

Bladder

Catheter

Chorion

Glucose challenge values in pregnancy

Shown here are normal values for pregnant patients taking the oral glucose challenge test to determine the risk of diabetes. These values are determined after a 100-g glucose load.

Normal blood glucose levels should remain between 90 and 120 mg/dl. If a pregnant woman's plasma glucose exceeds these levels, she should be treated as a potential diabetic.

Test type	Pregnancy glucose level (mg/dl)
Fasting	95
1 hour	180
2 hour	155
3 hour	140

Amniotic fluid analysis findings

Test component	Normal findings	Fetal implications of abnormal findings
Color	Clear, with white flecks of vernix caseosa in a mature fetus	Blood of maternal origin is usually harmless. "Port wine" fluid may signal abruptio placentae. Fetal blood may signal damage to fetal, placental, or umbilical cord vessels.
Bilirubin	Absent at term	High levels indicate hemolytic disease of the neonate.
Meconium	Absent (except in breech presentation)	Presence indicates fetal hypotension or distress.
Creatinine	More than 2 mg/dl (SI, 177 µmol/L), in a mature fetus	Decrease may indicate fetus less than 37 weeks.
Lecithin-sphingomyelin ratio	More than 2	Less than 2 indicates pulmonary immaturity.
Phosphatidyl glycerol	Present	Absence indicates pulmonary immaturity.
Glucose	Less than 45 mg/dl (SI, 2.3 mmol/L)	Excessive increases at term or near term indicate hypertrophied fetal pancreas.
Alpha fetoprotein	Variable, depending on gestational age and laboratory technique	Inappropriate increases indicate neural tube defects, impending fetal death, congenital nephrosis, or contamination of fetal blood.
Bacteria	Absent	Presence indicates chorioamnionitis.
Chromosome	Normal karyotype	Abnormal indicates fetal chromosome disorders.
Acetylcholinesterase	Absent	Presence may indicate neural tube defects, exomphalos, or other malformations.

Interpreting NST and OCT results

This chart lists the possible interpretations of results from a nonstress test (NST) and an oxytocin challenge test (OCT), commonly called a *stress test*. Appropriate actions are also included.

	Interpretation	Action
NST result		
Reactive	Two or more fetal heart rate (FHR) accelerations of 15 beats/minute lasting 15 seconds or more within 20 minutes; related to fetal movement	Repeat NST biweekly or weekly, depending on rationale for testing.
Nonreactive	Tracing without FHR accelerations or with accelerations of fewer than 15 beats/minute lasting less than 15seconds throughout fetal movement	Repeat test in 24 hours or perform a biophysical profile immediately.
Unsatisfactory	Quality of FHR recording inadequate for interpretation	Repeat test in 24 hours or perform a biophysical profile immediately.
OCT result		
Negative	No late decelerations; three contractions every 10 minutes; fetus would probably survive labor if it occurred within 1 week	No further action needed at this time.
Positive	Persistent and consistent late decelerations with more than half of contractions	Induce labor; fetus is at risk for perinatal morbidity and mortality.
Suspicious	Late decelerations with less than half of contractions after an adequate contraction pattern has been established	Repeat test in 24 hours.
Hyperstimulation	Late decelerations with excessive uterine activity (occurring more often than every 2 minutes or lasting longer than 90 seconds)	Repeat test in 24 hours.
Unsatisfactory	Poor monitor tracing or uterine contraction pattern	Repeat test in 24 hours.

Laboratory values for pregnant and nonpregnant patients

	Pregnant	Nonpregnant
Hemoglobin	11.5 to 14 g/dl	12 to 16 g/dl
Hematocrit	32% to 42%	36% to 48%
White blood cells	5,000 to 15,000/µl	4,500 to 10,000/µl
Neutrophils	60% ±10%	60%
Lymphocytes	34% ±10%	30%
Platelets	150,000 to 350,000/µl	150,000 to 350,000/µl
Serum calcium	7.8 to 9.3 mg/dl	8.4 to 10.2 mg/dl
Serum sodium	Increased retention	136 to 146 mmol/L
Serum chloride	Slight elevation	98 to 106 mmol/L
Serum iron	65 to 120 mcg/dl	75 to 150 mcg/dl
Fibrinogen	450 mg/dl	200 to 400 mg/dl
Red blood cells	1,500 to 1,900/mm^3	1,600/mm^3
Fasting blood glucose	Decreased	70 to 105 mg/dl
2-hour postprandial blood glucose	< 140 mg/dl (after a 100-g carbohydrate meal)	< 140 mg/dl
Blood urea nitrogen	Decreased	10 to 20 mg/dl
Serum creatinine	Decreased	0.5 to 1.1 mg/dl
Renal plasma flow	Increased by 25%	490 to 700 ml/minute
Glomerular filtration rate	Increased by 50%	88 to 128 ml/minute
Serum uric acid	Decreased	2 to 6.6 mg/dl
Erythrocyte sedimentation rate	Elevated during second and third trimesters	20 mm/hour
Prothrombin time	Decreased slightly	11 to 12.5 seconds
Partial thromboplastin time	Decreased slightly during pregnancy and again during second and third stages of labor (indicating clotting at placental site)	60 to 70 seconds

Biophysical profile

A biophysical profile combines data from two sources: real-time B-mode ultrasound imaging, which measures amniotic fluid volume (AFV) and fetal movement, and fetal heart rate monitoring.

A normal score is 8 to 10, a score of 4 to 6 indicates the fetus is in jeopardy, and 0 to 4 signals severe fetal compromise and delivery is indicated.

Biophysical variable	Normal (score = 2)	Abnormal (score = 0)
Nonstress test	Reactive	Nonreactive
Fetal breathing movements	One or more episodes in 30 minutes, each lasting 30 seconds or more	Episodes absent or no episode of 30 seconds or more in 30 minutes
Fetal body movements	Three discrete and definite movements of the arms, legs, or body	Less than three discrete movements of arms, legs, or body
Fetal muscle tone	One or more episodes of extension with return to flexion	Slow extension with return to flexion or fetal movement absent
AFV	Largest pocket of fluid is more than 1 cm in vertical diameter without containing loops of cord	Largest pocket is less than 1 cm in vertical diameter without loops of cord

Recommended daily allowances for pregnant women

Energy and calorie requirements increase during pregnancy; this is necessary to create new tissue and meet increased maternal metabolic needs. Nutrient requirements during pregnancy can be met by a diet that provides all of the essential nutrients, fiber, and energy in adequate amounts.

Calories	2,500 kcal
Protein	60 g

Fat-soluble vitamins

Vitamin A	800 mcg
Vitamin D	10 mcg
Vitamin E	10 mcg

Water-soluble vitamins

Ascorbic acid (vitamin C)	75 mg
Niacin	17 mg
Riboflavin	1.6 mg
Thiamine	1.5 mg
Folic acid	400 mcg
Vitamin B_6	2.2 mcg
Vitamin B_1	2.2 mcg

Minerals

Calcium	1,200 mg
Phosphorus	1,200 mg
Iodine	175 mcg
Iron	30 mg
Zinc	15 mg

The female pelvis

The female pelvis protects and supports the reproductive and other pelvic organs.

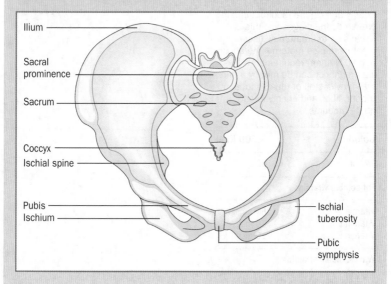

Head diameters at term

This illustration depicts three commonly used measurements of fetal head diameters. The measurements are averages for term neonates. Individual measurements vary with fetal size, attitude, and presentation.

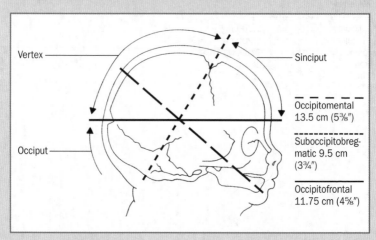

Distinguishing between true and false labor

True labor
- Regular contractions
- Back discomfort that spreads to the abdomen
- Progressive cervical dilation and effacement
- Gradually shortened intervals between contractions
- Increased intensity of contractions with ambulation
- Contractions that increase in duration and intensity

False labor
- Irregular contractions
- Discomfort that's localized in the abdomen
- No cervical change
- No change or irregular change
- Contractions may be relieved with ambulation
- Usually no change in contractions

Stages of labor

Stage 1
- Begins at onset of true labor
- Lasts until complete dilation, which is about 6 to 18 hours in the primipara and 2 to 20 in the multipara
- Divided into the latent, active, and transitional phases

  Latent phase
- Cervical dilation measures 0 to 3 cm.
- Contractions are irregular, short, and last 20 to 40 seconds.
- Phase lasts about 6 hours for a primipara and 4½ hours for a multipara.

  Active phase
- Cervical dilation measures 4 to 7 cm.
- Contractions are 5 to 8 minutes apart and last 45 to 60 seconds.
- Phase lasts about 3 hours for a primipara and 2 hours for a multipara.

  Transitional phase
- Cervical dilation measures 8 to 10 cm.
- Contractions are 1 to 2 minutes apart and last 60 to 90 seconds.
- At the end of this phase, the patient feels the urge to push.

Stage 2
- Extends from complete dilation to the delivery of the neonate
- Lasts from 1 to 3 hours for the primipara and 30 to 60 minutes for the multipara
- Occurs in seven cardinal movements
- Divided into the latent, active, and transitional phases

  Latent phase
- Begins at onset of contractions and ends when rapid cervical dilation begins.
- Phase lasts about 10 to 30 minutes.

  Active phase
- Cervical dilation rapidly moves from 4 to 7 cm.
- Phase duration varies.

  Transitional phase
- Maximum dilation is 8 to 10 cm.
- Average duration is 5 to 15 minutes.

Stage 3
- Extends from the delivery of the neonate to the delivery of the placenta
- Lasts from 5 to 30 minutes
- Divided into the placental separation and the placental expulsion phases

Stage 4
- Covers the time immediately after delivery of the placenta
- Typically, the first hour after delivery
- Referred to as the *recovery period*

Classifying fetal presentation

Fetal presentation may be broadly classified as cephalic, breech, shoulder, or compound. Cephalic presentations occur in almost all deliveries. Of the remaining three, breech deliveries are most common.

Cephalic
In the cephalic, or head-down, presentation, the fetus' position may be classified by the presenting skull landmark: vertex, brow, sinciput, or mentum (chin).

Vertex	Brow	Sinciput	Mentum
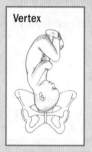	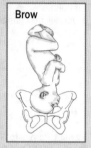	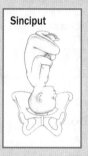	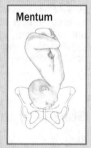

Breech
In the breech, or head-up, presentation, the fetus' position may be classified as complete, where the knees and hips are flexed; *frank*, where the hips are flexed and knees remain straight; *footling*, where neither the thighs nor lower legs are flexed; and *incomplete*, where one or both hips remain extended and one or both feet or knees lie below the breech.

Complete	Frank	Footling	Incomplete
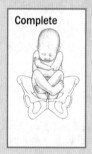	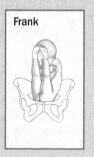	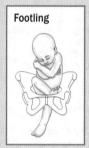	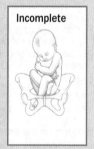

Shoulder
Although a fetus may adopt one of several shoulder presentations, examination can't differentiate among them; thus, all transverse lies are considered shoulder presentations.

Compound
In compound presentation, an extremity prolapses alongside the major presenting part so that two presenting parts appear in the pelvis at the same time.

Shoulder	Compound
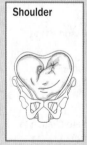	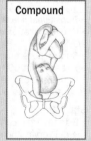

Fetal position abbreviations

These abbreviations, organized according to variations in presentation, are used when documenting fetal position.

Vertex presentation (occiput)
LOA, left occiput anterior
LOP, left occiput posterior
LOT, left occiput transverse
ROA, right occiput anterior
ROP, right occiput posterior
ROT, right occiput transverse

Breech presentation (sacrum)
LSaA, left sacrum anterior
LSaP, left sacrum posterior
LSaT, left sacrum transverse
RSaA, right sacrum anterior
RSaP, right sacrum posterior
RSaT, right sacrum transverse

Face presentation (mentum)
LMA, left mentum anterior
LMP, left mentum posterior
LMT, left mentum transverse
RMA, right mentum anterior
RMP, right mentum posterior
RMT, right mentum transverse

Shoulder presentation (acromion process)
LAA, left scapular anterior
LAP, left scapular posterior
RAA, right scapular anterior
RAP, right scapular posterior

Fetal positions

Right occiput anterior (ROA)

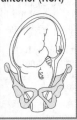

Right occiput transverse (ROT)

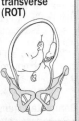

Left occiput anterior (LOA)

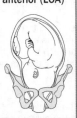

Left occiput transverse (LOT)

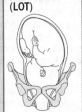

Right mentum anterior (RMA)

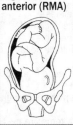

Right mentum posterior (RMP)

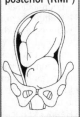

Left mentum anterior (LMA)

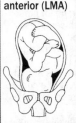

Left sacrum anterior (LSaA)

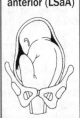

(continued)

Fetal positions *(continued)*

Left sacrum posterior (LSaP)	Right occiput posterior (ROP)	Left occiput posterior (LOP)
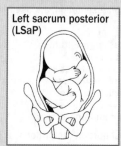	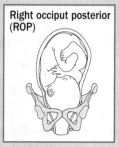	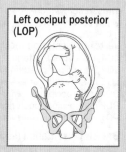

Fetal attitude

Fetal attitude refers to the relationship of fetal body parts to one another. It denotes whether presenting parts are in flexion or extension.

Complete flexion
• Most common
• Neck is completely flexed, with the head tucked down to the chest and the chin touching the sternum
• Arms are folded over the chest, with the elbows flexed
• Lower legs are crossed and the thighs are drawn up onto the abdomen, with the calf of each leg pressed against the thigh of the opposite leg

Moderate flexion
• Second most common
• Commonly known as the *military position* because the head's straightness makes the fetus appear to be "at attention"
• Involves sinciput (forehead) presentation through the birth canal
• Neck is slightly flexed
• Head is held straight but the chin doesn't touch the chest
• Many fetuses assume this attitude early in labor but convert to a complete flexion (vertex presentation) as labor progresses
• Birth usually isn't difficult because the second smallest anteroposterior diameter of the skull is presented through the pelvis during delivery

Partial extension
• Uncommon
• Involves brow presentation through the birth canal
• Neck is extended
• Head is moved backward slightly so that the brow is the first part of the fetus to pass through the pelvis during delivery
• Can cause a difficult delivery because the anteroposterior diameter of the skull may be equal to or larger than the opening in the pelvis

Complete extension
• Rare; considered abnormal
• Can result from various factors:
  – oligohydramnios (less than normal amniotic fluid)
  – neurologic abnormalities
  – multiparity or a large abdomen with decreased uterine tone
  – nuchal cord with multiple coils around the neck
  – fetal malformation (found in as many as 60% of cases)
• Involves a face presentation through the birth canal
• Head and neck of the fetus are hyperextended, with the occiput touching the upper back
• Back is usually arched, increasing the degree of hyperextension
• Usually requires cesarean birth

Cervical effacement and dilation

As labor advances, so do cervical effacement and dilation, which promote delivery. During effacement, the cervix shortens and its walls become thin, progressing from 0% effacement (palpable and thick) to 100% effacement (fully indistinct, or *effaced,* and paper-thin). Full effacement obliterates the constrictive uterine neck to create a smooth, unobstructed passageway for the fetus.

At the same time, dilation occurs. This progressive widening of the cervical canal—from the upper internal cervical os to the lower external cervical os—advances from 0 to 10 cm. As the cervical canal opens, resistance decreases; this further eases fetal descent.

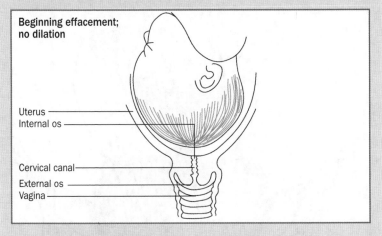

**Beginning effacement;
no dilation**

Uterus
Internal os
Cervical canal
External os
Vagina

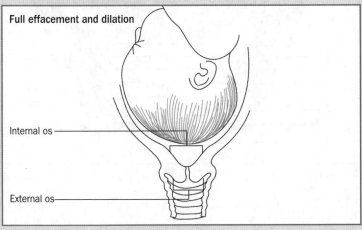

Full effacement and dilation

Internal os

External os

Assessing fetal engagement and station

During a vaginal examination, you'll assess the extent of the fetal presenting part into the pelvis. This is referred to as fetal engagement.

After you have determined fetal engagement, palpate the presenting part and grade the fetal station (where the presenting part lies in relation to the ischial spines of the maternal pelvis). If the presenting part isn't fully engaged into the pelvis, you won't be able to assess station.

Station grades range from −3 (3 cm above the maternal ischial spines) to +4 (4 cm below the maternal ischial spines, causing the perineum to bulge). A zero grade indicates that the presenting part lies level with the ischial spines.

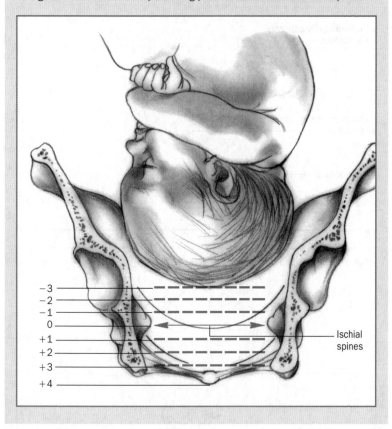

Systemic changes in the active phase of labor

System	Change
Cardiovascular	• Increased blood pressure • Increased cardiac output • Supine hypotension
Respiratory	• Increased oxygen consumption • Increased rate • Possible hyperventilation leading to respiratory alkalosis, hypoxia, and hypercapnia (if breathing isn't controlled)
Renal	• Difficulty voiding • Proteinuria (1 + normal)
Musculoskeletal	• Diaphoresis • Fatigue • Backache • Joint pain • Leg cramps
Neurologic	• Increased pain threshold and sedation caused by endogenous endorphins • Anesthetized perineal tissues caused by constant intense pressure on nerve endings
GI	• Dehydration • Decreased GI motility • Slow absorption of solid food • Nausea • Diarrhea
Endocrine	• Decreased progesterone level • Increased estrogen level • Increased prostaglandin level • Increased oxytocin level • Increased metabolism • Decreased blood glucose level

Reading a fetal monitor strip

Presented in two parallel recordings, the fetal monitor strip records the fetal heart rate (FHR) in beats per minute in the top recording and uterine activity (UA) in millimeters of mercury (mm Hg) in the bottom recording. You can obtain information on fetal status and labor progress by reading the strips horizontally and vertically.

Reading horizontally on the FHR or the UA strip, each small block represents 10 seconds. Six consecutive small blocks, separated by a dark vertical line, represent 1 minute. Reading vertically on the FHR strip, each block represents an amplitude of 10 beats/minute. Reading vertically on the UA strip, each block represents 5 mm Hg of pressure.

Assess the baseline FHR (the "resting" heart rate) between uterine contractions when fetal movement diminishes. This baseline FHR (normal range: 120 to 160 beats/minute) pattern serves as a reference for subsequent FHR tracings produced during contractions.

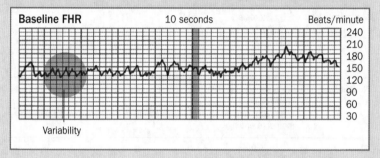

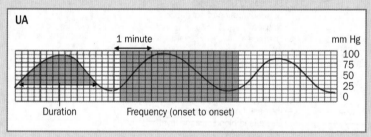

Identifying baseline FHR irregularities

When monitoring fetal heart rate (FHR), you need to be familiar with irregularities that may occur and their possible causes. Here's a guide to these irregularities.

Irregularity

Baseline tachycardia

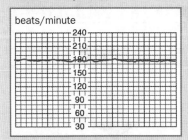

Possible causes: Early fetal hypoxia, maternal fever, parasympathetic agents such as atropine and scopolamine, beta-adrenergics such as terbutaline, amnionitis, maternal hyperthyroidism, fetal anemia, fetal heart failure, fetal arrhythmias

Baseline bradycardia

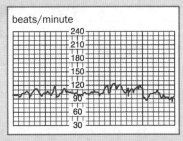

Possible causes: Late fetal hypoxia, beta-adrenergic blockers such as propranolol and anesthetics, maternal hypotension, prolonged umbilical cord compression, fetal congenital heart block

Early decelerations

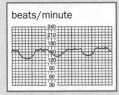

Possible causes: Fetal head compression

Late decelerations

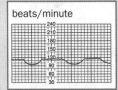

Possible causes: Uteroplacental circulatory insufficiency (placental hypoperfusion) caused by decreased intervillous blood flow during contractions or a structural placental defect such as abruptio placentae, uterine hyperactivity caused by excessive oxytocin infusion, maternal hypotension, maternal supine hypotension

Variable decelerations

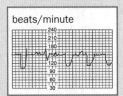

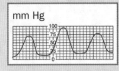

Possible causes: Umbilical cord compression causing decreased fetal oxygen perfusion

Evaluating FHR decelerations

Use this flowchart to determine how to proceed when you identify fetal heart rate (FHR) decelerations.

FHR decelerations

Deceleration inversely mirrors contraction.

YES
- Early deceleration.
- No interventions needed.
- Continue to monitor.

NO
Reevaluate.

Smooth waveforms inversely mirror contraction but late in onset.

YES
- Late deceleration.
- Reposition patient.
- Increase primary I.V. flow rate.
- Administer oxygen.
- Notify practitioner; if repetitive, discontinue oxytocin and prepare to assist with fetal scalp sampling.

NO
Reevaluate.

Onset, timing, and waveform vary.

YES
- Variable deceleration.
- Reposition patient.
- Continue to monitor.
- Administer oxygen by face mask.
- Notify practitioner.

NO
Continue to monitor, evaluating timing and waveform.

Comfort measures in labor

Nonpharmacologic ways to relieve pain
· Relaxation techniques—exercises to focus attention away from pain
· Focusing—concentration on an object
· Imagery—visualization of an object
· Effleurage—light abdominal massage
· Lamaze—patterns of controlled breathing
· Hypnosis—alteration in state of consciousness
· Acupuncture and acupressure—stimulation of trigger points with needles or pressure

· Yoga—deep-breathing exercises, body-stretching postures, and meditation to promote relaxation

Three key Lamaze techniques
· Slow breathing—inhaling through the nose and exhaling through the mouth or nose six to nine times per minute
· Accelerated-decelerated breathing—inhaling through the nose and exhaling through the mouth as contractions become more intense
· Pant-blow breathing—performing rapid, shallow breathing through the mouth only throughout contractions, particularly during the transitional phase

Understanding a pathologic retraction ring

A pathologic retraction ring, also called *Bandl's ring,* is the most common type of constriction ring responsible for dysfunctional labor. It's a key warning sign of impending uterine rupture.

A pathologic retraction ring appears as a horizontal indentation across the abdomen, usually during the second stage of labor (see arrow on illustration). The myometrium above the ring is considerably thicker than below the ring. When present, the ring prevents further passage of the fetus, holding the fetus in place at the point of the retraction. The placenta is also held at that point.

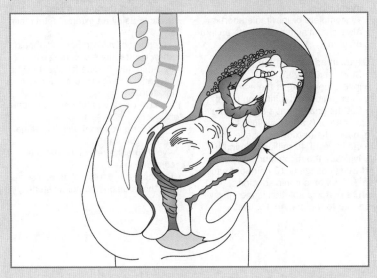

Primary indications for cesarean birth

Maternal
· Cephalopelvic disproportion
· Active genital herpes or papilloma
· Previous cesarean birth by classic incision
· Disabling condition, such as severe gestational hypertension or heart disease, that prevents pushing to accomplish the pelvic division of labor

Placental
· Complete or partial placenta previa
· Premature separation of the placenta

Fetal
· Transverse fetal lie
· Extremely low fetal size
· Fetal distress
· Compound conditions such as macrosomic fetus in a breech lie

Facts about oxytocin

· Synthetic oxytocin (Pitocin) is used to:
  – induce or augment labor
  – evaluate for fetal distress after 31 weeks' gestation
  – control bleeding and enhance uterine contractions after the placenta is delivered.
· May be used in patients with:
  – gestational hypertension
  – prolonged gestation
  – maternal diabetes
  – Rh sensitization
  – premature or prolonged rupture of membranes
  – incomplete or inevitable abortion.
· Always administered I.V. with an infusion pump.

Oxytocin administration
· Start a primary I.V. line.
· Insert the tubing of the administration set through the infusion pump.
· Set the drip rate at a starting infusion rate of 0.5 to 1 milliunits/minute. The maximum dosage of oxytocin is 20 to 40 milliunits/minute.
· Typically, the recommended labor-starting dosage is 10 units of oxytocin in 100 ml of isotonic solution.
· The oxytocin solution is then piggybacked to the primary I.V. line.

· If a problem occurs, such as decelerations of fetal heart rate or fetal distress, stop the piggyback infusion immediately and resume the primary line.
· Monitor uterine contractions immediately.
· Increase the oxytocin dosage as ordered but never increase it more than 1 to 2 milliunits/minute once every 15 to 60 minutes.
· Before each increase, assess:
  – contractions
  – maternal vital signs
  – fetal heart rhythm and rate.
· If you're using an external fetal monitor:
  – uterine activity strip or grid should show contractions occurring every 2 to 3 minutes, lasting for about 60 seconds, and followed by uterine relaxation.
· If you're using an internal fetal monitor:
  – look for an optimal baseline value of 5 to 15 mm Hg.
  – verify uterine relaxation between contractions.
· To manage hyperstimulation, discontinue the infusion and administer oxygen.

Complications of oxytocin administration

Uterine hyperstimulation
- May progress to tetanic contractions that last longer than 2 minutes.
- Signs of hyperstimulation include:
  - contractions that are less than 2 minutes apart and last 90 seconds or longer
  - uterine pressure that doesn't return to baseline between contractions
  - intrauterine pressure that rises above 75 mm Hg.

Other potential complications
- Fetal distress
- Abruptio placentae
- Uterine rupture
- Water intoxication

Stop signs
Watch for the following signs of oxytocin administration complications. If indications of potential complications exist, stop the oxytocin administration, administer oxygen via face mask, and notify the practitioner immediately.

Fetal distress
Signs of fetal distress include:
- late decelerations
- bradycardia.

Abruptio placentae
Signs of abruptio placentae include:
- sharp, stabbing uterine pain
- pain over and above the uterine contraction pain
- heavy bleeding
- hard, boardlike uterus.

Also watch for signs of shock, including rapid, weak pulse; falling blood pressure; cold and clammy skin; and dilation of the nostrils.

Uterine rupture
Signs of uterine rupture include:
- sudden, severe pain during a contraction
- tearing sensation
- absent fetal heart sounds.

Also watch for signs of shock.

Water intoxication
Signs of water intoxication include:
- headache and vomiting (usually seen first)
- hypertension
- peripheral edema
- shallow or labored breathing
- dyspnea
- tachypnea
- lethargy
- confusion
- change in level of consciousness.

Safety with magnesium

If your patient requires I.V. magnesium therapy, be cautious when administering the drug. Follow these guidelines to ensure safety during administration.

• Always administer the drug as a piggyback infusion so that if the patient develops signs and symptoms of toxicity, the drug can be discontinued immediately.

• Obtain a baseline serum magnesium level before initiating therapy and monitor the magnesium level frequently thereafter.

• Keep in mind that for I.V. magnesium to be effective as an anticonvulsant, the serum magnesium level should be 5 to 8 mg/dl. Levels above 8 mg/dl indicate toxicity and place the patient at risk for respiratory depression, cardiac arrhythmias, and cardiac arrest.

• Assess the patient's deep tendon reflexes—ideally by testing the patellar reflex. However, if the patient has received epidural anesthesia, test the biceps or triceps reflex. Diminished or hypoactive reflexes suggest magnesium toxicity.

• Assess for ankle clonus by rapidly dorsiflexing the patient's ankle three times in succession and then removing your hand, observing foot movement. If no further motion is noted, ankle clonus is absent; if the foot continues to move voluntarily, clonus is present. Moderate (3 to 5) or severe (6 or more) movements may suggest magnesium toxicity.

• Have calcium gluconate readily available at the patient's bedside. Anticipate administering this antidote for magnesium I.V. toxicity.

Administering terbutaline

I.V. terbutaline (Brethine) may be ordered for a patient in premature labor. When administering this drug, follow these steps:

- Obtain baseline maternal vital signs, fetal heart rate (FHR), and laboratory studies, including serum glucose and electrolyte levels and hematocrit.
- Institute external monitoring of uterine contractions and FHR.
- Prepare the drug with lactated Ringer's solution instead of dextrose and water to prevent additional glucose load and possible hyperglycemia.
- Administer the drug as an I.V. piggyback infusion into a main I.V. solution so that it can be discontinued immediately if the patient experiences adverse reactions.
- Use microdrip tubing and an infusion pump to ensure an accurate flow rate.
- Expect to adjust the infusion flow rate every 10 minutes until contractions cease or adverse reactions become problematic.
- Monitor maternal vital signs every 15 minutes while the infusion rate increases and then every 30 minutes until contractions cease; monitor the FHR every 15 to 30 minutes.
- Auscultate breath sounds for evidence of crackles or changes; monitor the patient for complaints of dyspnea and chest pain.
- Stay alert for maternal pulse rate greater than 120 beats/minute, blood pressure less than 90/60 mm Hg, or persistent tachycardia or tachypnea, chest pain, dyspnea, or abnormal breath sounds because these signs and symptoms could indicate developing pulmonary edema. Notify the practitioner immediately.
- Watch for fetal tachycardia or late or variable decelerations in the FHR pattern because they could indicate uterine bleeding or fetal distress, necessitating an emergency birth.
- Monitor input and output closely, every hour during the infusion and every 4 hours after the infusion.
- Expect to continue the infusion for 12 to 24 hours after contractions have ceased and then switch to oral therapy.
- Administer the first dose of oral therapy 30 minutes before discontinuing the I.V. infusion.
- Instruct the patient on how to take oral therapy. Tell her that therapy will continue until 37 weeks' gestation or until fetal lung maturity has been confirmed by amniocentesis; alternatively, if the patient is prescribed subcutaneous terbutaline via a continuous pump, teach her how to use the pump.
- Teach the patient how to measure her pulse rate before each dose of oral terbutaline, or at the recommended times with subcutaneous therapy; instruct the patient to call the practitioner if her pulse rate exceeds 120 beats/minute or if she experiences palpitations or severe nervousness.

Understanding perineal lacerations

Lacerations are tears in the perineum, vagina, or cervix that occur from stretching of tissues during delivery. Perineal lacerations are classified as first, second, third, or fourth degree.

• A first-degree laceration involves the vaginal mucosa and the skin of the perineum to the fourchette.

• A second-degree laceration involves the vagina, perineal skin, fascia, levator ani muscle, and perineal body.

• A third-degree laceration involves the entire perineum and the external anal sphincter.

• A fourth-degree laceration involves the entire perineum, rectal sphincter, and portions of the rectal mucous membrane.

Cardinal movements of labor

Engagement, descent, flexion

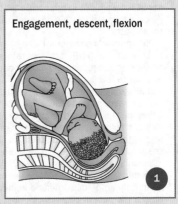

Internal rotation

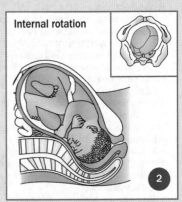

Extension beginning (rotation complete)

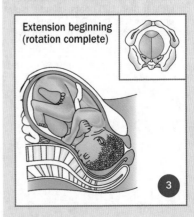

Extension complete

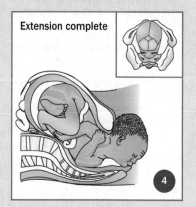

4

External rotation (shoulder rotation)

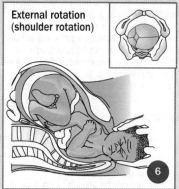

6

External rotation (restitution)

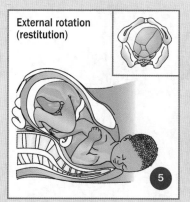

5

Expulsion

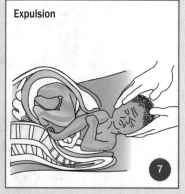

7

Umbilical cord prolapse

In umbilical cord prolapse, a loop of the umbilical cord slips down in front of the presenting fetal part. This prolapse may occur at any time after the membranes rupture, especially if the presenting part isn't fitted firmly into the cervix. Prolapse occurs in 1 out of 200 pregnancies. In a hidden prolapse, the cord remains within the uterus but is prolapsed.

Causes

Prolapse tends to occur more commonly with these conditions:

- premature rupture of membranes
- fetal presentation other than cephalic
- placenta previa
- intrauterine tumors that prevent the presenting part from engaging
- small fetus
- cephalopelvic disproportion that prevents firm engagement
- hydramnios
- multiple gestation.

Outward prolapse
The cord can be seen in the vagina.

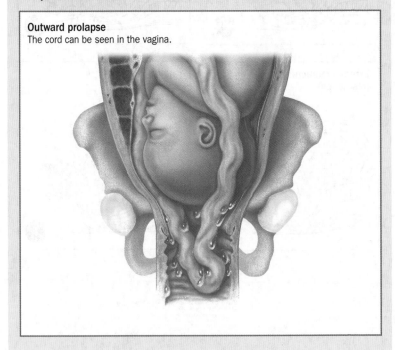

Highlighting the phases of the postpartum period

This chart summarizes the three phases of the postpartum period as identified by Reva Rubin.

Phase	Maternal behavior and tasks
Taking in 1 to 2 days after delivery	• Reflective time • Assumption of passive role and dependence on others for care • Verbalization about labor and birth • Sense of wonderment when looking at neonate
Taking hold 2 to 7 days after delivery	• Action-oriented time of increasing independence in care • Strong interest in caring for neonate; commonly accompanied by feelings of insecurity about ability to care for neonate
Letting go 7 days after delivery	• Ability to redefine new role • Acceptance of neonate's real image rather than fantasized image • Recognition of neonate as separate from herself • Assumption of responsibility for dependent neonate

Uterine involution

After delivery, the uterus begins its descent back into the pelvic cavity. It continues to descend about 1 cm per day until it isn't palpable above the symphysis at about 9 days after delivery.

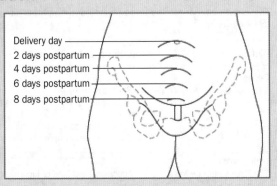

Delivery day
2 days postpartum
4 days postpartum
6 days postpartum
8 days postpartum

Assessing lochia flow

Use these guidelines when assessing a patient's lochia.

· *Character:* Lochia typically is described as lochia rubra, serosa, or alba, depending on the color of the discharge. Lochia should always be present during the first 3 weeks postpartum. The patient who has had a cesarean birth may have a scant amount of lochia; however, lochia is never absent.

· *Amount:* Although this varies, the amount can be compared to that of a menstrual flow. Saturating a perineal pad in less than 1 hour is considered excessive; the practitioner should be notified. Expect women who are breast-feeding to have less lochia. Lochia flow also increases with activity—for example, when the patient gets out of bed the first few times (due to pooled lochia being released) or when the patient engages in strenuous exercise, such as lifting a heavy object or walking up stairs (due to an actual increase in amount).

· *Color:* Depending on the postpartum day, lochia typically ranges from red to pinkish brown to creamy white or colorless. A sudden change in the color of lochia—for example, to bright red after having been pink—suggests new bleeding or retained placental fragments.

· *Odor:* Lochia has an odor similar to that of menstrual flow. A foul or offensive odor suggests infection.

· *Consistency:* Lochia should be clot-free. Evidence of large clots indicates poor uterine contraction, which requires intervention.

Breast-feeding positions

A breast-feeding position should be comfortable and efficient. By changing positions periodically, the patient can alter the neonate's grasp on the nipple, thereby avoiding contact friction on the same area. As appropriate, suggest these three typical positions.

Cradle position
The patient cradles the neonate's head in the crook of her arm.

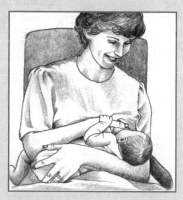

Side-lying position
The patient lies on her side with her stomach facing the neonate's. As the neonate's mouth opens, she pulls him toward the nipple.

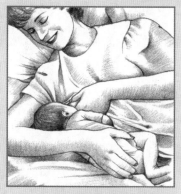

Football position
Sitting with a pillow under her arm, the patient places her hand under the neonate's head. As the neonate's mouth opens, she pulls the neonate's head near her breast. This position may be helpful for the patient who has had a cesarean birth.

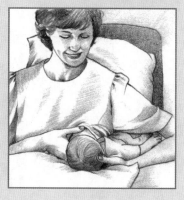

Assessing excessive vaginal bleeding

Use this flowchart to help guide your interventions when you determine that your patient has excessive vaginal bleeding.

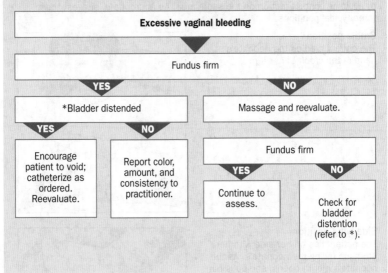

Assessing puerperal infection

Signs and symptoms of a puerperal infection depend on the extent and site of infection.

Localized perineal infection
- Pain
- Elevated temperature
- Edema
- Redness, firmness, and tenderness at the site of the wound
- Sensation of heat
- Burning on urination
- Discharge from the wound

Endometritis
- Heavy, sometimes foul-smelling lochia
- Tender, enlarged uterus
- Backache
- Severe uterine contractions persisting after childbirth

Parametritis (pelvic cellulitis)
- Vaginal tenderness
- Abdominal pain and tenderness (pain may become more intense as infection spreads)
- Inflammation may remain localized, may lead to abscess formation, or may spread through the blood or lymphatic system

Septic pelvic thrombophlebitis
- Caused by widespread inflammation
- Severe, repeated chills and dramatic swings in body temperature
- Lower abdominal or flank pain
- Possible palpable tender mass over the affected area, usually developing near the second postpartum week

Peritonitis
- Caused by widespread inflammation
- Elevated body temperature accompanied by tachycardia (heart rate greater than 140 beats/minute), weak pulse, hiccups, nausea, vomiting, and diarrhea
- Constant and possibly excruciating abdominal pain
- Rigid, boardlike abdomen with guarding (commonly the first manifestation)

Psychiatric disorders in the postpartum period

Disorder	Assessment findings	Treatment
Depression (most common)	• Commonly occurring within 4 to 6 weeks, with symptoms possibly lasting several months • Suicidal thinking • Feelings of failure • Exhaustion	• Psychotherapy • Drug therapy such as antidepressants
Mania	• Occurring 1 to 2 weeks after delivery, possibly after a brief period of depression • Agitation • Excitement possibly lasting 1 to 3 weeks	• Psychotherapy • Antimanic drugs
Schizophrenia	• Possibly occurring by the 10th postpartum day • Delusional thinking • Gross distortion of reality • Flight of ideas • Possible rejection of the father, infant, or both	• Antipsychotic drugs • Psychotherapy • Possible hospitalization
Psychosis	• Possibly appearing from 2 weeks to 12 months after delivery; more commonly seen within first month after delivery • Sleep disturbances • Restlessness • Depression • Indecisiveness progressing to bewilderment, perplexity, a dreamy state, impaired memory, confusion, and somatic delusion	• Antipsychotic drugs • Psychotherapy • Hospitalization

Postpartum maternal self-care

When teaching your patient about self-care for the postpartum period, include these topic areas and instructions.

Personal hygiene

- Change perineal pads frequently, removing them from the front to the back and disposing of them in a plastic bag.
- Perform perineal care each time that you urinate or move your bowels.
- Monitor your vaginal discharge; it should change from red to pinkish brown to clear or creamy white before stopping altogether.
- Notify your practitioner if the discharge returns to a previous color, becomes bright red or yellowish green, suddenly increases in amount, or develops an offensive odor.
- Follow your practitioner's instructions about using sitz baths or applying heat to your perineum.
- Shower daily.

Breasts

- Regardless of whether or not you're breast-feeding, wear a firm, supportive bra.
- If nipple leakage occurs, use clean gauze pads or nursing pads inside your bra to absorb the moisture.
- Inspect your nipples for cracking, fissures, or soreness, and report areas of redness, tenderness, or swelling.
- Wash breasts daily with clear water when showering and dry with a soft towel or allow to air dry.
- Don't use soap on your breasts; soap is drying.
- If you're breast-feeding and your breasts become engorged, allow your baby to suck at the breast or use warm compresses or stand under a warm shower for relief.
- If you aren't breast-feeding, apply cool compresses several times per day.

Activity and exercise

- Balance rest periods with activity, get as much sleep as possible at night, and take frequent rest periods or naps during the day.
- Check with your practitioner about when to begin exercising.
- If your vaginal discharge increases with activity, elevate your legs for about 30 minutes. If the discharge doesn't decrease with rest, call your practitioner.

Nutrition

- Increase your intake of protein and calories.
- Drink plenty of fluids throughout the day, including before and after breast-feeding.

Elimination

- If you have the urge to urinate or move your bowels, don't delay in doing so.
- Urinate at least every 2 to 3 hours. This helps keep the uterus contracted and decreases the risk of excessive bleeding.
- Report difficulty urinating, burning, or pain to your practitioner.
- Drink plenty of liquids and eat high-fiber foods to prevent constipation.
- Follow your practitioner's instructions about the use of stool softeners or laxatives.

Sexual activity and contraception

- Remember that breast-feeding isn't a reliable method of contraception.
- Discuss birth control options with your practitioner.
- Ask when you can resume sexual activity and contraceptive measures. Most couples can resume having sex within 3 to 4 weeks after delivery, or possibly as soon as lochia ceases.
- Use a water-based lubricant if necessary.
- Expect a decrease in intensity and rapidity of sexual response for about 3 months after delivery.
- Perform Kegel exercises to help strengthen your pelvic floor muscles. To do this, squeeze your pelvic muscles as if trying to stop urine flow and then release them.

(continued)

Postpartum maternal self-care *(continued)*

Sleeping positions
· To aid uterine involution, lie on your abdomen. This position tips the uterus into its natural forward position and provides support to the abdominal muscles.
· Avoid lying on your side in the knee-chest position until at least the third postpartal week or, better yet, until after the 6-week postpartal examination.

(Note: The knee-chest position may cause the vagina to open, possibly allowing air to enter through the still slightly open cervical os. The air can pass through the still open blood sinuses in the uterus and enter the circulatory system, placing the woman at risk for an air embolism. However, to avoid alarming the patient, simply tell her that the knee-chest position isn't as beneficial as lying on her abdomen.)

Preventing mastitis

If your patient is breast-feeding, include these instructions about breast care and preventing mastitis in your teaching plan.
· Wash your hands after using the bathroom, before touching your breasts, and before and after every breast-feeding.
· If necessary, apply a warm compress or take a warm shower to help facilitate milk flow.
· Position the neonate properly at the breast, and make sure that he grasps the nipple and entire areola area when feeding.
· Empty your breasts as completely as possible at feedings.
· Alternate feeding positions and rotate pressure areas.
· Release the neonate's grasp on the nipple before removing him from the breast.
· Expose your nipples to the air for part of each day.
· Drink plenty of fluids, eat a balanced diet, and get sufficient rest to enhance the breast-feeding experience.
· Don't wait too long between feedings or wean the infant abruptly.

Preventing DVT

Incorporate the instructions below in your teaching plan to reduce a woman's risk of developing deep vein thrombosis (DVT).
· Check with your practitioner about using a side-lying or back-lying position for birth instead of the lithotomy position to reduce the risk of blood pooling in the lower extremities.
· If you must use the lithotomy position, ask to have the stirrups padded so you put less pressure on your calves.
· Change positions frequently if on bed rest.
· Avoid deeply flexing your legs at the groin or sharply flexing your knees.
· Don't stand in one place for too long or sit with your knees bent or legs crossed. Elevate your legs to improve venous return.
· Don't wear garters or constrictive clothing.
· Wiggle your toes and perform leg lifts while in bed to minimize venous pooling and help increase venous return.
· Walk as soon as possible after delivery.
· Wear antiembolism or support stockings, as ordered. Put them on before getting out of bed in the morning.

Neonatal resuscitation algorithm

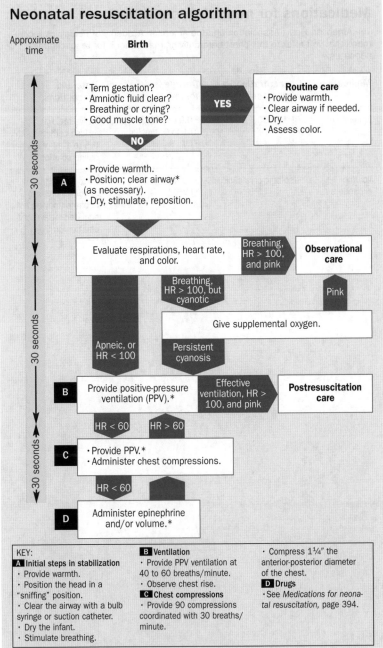

Approximate time

Birth

· Term gestation?
· Amniotic fluid clear?
· Breathing or crying?
· Good muscle tone?

YES

Routine care
· Provide warmth.
· Clear airway if needed.
· Dry.
· Assess color.

NO

30 seconds

A
· Provide warmth.
· Position; clear airway*
(as necessary).
· Dry, stimulate, reposition.

Evaluate respirations, heart rate, and color.

Breathing, HR > 100, and pink

Observational care

Breathing, HR > 100, but cyanotic

Pink

Give supplemental oxygen.

30 seconds

Apneic, or HR < 100

Persistent cyanosis

B
Provide positive-pressure ventilation (PPV).*

Effective ventilation, HR > 100, and pink

Postresuscitation care

HR < 60   HR > 60

C
· Provide PPV.*
· Administer chest compressions.

30 seconds

HR < 60

D
Administer epinephrine and/or volume.*

KEY:

A Initial steps in stabilization
· Provide warmth.
· Position the head in a "sniffing" position.
· Clear the airway with a bulb syringe or suction catheter.
· Dry the infant.
· Stimulate breathing.

B Ventilation
· Provide PPV ventilation at 40 to 60 breaths/minute.
· Observe chest rise.

C Chest compressions
· Provide 90 compressions coordinated with 30 breaths/minute.

· Compress 1¼" the anterior-posterior diameter of the chest.

D Drugs
· See *Medications for neonatal resuscitation*, page 394.

* Endotracheal intubation may be considered at several steps.
© American Heart Association.

Medications for neonatal resuscitation

The American Heart Association and the American Academy of Pediatrics recommend that you refer to this chart before giving medications for resuscitating neonates.

Medication	Concentration to administer	Dosage and route	Rate and precautions
Epinephrine	• 1:10,000	• 0.01 to 0.03 mg/kg (0.1 to 0.3 ml/kg) • I.V.	• Give rapidly. • Flush catheter with 0.5 to 1 ml of normal saline solution.
Volume expanders	• Isotonic crystalloid	• 10 ml/kg • I.V.	• Avoid giving too rapidly to preterm neonate (may be associated intraventricular hemorrhage)

Physiology of the neonate

Body system	Physiology after birth
Cardiovascular	• Functional closure of fetal shunts occurs. • Transition from fetal to postnatal circulation occurs.
Respiratory	• Onset of breathing occurs as air replaces the fluid that filled the lungs before birth.
Renal	• System doesn't mature fully until after the first year of life; fluid imbalances may occur.
GI	• System continues to develop. • Uncoordinated peristalsis of the esophagus occurs. • The neonate has a limited ability to digest fats.
Thermogenic	• The neonate is more susceptible to rapid heat loss because of an acute change in the environment and a thin layer of subcutaneous fat. • Nonshivering thermogenesis occurs. • The presence of brown fat (more in a mature neonate; less in a premature neonate) warms the neonate by increasing heat production.
Immune	• The inflammatory response of the tissues to localize infection is immature.
Hematopoietic	• Coagulation time is prolonged.
Neurologic	• Presence of primitive reflexes and time in which they appear and disappear indicate the maturity of the developing nervous system.
Hepatic	• The neonate may demonstrate jaundice.
Integumentary	• The epidermis and dermis are thin and bound loosely to each other. • Sebaceous glands are active.
Musculoskeletal	• More cartilage is present than ossified bone.
Reproductive	• Females may have a mucoid vaginal discharge and pseudomenstruation due to maternal estrogen levels. • Testes are descended in the scrotum in males. • Small, white, firm cysts called *epithelial pearls* may be visible at the tip of the prepuce. • Genitals may be edematous if the neonate is presented in the breech position.

Neonatal assessment

Initial neonatal assessment
• Ensure a proper airway via suctioning.
• Administer oxygen as needed.
• Dry the neonate under the warmer.
• Keep the neonate's head lower than the trunk to promote drainage of secretions.
• Help determine the Apgar score.
• Apply a cord clamp and monitor the neonate for abnormal bleeding from the cord.
• Analyze the umbilical cord. (Two arteries and one vein should be apparent.)
• Observe the neonate for voiding and meconium.
• Assess the neonate for gross abnormalities and signs of suspected abnormalities.
• Continue to assess the neonate by using the Apgar score criteria, even after the 5-minute score is received.
• Obtain clear footprints and fingerprints.
• Apply identification bands with matching numbers to the mother (one band) and neonate (two bands) before they leave the delivery room.
• Promote bonding between the mother and neonate.
• Review maternal prenatal and intrapartal data to determine factors that might impact neonatal well-being.

Ongoing assessment
• Assess the neonate's vital signs.
• Measure and record blood pressure.
• Measure and record the neonate's size and weight.
• Complete a gestational age assessment if indicated.

Categorizing gestational age
• Preterm neonate—Less than 37 weeks' gestation
• Term neonate—37 to 42 weeks' gestation
• Postterm neonate—Greater than or equal to 42 weeks' gestation

Average neonatal size and weight

Size
Average initial anthropometric ranges are:
• head circumference—13″ to 14″ (33 to 35.5 cm)
• chest circumference—12″ to 13″ (30.5 to 33 cm)
• head to heel—18″ to 21″ (46 to 53 cm)
• weight—2,500 to 4,000 g (5 lb, 8 oz to 8 lb, 13 oz).

Birth weight
• Normal: 2,500 g (5 lb, 8 oz) or greater
• Low: 1,500 g (3 lb, 5 oz) to 2,499 g
• Very low: 1,000 g (2 lb, 3 oz) to 1,499 g
• Extremely low: Less than 1,000 g

Preventing heat loss

Follow these steps to prevent heat loss in the neonate.

Conduction
· Preheat the radiant warmer bed and linen.
· Warm stethoscopes and other instruments before use.
· Before weighing the neonate, pad the scale with a paper towel or a preweighed, warmed sheet.

Convection
· Place the neonate's bed out of a direct line with an open window, fan, or air-conditioning vent.

Evaporation
· Dry the neonate immediately after delivery.
· When bathing, expose only one body part at a time; wash each part thoroughly, and then dry it immediately.

Radiation
· Keep the neonate and examining tables away from outside windows and air conditioners.

Normal neonatal vital signs

Respiration
· 30 to 50 breaths/minute

Temperature
· Rectal: 96° to 99.5° F (35.6° to 37.5° C)
· Axillary: 97.5° to 99° F (36.4° to 37.2° C)

Heart rate (apical)
· 110 to 160 beats/minute

Blood pressure
· Systolic: 60 to 80 mm Hg
· Diastolic: 40 to 50 mm Hg

Counting neonatal respirations

· Observe abdominal excursions rather than chest excursions.
· Auscultate the chest.
· Place the stethoscope in front of the mouth and nares.

Recording the Apgar score

Use this chart to determine the neonatal Apgar score at 1 minute and 5 minutes after birth. For each category listed, assign a score of 0 to 2, as shown. A total score of 7 or higher indicates that the neonate is in good condition; 4 to 6, fair condition (the neonate may have moderate central nervous system depression, muscle flaccidity, cyanosis, and poor respirations); 0 to 3, danger (the neonate needs immediate resuscitation, as ordered).

Sign	Apgar score		
	0	1	2
Heart rate	Absent	Less than 100 beats/minute	More than 100 beats/minute
Respiratory effort	Absent	Slow, irregular	Good crying
Muscle tone	Flaccid	Some flexion and resistance to extension of extremities	Active motion
Reflex irritability	No response	Grimace or weak cry	Vigorous cry
Color	Pallor, cyanosis	Pink body, blue extremities	Completely pink

Silverman-Anderson index

Used to evaluate the neonate's respiratory status, the Silverman-Anderson index assesses five areas: upper chest, lower chest, xiphoid retractions, nares dilation, and expiratory grunt. Each area is graded 0 (no respiratory difficulty), 1 (moderate difficulty), or 2 (maximum difficulty), with a total score ranging from 0 (no respiratory difficulty) to 10 (maximum respiratory difficulty).

	Grade 0	Grade 1	Grade 2
Upper chest	Synchronized	Lag on inspiration	Seesaw
Lower chest	No retractions	Just visible	Marked
Xiphoid retractions	None	Just visible	Marked
Nares dilation	None	Minimal	Marked
Expiratory grunt	None	Audible with stethoscope	Audible to naked ear

Adapted with permission from Silverman, W.A., and Anderson, D.H. "A Controlled Clinical Trial of Effects of Water Mist on Obstructive Respiratory Signs, Death Rate, and Necropsy Findings among Premature Infants," *Pediatrics* 17(1):1-10, 1956.

Neurologic assessment

Normal neonates display various reflexes. Abnormalities are indicated by absence, asymmetry, persistence, or weakness in these reflexes:

- *sucking*—begins when a nipple is placed in the neonate's mouth
- *Moro reflex*—when the neonate is lifted above the crib and suddenly lowered, his arms and legs symmetrically extend and then abduct while his fingers spread to form a "C"
- *rooting*—when the neonate's cheek is stroked, he turns his head in the direction of the stroke
- *tonic neck (fencing position)*— when the neonate's head is turned while he's lying in a supine position, his extremities on the same side straighten and those on the opposite side flex
- *Babinski's reflex*—when the sole on the side of the neonate's small toe is stroked, the toes fan upward
- *grasping*—when a finger is placed in each of the neonate's hands, his fingers grasp tightly enough that he can be pulled to a sitting position
- *stepping*—when the neonate is held upright with his feet touching a flat surface, he responds with dancing or stepping movements.

Common skin findings

The term neonate has beefy red skin for a few hours after birth before he turns his normal color. Other findings include:

- acrocyanosis (caused by vasomotor instability, capillary stasis, and high hemoglobin level) for the first 24 hours
- milia (clogged sebaceous glands) on the nose or chin
- lanugo (fine, downy hair) after 20 weeks' gestation on the entire body (except on palms and soles)
- vernix caseosa (a white, cheesy protective coating of desquamated epithelial cells and sebum)
- erythema toxicum neonatorum (a transient, maculopapular rash)
- telangiectasia (flat, reddened vascular areas) on the neck, eyelid, or lip
- port-wine stain (nevus flammeus), a capillary angioma below the dermis; commonly on the face
- strawberry hemangioma (nevus vasculosus), a capillary angioma in the dermal and subdermal skin layers indicated by a rough, raised, sharply demarcated birthmark
- sudamina or miliaria (distended sweat glands) that cause minute vesicles on the skin surface, especially on the face
- Mongolian spots (bluish black areas of pigmentation more commonly noted on the back and buttocks of dark-skinned neonates).

Assessing the neonate's head

The neonate's head may appear misshapen or asymmetrical. Caput succedaneum usually disappears in about 3 days. A cephalhematoma may take several weeks to resolve.

Caput succedaneum
· Swelling occurs below the scalp.
· Swelling can extend past the suture line.
· Usually disappears in about 3 days.

Cephalhematoma
· Swelling results from blood collecting under the periosteum of the skull bone.
· Swelling doesn't cross the suture line.
· May take several weeks to resolve.

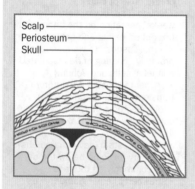

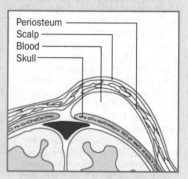

Neonatal sutures and fontanels

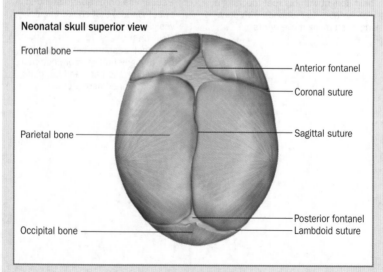

Assessing hip abduction

Assessing hip abduction helps identify whether the neonate's hip joint, including the acetabulum, is properly formed. Follow these steps:

· Place the neonate in the supine position on a bed or examination table.
· Flex the neonate's knees to 90 degrees at the hip.
· Apply upward pressure over the greater trochanter area while abducting the hips; typically, the hips should abduct to about 180 degrees, almost touching the surface of the bed or examination table.
· Listen for any sounds; normally this motion should produce no sound; evidence of a clicking or clunking sound denotes the femoral head hitting the acetabulum as it slips back into it. This sound is considered a positive Ortolani sign, suggesting hip subluxation.
· Flex the neonate's knees and hips to 90 degrees.

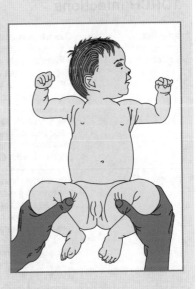

· Apply pressure down and laterally while adducting the hips.
· Feel for any slipping of the femoral head out of the hip socket. Evidence of slipping denotes a positive Barlow's sign, suggesting hip instability and possible developmental dysplasia of the hip.

TORCH infections

Infection	Description and implications
Toxoplasmosis	• Toxoplasmosis is transmitted to the fetus primarily via the mother's contact with contaminated cat box filler. • Effects include increased frequency of stillbirths, neonatal deaths, severe congenital anomalies, deafness, retinochoroiditis, seizures, and coma. • A therapeutic abortion is recommended if the diagnosis is made before 20 weeks' gestation. • Maternal treatment involves anti-infective therapy—for example, with a sulfa drug or clindamycin.
Rubella	• Rubella, a chronic viral infection, lasts from the first trimester to months after delivery. • The greatest risk occurs within the first trimester. • Effects include congenital heart disease, intrauterine growth retardation, cataracts, mental retardation, and hearing impairment. • Management includes therapeutic abortion if the disease occurs during the first trimester, and emotional support for the parents. • Women of childbearing age should be tested for immunity and vaccinated if necessary. • The neonate may persistently shed the virus for up to 1 year.
Cytomegalovirus (CMV)	• CMV is a herpesvirus that can be transmitted from an asymptomatic mother transplacentally to the fetus or via the cervix to the neonate at delivery. • It's the most common cause of viral infections in fetuses. • Principal sites of damage are the brain, liver, and blood. • CMV is a common cause of mental retardation. • Other effects include auditory difficulties and a birth weight that's small for gestational age. • The neonate may also demonstrate a characteristic pattern of petechiae called *blueberry muffin syndrome.* • Antiviral drugs can't prevent CMV and aren't effective in treating the neonate.
Herpesvirus type II	• The fetus can be exposed to the herpesvirus through indirect contact with infected genitals or via direct contact with those tissues during delivery. • Affected neonates may be asymptomatic for 2 to 12 days but then may develop jaundice, seizures, increased temperature, and characteristic vesicular lesions. • A cesarean birth can protect the fetus from infection. • Pharmacologic treatment may include acyclovir and vidarabine I.V. after exposure.

Administering vitamin K

Vitamin K (AquaMEPHYTON) is administered prophylactically to prevent a transient deficiency of coagulation factors II, VII, IX, and X.
· Dosage is 0.5 to 1 mg I.M. up to 1 hour after birth.
· Administer in a large leg muscle such as the vastus lateralis (as shown).

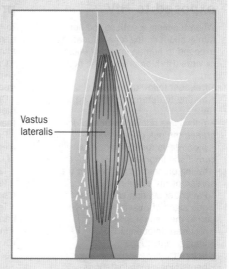

Vastus lateralis

Erythromycin treatment

Description
· Involves instilling 0.5% erythromycin ointment into the neonate's eyes
· Prevents gonorrheal conjunctivitis caused by *Neisseria gonorrhoeae,* which the neonate may have acquired from the mother as he passed through the birth canal (Erythromycin is also effective against chlamydial infection.)
· Required by law in all 50 states
· May be administered in the birthing room
· Can be delayed for up to 1 hour to allow initial parent-child bonding
· May not be effective if the infection was acquired in utero from premature rupture of membranes

Procedure
· Wash your hands and put on gloves.
· Using your nondominant hand, gently raise the neonate's upper eyelid with your index finger.
· Pull down the lower lid with your thumb.
· Using your dominant hand, apply the ointment in a line along the lower conjunctival sac (as shown here).
· Close the eye to allow ointment to spread across the conjunctiva.
· Repeat the procedure for the other eye.

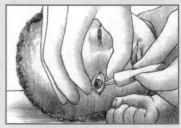

Caring for a neonate exposed to HIV

When teaching a patient and her family about caring for a neonate exposed to human immunodeficiency virus (HIV), emphasize the need for:
• frequent follow-up
• testing to determine infection status
• zidovudine administration to decrease the risk of infection
• prophylaxis for *Pneumocystis carinii* pneumonia
• taking precautions to prevent the spread of HIV infection.

Patient education should also include signs of possible HIV infection in the neonate, including:
• recurrent infections
• unusual infections
• failure to thrive
• hematologic manifestations
• renal disease
• neurologic manifestations.

Teaching parents of a premature neonate

To help the parents of a premature neonate cope with this difficult situation, follow these guidelines.
• Orient them to the neonatal intensive care unit environment and introduce them to all caregivers.
• Orient them to the machinery and monitors that may be attached to their neonate.
• Reassure them that the staff is alert to alarms as well as the cues of their child.
• Tell them what to expect.
• Teach them the characteristics of a premature neonate.
• Teach them how to handle their neonate.
• Instruct them on feeding, whether it's through gavage, breast, or bottle.
• Inform them of potential complications.
• Offer discharge planning.
• Make appropriate referrals.

Teaching parents about PKU

Phenylketonuria (PKU) is an inborn error of metabolism characterized by the body's inability to metabolize the essential amino acid phenylalanine. Teach parents how to limit phenylalanine intake by:
• providing a basic understanding of the disorder
• offering practical suggestions for meal planning
• instructing the family on how to:
  – eliminate or restrict foods high in phenylalanine
  – determine if foods are low in phenylalanine by reading food labels
  – avoid using artificial sweeteners containing aspartame (such as NutraSweet).

Teaching proper care of a circumcision

Be sure to show parents the circumcision before discharge so that they can ask questions. Teach them these tips for proper care of a circumcision.
• Reapply fresh petroleum gauze after each diaper change, if applicable.
• Don't use premoistened towelettes to clean the penis because they contain alcohol, which can delay healing and cause discomfort.
• Don't attempt to remove exudate that forms around the penis. Removing exudate can cause bleeding.
• Change the neonate's diaper at least every 4 hours to prevent it from sticking to the penis.
• Check to make sure that the neonate urinates after being circumcised. He should have 6 to 10 wet diapers in a 24-hour period. If he doesn't, notify the pediatrician.
• Wash the penis with warm water to remove urine or stools until the circumcision is healed. Soap can be used after the circumcision has healed.
• Notify the pediatrician if redness, swelling, or discharge is present on the penis. These signs may indicate infection. Note that the penis is dark red after circumcision and then becomes covered with a yellow exudate in 24 hours.

Performing phototherapy

To perform phototherapy, follow these steps:

· Set up the phototherapy unit about 18″ (46 cm) above the neonate's crib and verify placement of the lightbulb shield. If the neonate is in an incubator, place the phototherapy unit at least 3″ (7.5 cm) above the incubator and turn on the lights. Place a photometer probe in the middle of the crib to measure the energy emitted by the lights.

· Explain the procedure to the parents.

· Record the neonate's initial bilirubin level and his axillary temperature.

· Place the opaque eye mask over the neonate's closed eyes and fasten securely.

· Undress the neonate and place a diaper under him. Cover male genitalia with a surgical mask or small diaper to catch urine and prevent possible testicular damage from the heat and light waves.

· Take the neonate's axillary temperature every 2 hours and provide additional warmth by adjusting the warming unit's thermostat.

· Monitor elimination and weigh the neonate twice daily. Watch for signs of dehydration (dry skin, poor turgor, depressed fontanels) and check urine specific gravity with a urinometer to gauge hydration status.

· Take the neonate out of the crib, turn off the phototherapy lights, and unmask his eyes at least every 3 to 4 hours with feedings. Assess his eyes for inflammation or injury.

· Reposition the neonate every 2 hours to expose all body surfaces to the light and to prevent head molding and skin breakdown from pressure.

· Check the bilirubin level at least once every 24 hours—more often if levels rise significantly. Turn off the phototherapy unit before drawing venous blood for testing because the lights may degrade bilirubin in the blood. Notify the pediatrician if the bilirubin level nears 20 mg/dl in full-term neonates or 15 mg/dl in premature neonates.

Normal neonatal laboratory values

This chart shows laboratory tests that may be ordered for neonates, including the normal ranges for full-term neonates. Note that ranges may vary among facilities. Because test results for preterm neonates usually reflect weight and gestational age, ranges for preterm neonates vary.

Test	Normal range
Blood	
Acid phosphatase	7.4 to 19.4 units/L
Albumin	3.6 to 5.4 g/dl
Alkaline phosphatase	40 to 300 units/L (1 week)
Alpha fetoprotein	Up to 10 mg/L, with none detected after 21 days
Ammonia	90 to 150 mcg/dl
Amylase	0 to 1,000 international units/hour
Bicarbonate	20 to 26 mmol/L
Bilirubin, direct	< 0.5 mg/dl
Bilirubin, total	< 2.8 mg/dl (cord blood)
0 to 1 day	2.6 mg/dl (peripheral blood)
1 to 2 days	6 to 7 mg/dl (peripheral blood)
3 to 5 days	4 to 6 mg/dl (peripheral blood)
Bleeding time	2 minutes
Arterial blood gases	
pH	7.35 to 7.45
$Paco_2$	35 to 45 mm Hg
Pao_2	50 to 90 mm Hg
Venous blood gases	
pH	7.35 to 7.45
Pco_2	41 to 51 mm Hg
Po_2	20 to 49 mm Hg
Calcium, ionized	2.5 to 5 mg/dl
Calcium, total	7 to 12 mg/dl
Chloride	95 to 110 mEq/L
Clotting time (2 tubes)	5 to 8 minutes
Creatine kinase	10 to 300 international units/L
Creatinine	0.3 to 1 mg/dl
Digoxin level	> 2 ng/ml possible; > 30 ng/ml probable
Fibrinogen	0.18 to 0.38 g/dl
Glucose	30 to 125 mg/dl
Glutamyltransferase	14 to 331 units/L
Hematocrit	52% to 58% 53% (cord blood)
Hemoglobin	17 to 18.4 g/dl 16.8 g/dl (cord blood)
Immunoglobulins (Ig), total	660 to 1,439 mg/dl
IgG	398 to 1,244 mg/dl
IgM	5 to 30 mg/dl
IgA	0 to 2.2 mg/dl
Iron	100 to 250 mcg/dl
Iron-binding capacity	100 to 400 mcg/dl

(continued)

Normal neonatal laboratory values *(continued)*

Test	Normal range
Blood *(continued)*	
Lactate dehydrogenase	357 to 953 international units/L
Magnesium	1.5 to 2.5 mEq/L
Osmolality	270 to 294 mOsm/kg H_2O
Partial thromboplastin time	40 to 80 seconds
Phenobarbital level	15 to 40 mcg/dl
Phosphorus	5 to 7.8 mg/dl (birth)
	4.9 to 8.9 mg/dl (7 days)
Platelets	100,000 to 300,000/µl
Potassium	4.5 to 6.8 mEq/L
Protein, total	4.6 to 7.4 g/dl
Prothrombin time	12 to 21 seconds
Red blood cell (RBC) count	5.1 to 5.8 (1,000,000/µl)
Reticulocytes	3% to 7% (cord blood)
Sodium	136 to 143 mEq/L
Theophylline level	5 to 10 mcg/ml
Thyroid-stimulating hormone	< 7 microunits/ml
Thyroxine	10.2 to 19 mcg/dl
Transaminase	
glutamic-oxaloacetic (aspartate)	24 to 81 units/L
glutamic-pyruvic (alanine)	10 to 33 units/L
Triglycerides	36 to 233 mg/dl
Urea nitrogen	5 to 25 mg/dl
White blood cell (WBC) count	18,000/µl
eosinophils-basophils	3%
immature WBCs	10%
lymphocytes	30%
monocytes	5%
neutrophils	45%
Urine	
Casts, WBCs	Present first 2 to 4 days
Osmolality	50 to 600 mOsm/kg
pH	5 to 7
Phenylketonuria	No color change
Protein	Present first 2 to 4 days
Specific gravity	1.006 to 1.008

Normal neonatal laboratory values *(continued)*

Test	Normal range
Cerebrospinal fluid	
Calcium	4.2 to 5.4 mg/dl
Cell count	0 to 15 WBCs/µl
	0 to 500 RBCs/µl
Chloride	110 to 120 mg/L
Glucose	32 to 62 mg/dl
pH	7.33 to 7.42
Pressure	50 to 80 mm Hg
Protein	32 to 148 mg/dl
Sodium	130 to 165 mg/L
Specific gravity	1.007 to 1.009

Pediatric care

Stages of childhood development

- *Infancy:* Birth to age 1
- *Toddler stage:* Ages 1 to 3
- *Preschool stage:* Ages 3 to 6
- *School age:* Ages 6 to 12
- *Adolescence:* Ages 12 to 19

Patterns of development

This chart shows the patterns of development and their progression and gives examples of each.

Pattern	Path of progression	Examples
Cephalocaudal	From head to toe	Head control precedes the ability to walk.
Proximodistal	From the trunk to the tips of the extremities	The infant can move his arms and legs but can't pick up objects with his fingers.
General to specific	From simple tasks to more complex tasks (mastering simple tasks before advancing to those that are more complex)	The child progresses from crawling to walking to skipping.

Theories of development

The child development theories discussed in this chart shouldn't be compared directly because they measure different aspects of development. Erik Erikson's psychosocial-based theory is the most commonly accepted model for child development, although it can't be empirically tested.

Age-group	Psychosocial theory	Cognitive theory	Psychosexual theory	Moral development theory
Infancy (birth to age 1)	Trust versus mistrust	Sensorimotor	Oral	Not applicable
Toddlerhood (ages 1 to 3)	Autonomy versus shame and doubt	Sensorimotor to preoperational	Anal	Preconventional
Preschool age (ages 3 to 6)	Initiative versus guilt	Preoperational	Phallic	Preconventional
School age (ages 6 to 12)	Industry versus inferiority	Concrete operational	Latency	Conventional
Adolescence (ages 12 to 19)	Identity versus role confusion	Formal operational thought	Genitalia	Postconventional

A closer look at theories of development

Psychosocial theory (Erik Erikson)

• Trust versus mistrust: Develops trust as the primary caregiver meets his needs.

• Autonomy versus shame and doubt: Learns to control body functions; becomes increasingly independent.

• Initiative versus guilt: Learns about the world through play; develops a conscience.

• Industry versus inferiority: Enjoys working with others; tends to follow rules; forming social relationships takes on greater importance.

• Identity versus role confusion: Is preoccupied with how he looks and how others view him; tries to establish his own identity while meeting the expectations of his peers.

Cognitive theory (Jean Piaget)

• Sensorimotor stage: Progresses from reflex activity, through simple repetitive behaviors, to imitative behaviors; concepts to be mastered include object permanence, causality, and spatial relationships.

• Preoperational stage: Is egocentric and employs magical thinking; concepts to be mastered include representational language and symbols and transductive reasoning.

• Concrete operational stage: Thought processes become more logical and coherent; can't think abstractly; concepts to be mastered include sorting, ordering, and classifying facts to use in problem solving.

• Formal operational thought stage: Is adaptable and flexible; concepts to be mastered include abstract ideas and concepts, possibilities, inductive reasoning, and complex deductive reasoning.

Psychosexual theory (Sigmund Freud)

• Involves the *id* (primitive instincts; requires immediate gratification), *ego* (conscious, rational part of the personality), and *superego* (a person's conscience and ideals).

• Oral stage: Seeks pleasure through sucking, biting, and other oral activities.

• Anal stage: Goes through toilet training, learning how to control his excreta.

• Phallic stage: Interested in his genitalia; discovers the difference between boys and girls.

• Latency period: Concentrates on playing and learning (not focused on a particular body area).

• Genitalia stage: At maturation of the reproductive system, develops the capacity for object love and maturity.

Moral development theory (Lawrence Kohlberg)

• Preconventional level of morality: Attempts to follow rules set by authority figures; adjusts behavior according to good and bad, right and wrong.

• Conventional level of morality: Seeks conformity and loyalty; follows fixed rules; attempts to maintain social order.

• Postconventional autonomous level of morality: Strives to construct a value system independent of authority figures and peers.

Expected growth rates

Age-group	Weight	Height or length	Head circumference
Infancy (birth to age 1)	• Birth weight doubles by age 5 months • Birth weight triples by age 1 • Gains 1½ lb (680 g)/month for first 5 months • Gains ¾ lb (340 g)/month during second 6 months	• Birth length increases by 50% by age 1, with most growth occurring in the trunk rather than the legs • Grows 1" (2.5 cm)/month during first 6 months • Grows ½" (1.3 cm)/month during second 6 months	• Increases by almost 33% by age 1 • Increases ¾" (1.9 cm)/month during the first 3 months • Increases ⅓" (0.86 cm)/month from ages 4 to 6 months • Increases ¼" (0.6 cm)/month during second 6 months
Toddlerhood (ages 1 to 3)	• Birth weight quadruples by age 2½ • Gains 8 oz (227 g)/month from ages 1 to 2 • Gains 3 to 5 lb (1.5 to 2.5 kg) from ages 2 to 3	• Growth occurs mostly in legs rather than trunk • Grows 3½" to 5" (9 to 12.5 cm) from ages 1 to 2 • Grows 2" to 2½" (5 to 6.5 cm) from ages 2 to 3	• Increases 1" (2.5 cm) from ages 1 to 2 • Increases less than ½" (1.3 cm)/year from ages 2 to 3
Preschool age (ages 3 to 6)	• Gains 3 to 5 lb (1.5 to 2.5 kg)/year	• Growth occurs mostly in legs rather than trunk • Grows 2½" to 3" (6.5 to 7.5 cm)/year	• Increases less than ½"/year from ages 3 to 5
School age (ages 6 to 12)	• Gains 6 lb (2.7 kg)/year	• Grows 2" (5.1 cm)/year • Girls: Grow 3" to 6" (7.5 to 15 cm)/year until age 16	• Not applicable
Adolescence (ages 12 to 19)	• Girls: Gain 15 to 55 lb (7 to 25 kg) • Boys: Gain 15 to 65 lb (7 to 29.5 kg)	• Boys: Grow 3" to 6"/year until age 18	• Not applicable

Height measurements for boys, ages 2 through 18 years

| Age | Height by percentiles | | | | | |
	10%		50%		90%	
	cm	*inches*	*cm*	*inches*	*cm*	*inches*
2 years	84.7	33.3	91.0	35.8	97.6	38.4
3 years	92.5	36.4	98.8	38.9	103.9	40.9
4 years	100.7	39.6	106.5	41.9	112.1	44.1
5 years	105.8	41.7	114.2	45.0	119.1	46.9
6 years	111.6	43.9	119.3	47.0	125.9	49.6
7 years	117.7	46.3	126.6	49.8	135.0	53.1
8 years	123.8	48.7	132.5	52.2	140.9	55.5
9 years	130.1	51.2	137.5	54.1	145.4	57.2
10 years	133.4	52.5	141.1	55.6	149.1	58.7
11 years	139.7	55.0	148.8	58.6	157.4	62.0
12 years	143.0	56.3	153.9	60.6	167.8	66.0
13 years	147.2	58.0	160.5	63.2	171.6	67.6
14 years	155.1	61.1	169.1	66.6	179.0	70.5
15 years	163.5	64.4	174.2	68.6	182.8	72.0
16 years	165.7	65.2	175.3	69.0	183.4	72.2
17 years	166.6	65.6	175.6	69.1	184.2	72.5
18 years	168.1	66.2	176.1	69.3	184.9	72.8

Adapted from McDowell, M.A., et al. *Anthropometric Reference Data for Children and Adults: U.S. Population, 1999–2002.* U.S. Department of Health and Human Services, Centers for Disease Control and Prevention, National Center for Health Statistics, 2005.

Weight measurements for boys, ages 1 through 18 years

| Age | Weight by percentiles | | | | | |
| | 10% | | 50% | | 90% | |
	kg	lb	kg	lb	kg	lb
1 year	9.5	20.9	11.1	24.5	13.1	28.9
2 years	11.5	25.4	13.7	30.2	15.9	35.1
3 years	12.9	28.4	16.0	35.3	18.8	41.4
4 years	15.4	34.0	18.2	40.1	21.4	47.2
5 years	17.0	37.5	20.7	45.6	26.0	57.3
6 years	18.2	40.1	22.7	50.0	29.0	63.9
7 years	21.6	47.6	25.7	56.7	33.1	73.0
8 years	23.5	51.8	30.4	67.0	45.8	101.0
9 years	26.5	58.4	34.1	75.2	49.6	109.3
10 years	27.8	61.3	36.1	79.6	50.2	110.7
11 years	31.2	68.8	42.1	92.9	57.2	126.1
12 years	35.0	77.1	46.3	102.1	71.8	158.3
13 years	34.2	75.4	53.0	116.9	75.3	166.0
14 years	45.4	100.0	61.0	134.5	90.1	198.6
15 years	51.7	114.0	64.0	141.1	93.1	205.3
16 years	54.9	121.0	69.4	153.0	97.6	215.2
17 years	55.6	122.6	70.6	155.6	98.1	216.3
18 years	58.3	128.5	72.9	160.7	98.9	218.0

Adapted from McDowell, M.A., et al. *Anthropometric Reference Data for Children and Adults: U.S. Population, 1999–2002*. U.S. Department of Health and Human Services, Centers for Disease Control and Prevention, National Center for Health Statistics, 2005.

Height measurements for girls, ages 2 through 18 years

| Age | Height by percentiles | | | | | |
	10%		50%		90%	
	cm	inches	cm	inches	cm	inches
2 years	84.9	33.4	89.7	35.3	95.3	37.5
3 years	92.6	36.5	98.1	38.6	102.2	40.2
4 years	100.3	39.5	105.8	41.6	111.7	44.0
5 years	106.5	41.9	111.9	44.1	119.5	47.0
6 years	110.2	43.4	117.2	46.1	124.0	48.8
7 years	117.5	46.3	124.2	48.9	131.6	51.8
8 years	123.0	48.4	131.0	51.6	138.5	54.5
9 years	128.2	50.5	137.2	54.0	146.5	57.7
10 years	*	*	142.8	56.2	*	*
11 years	141.1	55.6	151.3	59.6	161.1	63.4
12 years	146.5	57.7	156.6	61.7	164.8	64.9
13 years	149.9	59.0	158.4	62.4	168.6	66.4
14 years	154.1	60.7	161.6	63.6	169.2	66.6
15 years	153.2	60.3	162.5	64.0	169.3	66.7
16 years	154.0	60.6	161.3	63.5	169.6	66.8
17 years	154.6	60.9	163.5	64.4	172.1	67.8
18 years	155.4	61.2	163.1	64.2	171.2	67.4

* Figure doesn't meet the standard of reliability or precision.
Adapted from McDowell, M.A., et al. *Anthropometric Reference Data for Children and Adults: U.S. Population, 1999-2002.* U.S. Department of Health and Human Services, Centers for Disease Control and Prevention, National Center for Health Statistics, 2005.

Weight measurements for girls, ages 1 through 18 years

| Age | Weight by percentiles | | | | | |
| | 10% | | 50% | | 90% | |
	kg	lb	kg	lb	kg	lb
1 year	9.1	20.1	10.6	23.4	12.9	28.4
2 years	11.1	24.5	12.9	28.4	15.6	34.4
3 years	12.9	28.4	15.0	33.1	17.5	38.6
4 years	14.7	32.4	17.2	38.0	20.8	45.9
5 years	16.6	36.6	19.2	42.3	26.9	59.3
6 years	17.9	39.5	21.5	47.4	27.7	61.1
7 years	20.3	44.8	24.7	54.5	32.9	72.5
8 years	22.3	49.2	29.1	64.2	44.1	97.2
9 years	25.6	56.4	34.1	75.2	48.4	106.7
10 years	27.8	61.3	38.3	84.5	53.9	118.8
11 years	32.9	72.6	44.9	99.0	69.0	152.1
12 years	36.3	80.0	49.7	109.6	69.3	152.8
13 years	41.0	90.4	55.5	122.4	79.7	175.7
14 years	46.2	101.9	56.3	124.1	80.9	178.4
15 years	45.7	100.8	57.6	127.0	83.3	183.6
16 years	47.7	105.2	59.1	130.3	84.1	185.4
17 years	46.7	103.0	59.3	130.8	87.3	192.4
18 years	47.0	103.6	60.9	134.3	93.2	205.5

Adapted from McDowell, M.A., et al. *Anthropometric Reference Data for Children and Adults: U.S. Population, 1999–2002.* U.S. Department of Health and Human Services, Centers for Disease Control and Prevention, National Center for Health Statistics, 2005.

Infant gross and fine motor development

Age	Gross motor skills
1 month	• Can hold head parallel momentarily but still has marked head lag • Back is rounded in sitting position, with no head control
2 months	• In prone position, can lift head 45 degrees off table • In sitting position, back is still rounded but with more head control
3 months	• Displays only slight head lag when pulled to a seated position • In prone position, can use forearms to lift head and shoulders 45 to 90 degrees off table • Can bear slight amount of weight on legs in standing position
4 months	• No head lag • Holds head erect in sitting position, back less rounded • In prone position, can lift head and chest 90 degrees off table • Can roll from back to side
5 months	• No head lag • Holds head erect and steady when sitting • Back is straight • Can put feet to mouth when supine • Can roll from stomach to back
6 months	• Can lift chest and upper abdomen off table, bearing weight on hands • Can roll from back to stomach • Can bear almost all of weight on feet when held in standing position • Sits with support
7 months	• Can sit, leaning forward on hands for support • When in standing position, can bear full weight on legs and bounce
8 months	• Can sit alone without assistance • Can move from sitting to kneeling position
9 months	• Creeps on hands and knees with belly off of floor • Pulls to standing position • Can stand while holding on to furniture
10 months	• Can move from prone to sitting position • Stands with support; may lift a foot as if to take a step
11 months	• Can cruise (take side steps while holding on to furniture) or walk with both hands held
12 months	• Cruises well; may walk with one hand held • May try to stand alone

Fine motor skills

- Strong grasp reflex
- Hands remain mostly closed in a fist

- Diminishing grasp reflex
- Hands open more often

- Grasp reflex now absent
- Hands remain open
- Can hold a rattle and clutch own hand

- Regards own hand
- Can grasp objects with both hands
- May try to reach for an object without success
- Can move objects toward mouth

- Can voluntarily grasp objects
- Can move objects directly to mouth

- Can hold bottle
- Can voluntarily grasp and release objects

- Transfers objects from hand to hand
- Rakes at objects
- Can bang objects on table

- Has beginning pincer grasp
- Reaches for objects out of reach

- Refining pincer grasp
- Use of dominant hand evident

- Refining pincer grasp

- Can move objects into containers
- Deliberately drops object to have it picked up
- Neat pincer grasp

- May attempt to build a two-block tower
- Can crudely turn pages of a book
- Feeds self with cup and spoon

Infant language and social development

Age	Behaviors
0 to 2 months	• Listens to voices; quiets to soft music, singing, or talking • Distinguishes mother's voice after 1 week, father's by 2 weeks • Prefers human voices to other sounds • Produces vowel sounds "ah," "eh," and "oh"
3 to 4 months	• Coos and gurgles • Babbles in response to someone talking to him • Babbles for own pleasure with giggles, shrieks, and laughs • Says "da," "ba," "ma," "pa," and "ga" • Vocalizes more to a real person than to a picture • Responds to caregiver with a social smile by 3 months
5 to 6 months	• Notices how his speech influences the actions of others • Makes "raspberries" and smacks lips • Begins learning to take turns in conversation • Talks to toys and self in mirror • Recognizes names and familiar sounds
7 to 9 months	• Tries to imitate more sounds; makes several sounds in one breath • Begins learning the meaning of "no" by tone of voice and actions • Experiences early literacy; enjoys listening to simple books being read • Enjoys pat-a-cake • Recognizes and responds to his name and names of familiar objects
10 to 12 months	• May have a few word approximations, such as "bye-bye" and "hi" • Follows one-step instructions such as "go to daddy" • Recognizes words as symbols for objects • Says "ma-ma-ma" and "da-da-da"

Infant cognitive development and play

This table shows the infant's development of two cognitive skills: object permanence and causality. It includes play, an integral part of infant development.

Age	Object permanence	Causality	Play
0 to 4 months	• Doesn't think of objects once they are out of sight • Continues to look at hand after object is dropped out of it	• Creates bodily sensations by actions (for example, thumb-sucking)	• Grasps and moves objects such as a rattle • Looks at contrasting colors
4 to 8 months	• Can locate a partially hidden object • Visually tracks dropped objects	• Uses causal behaviors to re-create accidentally discovered interesting effects (for example, kicking the bed after the chance discovery that this will set in motion a mobile above the bed)	• Reaches and grasps an object and then will mouth, shake, bang, and drop the object (in this order)
9 to 12 months	• Develops object permanence • Can find an object when hidden but can't retrieve an object that's moved in plain view from one hiding place to another • Knows parents still exist when out of view but can't imagine where they might be (separation anxiety may arise)	• Understands cause and effect, which leads to intentional behavior aimed at getting specific results	• Manipulates objects to inspect with eyes and hands • Has ability to process information simultaneously instead of sequentially • Demonstrates object permanence via ability to play peek-a-boo

Toddler gross and fine motor development

Age	Gross motor skills	Fine motor skills
1 year	• Walks alone using a wide stance • Begins to run but falls easily	• Grasps a very small object (but can't release it until about 15 months)
2 years	• Runs without falling most of the time • Throws a ball overhand without losing balance • Jumps with both feet • Walks up and down stairs • Uses push and pull toys	• Builds a tower of four blocks • Scribbles on paper • Drops a small pellet into a small, narrow container • Uses a spoon well and drinks well from a covered cup • Undresses himself

Toddler language development

During toddlerhood, the ability to understand speech is much more developed than the ability to speak. This table highlights language development during the toddler years.

Age	Language skills
1 year	• The toddler uses one-word sentences or holophrases (real words that are meant to represent entire phrases or ideas). • The toddler has learned about four words. • About 25% of a 1-year-old's vocalization is understandable.
2 years	• The number of words learned has increased from about 4 (at age 1) to approximately 300. • The toddler uses multiword (two- to three-word) sentences. • About 65% of speech is understandable. • Frequent, repetitive naming of objects helps toddlers learn appropriate words for objects.

Toddler socialization

Toddlers develop social skills that determine the way they interact with others. As the toddler develops psychologically, he can:
• differentiate himself from others
• tolerate being separated from a parent
• withstand delayed gratification
• control his bodily functions
• acquire socially acceptable behaviors
• communicate verbally
• become less egocentric.

Toddler psychosocial development

According to Erikson, the developmental task of toddlerhood is autonomy versus doubt and shame. Toddlers:
• are in the final stages of developing a sense of trust (the task from infancy) and start asserting control, independence, and autonomy
• display negativism in their quest for autonomy
• need to maintain sameness and reliability for comfort; employ ritualism
• view the "paternal" person in their life as a significant other
• develop an ego, which creates conflict between the impulses of the id (which requires immediate gratification) and socially acceptable actions
• begin to develop a superego, or conscience, which starts to incorporate the morals of society.

Toddler cognitive development

According to Piaget, a child moves from the sensorimotor stage of infancy and early toddlerhood (birth to age 2) to the longer, preoperational stage (ages 2 to 7). In these stages, toddlers:
• employ tertiary circular reactions (use of active experimentation; also called *trial and error* [in the 13- to 18-month-old])
• may be aware of the relationship between two events (cause and effect) but may be unable to transfer that knowledge to a new situation
• look for new ways to accomplish tasks through mental calculations (ages 18 to 24 months)
• advance in understanding object permanence and gain awareness of the existence of objects or people that are out of sight
• engage in imitative play, which indicates a deeper understanding of their role in the family
• begin to use preoperational thought with increasing use of words as symbols, problem solving, and creative thinking.

Toddler play

• Play changes considerably as the toddler's motor skills develop; he uses his physical skills to push and pull objects; to climb up, down, in, and out; and to run or ride on toys.

• A short attention span requires frequent changes in toys and play media.

• Toddlers increase their cognitive abilities by manipulating objects and learning about their qualities, which makes tactile play (with water, sand, finger paints, clay) important.

• Many play activities involve imitating behaviors the child sees at home, which helps him learn new actions and skills.

• Toddlers engage in parallel play—playing with others without actually interacting. In this type of play, children play side-by-side, commonly with similar objects. Interaction is limited to the occasional comment or trading of toys.

Safe toddler toys

• Play dough and modeling clay
• Building blocks
• Plastic, pretend housekeeping toys, such as pots, pans, and play food
• Stackable rings and blocks of varying sizes
• Toy telephones
• Wooden puzzles with big pieces
• Textured or cloth books
• Plastic musical instruments and noise-makers
• Toys that roll, such as cars and trains
• Tricycles or riding cars
• Fat crayons and coloring books
• Stuffed animals with painted faces (button eyes are a choking hazard)

Preschool gross and fine motor development

Age	Gross motor skills	Fine motor skills
3 years	• Stands on one foot for a few seconds • Climbs stairs with alternating feet • Jumps in place • Performs a broad jump • Dances but with somewhat poor balance • Kicks a ball • Rides a tricycle	• Builds a tower of nine or 10 blocks and a three-block bridge • Copies a circle and imitates a cross and vertical and horizontal lines • Draws a circle as a head, but not a complete stick figure • Uses a fork well
4 years	• Hops, jumps, and skips on one foot • Throws a ball overhand • Rides a tricycle or bicycle with training wheels	• Copies a square and traces a cross • Draws recognizable familiar objects or human figures
5 years	• Skips, using alternate feet • Jumps rope • Balances on each foot for 4 or 5 seconds	• Copies a triangle and a diamond • Draws a stick figure with several body parts, including facial features

Preschool language development and socialization

By the time a child reaches pre-school age:
· his vocabulary increases to about 900 words by age 3 and 2,100 words by age 5
· he may talk incessantly and ask many "why" questions
· he usually talks in three- or four-word sentences by age 3; by age 5, he speaks in longer sentences that contain all parts of speech.

Socialization continues to develop as the preschooler's world expands beyond himself and his family (although parents remain central). Regular interaction with same-age children is necessary to further develop social skills.

Preschool psychosocial development

According to Erik Erikson, children ages 3 to 5 have mastered a sense of autonomy and face the task of initiative versus guilt. During this time, the child's:
· significant other is the family
· conscience begins to develop, introducing the concept of right and wrong
· sense of guilt arises when he feels that his imagination and activities are unacceptable or clash with his parents' expectations
· simple reasoning develops and longer periods of delayed gratification are tolerated.

Preschool play

In the preschool stage, the parallel play of toddlerhood is replaced by more interactive, cooperative play, including:
· more associative play, in which children play together
· better understanding of the concept of sharing
· enjoyment of large motor activities, such as swinging, riding tricycles or bicycles, and throwing balls
· more dramatic play, in which the child lives out the dramas of human life (in preschool years) and may have imaginary playmates.

Preschool cognitive development

Jean Piaget's theory divides the pre-operational phase of the preschool years into two stages.

Preconceptual phase
During the preconceptual phase (from ages 2 to 4), the child can:
· form beginning concepts that aren't as complete or logical as an adult's
· make simple classifications
· rationalize specific concepts but not the idea as a whole
· exhibit egocentric thinking (evaluating each situation based on his feelings or experiences, rather than those of others).

Intuitive thought phase
During the intuitive thought phase (from ages 4 to 7), the child:
· can classify, quantify, and relate objects (but can't yet understand the principles behind these operations)
· uses intuitive thought processes (but can't fully see the viewpoints of others)
· uses many words appropriately (but without true understanding of their meaning).

Preschool moral and spiritual development

Lawrence Kohlberg's preconventional phase spans the preschool years and more, extending from ages 4 to 10. During this phase:
· the preschooler's conscience emerges and its emphasis is on control
· the preschooler's moral standards are those of others, and he understands that these standards must be followed to avoid punishment for inappropriate behavior or gain rewards for good or desired behavior
· the preschooler behaves according to what freedom is given or what restriction is placed on his actions.

Preschoolers can understand the basic plot of simple religious stories but typically don't grasp the underlying meanings. Religious principles are best learned from concrete images in picture books and small statues such as those seen at a place of worship.

During this stage, children may view an illness or hospitalization as a punishment from a higher being for some real or perceived bad behavior.

School-age fine motor development

· Development of small-muscle and eye-hand coordination increases during the school-age years, leading to the skilled handling of tools, such as pencils and papers for drawing and writing.
· During the remainder of this period, the child refines physical and motor skills and coordination.

School-age language development and socialization

· The school-age child has an efficient vocabulary and begins to correct previous mistakes in usage.
· Peers become increasingly significant; his need to find his place within a group is important.
· The child may be overly concerned with peer rules; however, parental guidance continues to play an important role in his life.
· The school-age child typically has two or three best friends (although choice of friends may change frequently).

School-age psychosocial development

The school-age child enters Erik Erikson's stage of industry versus inferiority. In this stage:
· the child wants to work and produce, accomplishing and achieving tasks
· the child may display negative attributes of inadequacy and inferiority if too much is expected of him or if he feels unable to measure up to set standards.

School-age cognitive development

The school-age child is in Jean Piaget's concrete-operational period. In this period:

- magical thinking diminishes and the child has a much better understanding of cause and effect
- the child begins to accept rules but may not necessarily understand them
- the child is ready for basic reading, writing, and arithmetic
- abstract thinking begins to develop during the middle elementary school years
- parents remain very important and adult reassurance of the child's competence and basic self-worth is essential.

Pubertal changes

- The pubertal growth spurt begins in girls at about age 10 and in boys at about age 12.
- The feet are the first part of the body to experience a growth spurt.
- Increased foot size is followed by a rapid increase in leg length and then trunk growth.
- In addition to bones, gonadal hormone levels increase and cause the sexual organs to mature.

Preparation for menses

- The first menstruation (called *menarche*) can occur as early as age 9 or as late as age 17 and still be considered normal.
- The menstrual cycle may be irregular at first.
- Secondary sexual characteristics may start to develop (breasts, hips, and pubic hair), and the girl may experience a sudden increase in height.

School-age moral and spiritual development

The school-age child is in Lawrence Kohlberg's conventional level. During this time, the child behaves according to socially acceptable norms because an authority figure tells him to do so. As the child approaches adolescence, school and parental authority is questioned, and even challenged or opposed. The importance of the peer group intensifies, and it eventually becomes the source of behavior standards and models.

Spiritual lessons should be taught in concrete terms during this time. Children have a hard time understanding supernatural religious symbols.

Adolescent psychosocial development

According to Erik Erikson, adolescents enter the stage of identity versus role confusion. During this stage, they:
• experience rapid changes in their bodies
• have a preoccupation with looks and others' perceptions of them
• feel pressure to meet expectations of peers and conform to peer standards (diminishes by late adolescence as young adults become more aware of who they are)
• try to establish their own identities.

Adolescent cognitive development

Teenagers move from the concrete thinking of childhood into Jean Piaget's stage of formal operational thought, which is characterized by:
• logical reasoning about abstract concepts
• derivation of conclusions from hypothetical premises
• forethought of future events instead of focus on the present (as in childhood).

Adolescent moral and spiritual development

Kohlberg's conventional level of moral development continues into early adolescence. At this level, adolescents do what is right because it's the socially acceptable action.

As adolescence ends, teenagers enter the postconventional, or *principled,* level of moral development. During this time, adolescents:
• form moral decisions independent of their peer group
• choose values for themselves instead of letting values be dictated by peers
• develop solidified worldviews
• formulate questions about the larger world as they consider religion, philosophy, and the values held by parents, friends, and others
• sort through and adopt religious beliefs that are consistent with their own moral character.

Development of secondary sex characteristics

The pituitary gland is stimulated at puberty to produce androgen steroids responsible for secondary sex characteristics. The hypothalamus produces gonadotropin-releasing hormone, which triggers the anterior pituitary gland to produce follicle-stimulating hormone (FSH) and luteinizing hormone (LH). FSH and LH promote testicular maturation and sperm production in boys and initiate the ovulation cycle in girls.

Male secondary sexual development

· Male secondary sexual development consists of genital growth and the appearance of pubic and body hair.

· Most boys achieve active spermatogenesis at ages 12 to 15.

Female secondary sexual development

· Female secondary sexual development involves increases in the size of the ovaries, uterus, vagina, labia, and breasts.

· The first visible sign of sexual maturity is the appearance of breast buds.

· Body hair appears in the pubic area and under the arms, and menarche occurs.

· The ovaries, present at birth, become active at puberty.

Sexual maturity in boys

Genital development and pubic hair growth are the first signs of sexual maturity in boys. These illustrations show the development of the male genitalia and pubic hair in puberty.

Stage 1
No pubic hair is present.

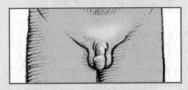

Stage 2
Downy hair develops laterally and later becomes dark; the scrotum becomes more textured, and the penis and testes may become larger.

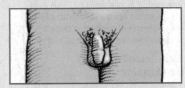

Stage 3
Pubic hair extends across the pubis; the scrotum and testes are larger; and the penis elongates.

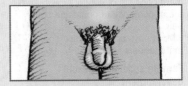

Stage 4
Pubic hair becomes more abundant and curls, and the genitalia resemble those of adults; the glans penis has become larger and broader, and the scrotum becomes darker.

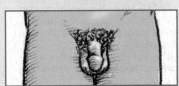

Stage 5
Pubic hair resembles an adult's in quality and pattern, and the hair extends to the inner borders of the thighs; the testes and scrotum are adult in size.

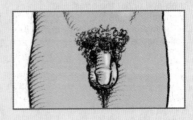

Sexual maturity in girls

Breast development and pubic hair growth are the first signs of sexual maturity in girls. These illustrations show the development of the female breast and pubic hair in puberty.

Breast development

Stage 1
Only the *papilla* (nipple) elevates (not shown).

Stage 2
Breast buds appear; the areola is slightly widened and appears as a small mound.

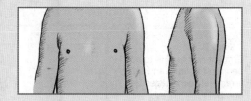

Stage 3
The entire breast enlarges; the nipple doesn't protrude.

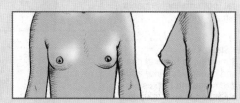

Stage 4
The breast enlarges; the nipple and the papilla protrude and appear as a secondary mound.

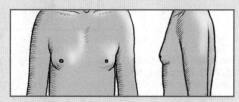

Stage 5
The adult breast has developed; the nipple protrudes and the areola no longer appears separate from the breast.

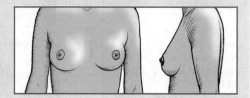

(continued)

Sexual maturity in girls *(continued)*

Pubic hair growth

Stage 1
No pubic hair is present.

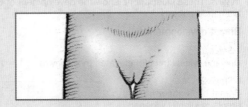

Stage 2
Straight hair begins to appear on the labia and extends between stages 2 and 3.

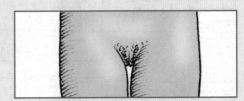

Stage 3
Pubic hair increases in quantity; it appears darker, curled, and more dense and begins to form the typical (but smaller in quantity) female triangle.

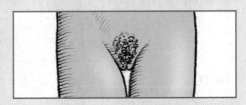

Stage 4
Pubic hair is more dense and curled; it's more adult in distribution but less abundant than in an adult.

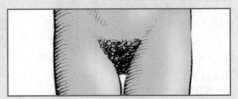

Stage 5
Pubic hair is abundant, appears in an adult female pattern, and may extend onto the medial part of the thighs.

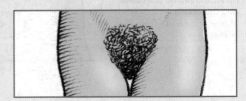

Minimizing the trauma of hospitalization

• Prepare a child for hospitalization and procedures to help him cope more effectively and make it easier for him to trust the health care professionals responsible for his care.
• Consider the child's age, developmental stage, and personality and the length of the procedure or treatment when preparing him.
• Use child life specialists, who can explain procedures step-by-step and can also stay with the child during those procedures.
• Help the child and his family cope with fears associated with hospitalization by:
  – explaining procedures
  – answering questions openly and honestly
  – minimizing separation from the parents
  – structuring the environment to allow the child to retain as much control as possible.
• Foster family-centered care, which permits the family to remain as involved as possible and helps give the child and his family a sense of control in a difficult and unfamiliar situation.
• Use developmentally appropriate activities to help the child cope with the stress of hospitalization.

The importance of play

• Play is an excellent stress reducer and tension reliever. It allows the child freedom of expression to act out his fears, concerns, and anxieties.
• Play provides a source of diversion, alleviating separation anxiety.
• Play provides the child with a sense of safety and security because, while he's engaging in play, he knows that no painful procedures will occur.
• Developmentally appropriate play fosters the child's normal growth and development, especially for a child who's repeatedly hospitalized for a chronic condition.
• Play puts the child in the driver's seat, allowing him to make choices and giving him a sense of control.

Concepts of death in childhood

Developmental stage	Concept of death	Nursing considerations
Infancy	• None	• Be aware that the older infant will experience separation anxiety. • Help the family cope with death so they can be available to the infant.
Early childhood	• Knows the words *dead* and *death* • Reactions influenced by the attitudes of his parents	• Help the family members (including siblings) cope with their feelings. • Allow the child to express his own feelings in an open and honest manner.
Middle childhood	• Understands universality and irreversibility of death • May have a fear of his parents dying	• Use play to facilitate the child's understanding of death. • Allow siblings to express their feelings.
Late childhood	• Begins to incorporate family and cultural beliefs about death • Explores views of an afterlife • Faces the reality of own mortality	• Provide opportunities for the child to verbalize his fears. • Help the child discuss his concerns with his family.
Adolescence	• Has adult perception of death but still focuses on the "here and now"	• Use opportunities to open discussion about death. • Allow expression of feelings of guilt, confusion, and anxiety. • Support and maintain the child's self-esteem.

Preparing children for surgery

What a child imagines about surgery is likely much more frightening than the reality. A child who knows what to expect ahead of time will be less fearful and more cooperative and will learn to trust his caregivers.

Before surgery
· Begin by asking the child to tell you what he thinks is going to happen during his surgery.
· Ask the child about worries or fears.
· Provide honest, age-appropriate explanations.
· Involve the parents.
· Focus on what the child will see, hear, and feel; where his parents will be waiting for him; and when they'll be reunited.
· Encourage him to ask questions.

· Reassure the child that he won't wake up during the surgery but that the doctor knows how and when to wake him up afterward.
· Show the child an induction mask (if it will be used) and allow him to "practice" by placing it on his face (or yours).
· Prepare the child for equipment he'll wake up with.
· Tell the child it's perfectly fine to be afraid and to cry.
· After the surgery, encourage the child to talk about the experience; he may also express his feelings through art or play.

Many of the concerns that children have about hospitalization and surgery relate to their particular stage of development, as shown in this table.

Age	Considerations
Infants, toddlers, and preschoolers	· Infants and toddlers are most concerned about separation from their parents, making separation during surgery difficult. · Because toddlers think concretely, showing is as important as telling when preparing toddlers for surgery. · Preschoolers may view medical procedures, including surgeries, as punishments for perceived bad behavior. · Preschoolers are also likely to have many misconceptions about what will happen during surgery.
School-age children	· School-age children have concerns about fitting in with peers and may view surgery as something that sets them apart. · A desire to appear "grown up" may make the school-age child reluctant to express his fears. · Despite a reluctance to express fear, school-age children are especially curious and interested in learning, are very receptive to preoperative teaching, and will likely ask many important questions (although they may need to be given "permission" to do so).
Adolescents	· Adolescents struggle with the conflict between wanting to assert their independence and needing their parents (and other adults) to take care of them during illness and treatment. · Adolescents may want to discuss their illness and treatment without a parent present. · In addition, adolescents may have a hard time admitting that they're afraid or experiencing pain or discomfort.

Recommended immunization schedule for persons age 0 to 6 years

Vaccine	Age				
	Birth	1 month	2 months	4 months	
Hepatitis B	HepB	HepB		*	
Rotavirus			Rota	Rota	
Diphtheria, tetatus, pertussis			DTaP	DTaP	
Haemophilus influenzae type b			Hib	Hib	
Pneumococcal			PCV	PCV	
Inactivated poliovirus			IPV	IPV	
Influenza					
Measles, mumps, rubella					
Varicella					
Hepatitis A					
Meningoccocal					

*For complete information, go to www.cdc.gov/nip/cecs/child-schedule.htm.

Recommended immunization schedule for persons age 7 to 18 years

Vaccine	Age				
	7 to 10 years	11 to 12 years	13 to 14 years	15 years	16 to 18 years
Tetanus, diphtheria, pertussis	*	Tdap	Tdap		
Human papillomavirus	*	HPV (3 doses)	HPV Series		
Meningococcal	MPSV4	MCV4		MCV4 / MCV4	
Pneumococcal	PPV				
Influenza	Influenza (yearly)				
Hepatitis A	HepA series				
Hepatitis B	HepB series				
Inactivated poliovirus	IPV series				
Measles, mumps, rubella	MMR series				
Varicella	Varicella series				

*For complete information, go to www.cdc.gov/nip/cecs/child-schedule.htm.

Range of recommended ages   Catch-up immunization   Certain high-risk groups

				Age			
6 months	**12 months**	**15 months**	**18 months**	**19 to 23 months**	**2 to 3 years**	**4 to 6 years**	
HepB				HepB series			
Rota							
DTaP		DTaP				DTaP	
Hib	Hib			Hib			
PCV	PCV				PCV		
					PPV		
IPV						IPV	
Influenza (yearly)							
	MMR					MMR	
	Varicella					Varicella	
	HepA (2 doses)				HepA series		
					MPSV4		

Range of recommended ages   Catch-up immunization   Certain high-risk groups

Catch-up immunization schedule

Vaccine	Minimum age for dose 1	Minimum interval between doses
		Dose 1 to Dose 2
Catch-up schedule for persons age 4 months to 6 years		
Hepatitis B	Birth	4 weeks
Rotavirus	6 weeks	4 weeks
Diphtheria, tetanus, pertussis	6 weeks	4 weeks
Haemophilus influenzae type b	6 weeks	4 weeks (if first dose administered at age < 12 months) 8 weeks (as final dose) (if first dose administered at age 12 to 14 months) No further doses needed (if first dose administered at age ≥ 15 months)
Pneumococcal	6 weeks	4 weeks (if first dose administered at age < 12 months and current age < 24 months) 8 weeks (as final dose) (if first dose administered at age ≥ 12 months or current age 24 to 59 months) No further doses needed (for healthy children if first dose administered at age ≥ 24 months)
Inactivated poliovirus	6 weeks	4 weeks
Measles, mumps, rubella	12 months	4 weeks
Varicella	12 months	3 months
Hepatitis A	12 months	6 months
Catch-up schedule for persons age 7 to 18 years		
Tetanus, diphtheria/tetanus, diphtheria, pertussis	7 years	4 weeks

For complete information, go to *www.cdc.gov/nip/cecs/child-schedule.htm*.

Minimum interval between doses

Dose 2 to Dose 3	Dose 3 to Dose 4	Dose 4 to Dose 5
8 weeks (and 16 weeks after first dose)		
4 weeks		
4 weeks	6 months	6 months
4 weeks (if current age < 12 months) 8 weeks (as final dose) (if current age ≥ 12 months and second dose administered at age < 15 months) No further doses needed (if previous dose administered at age ≥ 15 months)	8 weeks (as final dose) (this dose only necessary for children age 12 months to 5 years who received 3 doses before age 12 months)	
4 weeks (if current age < 12 months) 8 weeks (as final dose) (if current age ≥ 12 months) No further doses needed (for healthy children if previous dose administered at age ≥ 24 months)	8 weeks (as final dose) (this dose only necessary for children age 12 months to 5 years who received 3 doses before age 12 months)	
4 weeks	4 weeks	
8 weeks (if first dose administered at age < 12 months) 6 months (if first dose administered at age ≥ 12 months)	6 months (if first dose administered at age < 12 months)	

(continued)

Catch-up immunization schedule *(continued)*

Vaccine	Minimum age for dose 1	Minimum interval between doses
		Dose 1 to Dose 2
Catch-up schedule for persons aged 7 to 18 years *(continued)*		
Human papillomavirus	9 years	4 weeks
Hepatitis A	12 months	6 months
Hepatitis B	Birth	4 weeks
Inactivated polivirus	6 weeks	4 weeks
Measles, mumps, rubella	12 months	4 weeks
Varicella	12 months	4 weeks (if first dose administered at age ≥ 13 years) 3 months (if first dose administered at age < 13 years)

* For complete information, go to *www.cdc.gov/nip/cecs/child-schedule.htm.*

Pediatric health history

Birth history and early development
• Did the child's mother have a disease or another problem during the pregnancy?
• Was there birth trauma or a difficult delivery?
• Did the child arrive at developmental milestones—such as sitting up, walking, and talking—at the usual ages?
• Ask about childhood diseases and injuries and the presence of known congenital abnormalities.
• More specific questions will depend on which body system is being assessed.

Eyes and ears
• Look for clues to familial eye disorders, such as refractive errors and retinoblastoma (such as a family history of glaucoma).

• Does the child hold reading materials too close to his face while reading?
• Ask about behavior problems or poor performance in school.
• Ask about the child's birth history for risk of congenital hearing loss. (Maternal infection, maternal or infant use of ototoxic drugs, hypoxia, and trauma are all risk factors.)
• Ask the parents about behaviors that indicate possible hearing loss, such as delayed speech development.

Respiratory system
• Ask the parents how often the child has upper respiratory tract infections.
• Find out if the child has had other respiratory signs and symptoms, such as a cough, dyspnea, wheezing, rhinorrhea, and a stuffy nose. Ask whether these symptoms appear to be related

Minimum interval between doses

Dose 2 to Dose 3	Dose 3 to Dose 4	Dose 4 to Dose 5
12 weeks		
8 weeks (and 16 weeks after first dose)		
4 weeks	4 weeks	

to the child's activities or to seasonal changes.

Cardiovascular system

· Ask the parents whether the child has difficulty keeping up physically with other children his age.

· Ask whether the child experiences cyanosis on exertion, dyspnea, or orthopnea.

· Find out whether the child assumes a squatting position or sleeps in the knee-chest position (either sign may indicate tetralogy of Fallot or another congenital heart defect).

GI system

· If the child has abdominal pain, ask him questions to help determine the pain's nature and severity.

· Determine the frequency and consistency of bowel movements and whether the child suffers from constipation or diarrhea.

· Determine the characteristics of nausea and vomiting, especially projectile vomiting.

Urinary system

· Ask about a history of urinary tract malformations.

· Explore a history of discomfort with voiding and persistent enuresis after age 5.

Nervous system

· Find out whether the child has experienced head or neck injuries, headaches, tremors, seizures, dizziness, fainting spells, or muscle weakness.

· Ask the parents whether the child is overly active.

(continued)

Pediatric health history (continued)

Musculoskeletal system
• Determine the ages at which the child reached major motor development milestones:
– For an infant, these milestones include the age at which he held up his head, rolled over, sat unassisted, and walked alone.
– For an older child, these milestones include the age at which the child first ran, jumped, walked up stairs, and pedaled a tricycle.
• Ask about a history of repeated fractures, muscle strains or sprains, painful joints, clumsiness, lack of coordination, abnormal gait, or restricted movement.

Hematologic and immune systems
• Check for anemia:
– Ask the parents whether the child has exhibited the common signs and symptoms of pallor, fatigue, failure to gain weight, malaise, and lethargy.
– Ask the mother who's bottle-feeding whether she uses an iron-fortified infant formula.
• Ask about the patient's history of infections. For an infant, five to six viral infections per year are normal; eight to 12 are average for school-age children.
• Obtain a thorough history of allergic conditions.

Age-specific interview and assessment tips

Infant
• Before performing a procedure, talk to and touch the infant.
• Use a gentle touch.
• Speak softly.
• Allow the infant to hold a favorite toy during the assessment.
• Let an older infant hold a small block in each hand.
• Remember that an older infant may be wary of strangers.
• Be alert to infant cues, such as crying, kicking, or waving arms.
• Perform traumatic procedures last when the infant is crying.
• Use distractions, such as bright objects, rattles, and talking.
• Enlist the parent's aid when examining the ears and mouth.
• Avoid abrupt, jerky movements.
• When the child is quiet, auscultate the heart, lungs, and abdomen.

Toddler
• Encourage the parents to be with you during the interview.
• Allow the toddler to be close to his parents.
• Provide simple explanations and use simple language.

• Use play as a communication tool.
• Tell the toddler that it's OK to cry.
• Watch for separation anxiety.
• Use the toddler's favorite toy as a tool during the interview. Encourage the toddler to use the toy for communication.
• Use play (count fingers or tickle toes) to assess body parts.
• Use parent assistance during the examination. For example, ask the parents to remove the toddler's outer clothing and help restrain the child during eye and ear examination.
• Use encouraging words during the examination.

Preschool child
• Ask simple questions.
• Allow the child to ask questions.
• Provide simple explanations.
• Avoid using words that sound threatening or have double meanings.
• Avoid slang words.
• Validate the child's perception.
• Use toys for expression.
• Use simple visual aids.
• Enlist the child's help during the examination, such as by allowing him to give you the stethoscope.

• Ask about the family's history of infections and allergic or autoimmune disorders.

Endocrine system
• Obtain a thorough family history from one or both parents. Many endocrine disorders, such as diabetes mellitus and thyroid problems, can be hereditary. Others, such as delayed or precocious puberty, sometimes show a familial tendency.
• Ask about a history of poor weight gain, feeding problems, constipation, jaundice, hypothermia, or somnolence.

• Allow the child to touch and operate the diagnostic equipment.
• Explain what the child is going to feel before it happens. For example, explain that the stethoscope will be cold before using it on the child.
• Utilize the child's imagination through puppets and play.
• Give the child choices when possible.

School-age child
• Provide explanations for procedures.
• Explain the purpose of equipment such as an ophthalmoscope to see inside the eye.
• Avoid abstract explanations.
• Help the child vocalize his needs.
• Allow the child to engage in the conversation.
• Perform demonstration.
• Allow the child to undress himself.
• Respect the child's need for privacy.

Adolescent
• Give the adolescent control whenever possible.
• Facilitate trust, and stress confidentiality.

• Encourage honest and open communication.
• Be nonjudgmental.
• Use clear explanations.
• Ask open-ended questions.
• Anticipate that the adolescent may be angry or upset.
• Ask whether you can speak to the adolescent without the parent present.
• Ask the adolescent about parental involvement before initiating it.
• Give your undivided attention to the adolescent.
• Respect the adolescent's views, feeling, and differences.
• Allow the adolescent to undress in private, and provide the child with a gown.
• Expose only the area to be examined.
• Explain findings during the examination.
• Emphasize the normalcy of the adolescent's development.
• Examine genitalia last, but examine them as you would examine any other body part.

Normal heart rates in children

Age	Awake (beats/minute)	Asleep (beats/minute)	Exercise or fever (beats/minute)
Neonate	100 to 160	80 to 140	< 220
1 week to 3 months	100 to 220	80 to 200	< 220
3 months to 2 years	80 to 150	70 to 120	< 200
2 to 10 years	70 to 110	60 to 90	< 200
> 10 years	55 to 100	50 to 90	< 200

Normal blood pressure in children

Age	Weight (kg)	Systolic BP (mm Hg)	Diastolic BP (mm Hg)
Neonate	1	40 to 60	20 to 36
Neonate	2 to 3	50 to 70	30 to 45
1 month	4	64 to 96	30 to 62
6 months	7	60 to 118	50 to 70
1 year	10	66 to 126	41 to 91
2 to 3 years	12 to 14	74 to 124	39 to 89
4 to 5 years	16 to 18	79 to 119	45 to 85
6 to 8 years	20 to 26	80 to 124	45 to 85
10 to 12 years	32 to 42	85 to 135	55 to 88
> 14 years	> 50	90 to 140	60 to 90

Normal respiratory rates in children

Age	Breaths per minute
Birth to 6 months	30 to 60
6 months to 2 years	20 to 30
3 to 10 years	20 to 28
10 to 18 years	12 to 20

Normal temperature ranges in children

Age	Temperature	
	°F	°C
Neonate	98.6 to 99.8	37 to 37.7
3 years	98.5 to 99.5	36.9 to 37.5
10 years	97.5 to 98.6	36.4 to 37
16 years	97.6 to 98.8	36.4 to 37.1

Cardiovascular assessment

Findings for a cardiovascular assessment are described here.

Inspection

· Skin is pink, warm, and dry.
· Chest is symmetrical.
· Pulsations may be visible in children with thin chest walls. The point of maximal impulse is commonly visible.
· Capillary refill is no more than 2 seconds.
· Cyanosis may be an early sign of a cardiac condition in an infant or a child.
· Dependent edema is a late sign of heart failure in children.

Palpation

· Pulses should be regular in rhythm and strength:
    4 + = bounding
    3 + = increased
    2 + = normal
    1 + = weak
    0 = absent
· No thrills or rubs are evident.

Auscultation

· Heart sounds are regular in rhythm, clear, and distinct (not weak or pounding, muffled, or distant).
· First heart sound (S_1) is heard best with the stethoscope diaphragm over the mitral and tricuspid areas.
· Second heart sound (S_2) is heard best with the stethoscope diaphragm over the pulmonic and aortic areas.
· Third heart sound (S_3) is heard best with the stethoscope bell over the mitral area. This sound is considered normal in some children and young adults but is abnormal when heard in older adults.
· Fourth heart sound (S_4) if present, indicates the need for further cardiac evaluation because it's rarely heard as a normal heart sound.
· Murmurs in children may be innocent, functional, or organic. If a murmur is heard, note its location, timing within the cardiac cycle, intensity in relation to the child's position, and loudness.

Heart sound sites

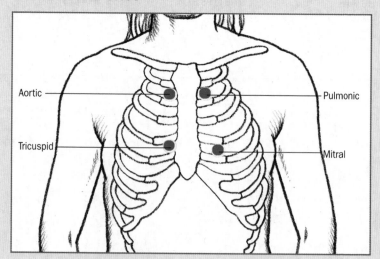

Respiratory assessment

Findings for a respiratory assessment are described here.

Inspection
· Respirations are regular and effortless.
· No nasal flaring, grunting, or retractions are present. Nasal flaring, expiratory grunting, and retractions are signs of respiratory distress in children.

Palpation
· Chest wall expands symmetrically on inspiration.
· Tactile fremitus is palpable.
· No rubs or vibrations are present.

Percussion
· Resonance is heard over most lung tissue.
· Dullness is normal over the heart area.

Auscultation
· Breath sounds normally sound louder and harsher than in adults because of the closeness of the stethoscope to the origins of the sound.
· Breath sounds are clear and equal; adventitious breath sounds are absent. Absent or diminished breath sounds are always abnormal and require further evaluation.

Looking for retractions

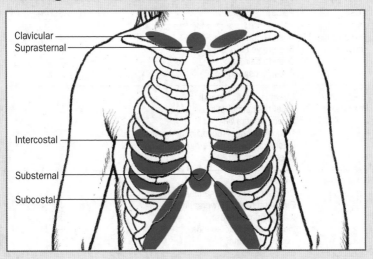

Qualities of normal breath sounds

Breath sound	Quality	Location
Tracheal	Harsh, high-pitched	Over trachea
Bronchial	Loud, high-pitched	Next to trachea
Bronchovesicular	Medium loudness and pitch	Next to sternum
Vesicular	Soft, low-pitched	Remainder of lungs

Pediatric coma scale

To quickly assess a patient's level of consciousness and to uncover baseline changes, use the pediatric coma scale (modified Glasgow Coma Scale). This assessment tool grades consciousness in relation to eye opening and motor response and responses to auditory or visual stimuli. Children under age 5 may have a lower score than adults because of verbal and motor responses. A score of 15 (the maximum) relates the best prognosis. A score of 7 or above relates good prognosis for the child's recovery. A score of 5 or lower is potentially fatal.

Test	Patient's reaction	Score
Eye opening response	Open spontaneously	4
	Open to verbal stimuli	3
	Open to pain	2
	Doesn't respond	1
Best motor response	Obeys verbal command	6
	Localizes painful stimuli	5
	Flexion-withdrawal	4
	Flexion-abnormal (decorticate rigidity)	3
	Extension (decerebrate rigidity)	2
	Doesn't respond	1
Best verbal response	**Verbal child**	
	Oriented and conversational	5
	Disoriented and conversational	4
	Inappropriate words	3
	Incomprehensible sounds	2
	Doesn't respond	1
	or	
	Nonverbal child	
	Smiles, oriented to sound, follows object, interacts	5
	Cries, consolable, interacts	4
	Inappropriate persistent cry, moans, inconsistently consolable	3
	Inconsolable, agitated, restless, cries	2
	Doesn't respond	1

Total possible score: 3 to 15

Infant reflexes

Reflex	How to elicit	Age at disappearance
Trunk incurvature	When a finger is run laterally down the neonate's spine, the trunk flexes and the pelvis swings toward the stimulated side.	2 months
Tonic neck (fencing position)	When the neonate's head is turned while he's lying supine, the extremities on the same side extend outward while those on the opposite side flex.	2 to 3 months
Grasping	When a finger is placed in each of the neonate's hands, his fingers grasp tightly enough to be pulled to a sitting position.	3 to 4 months
Rooting	When the cheek is stroked, the neonate turns his head in the direction of the stroke.	3 to 4 months
Moro (startle reflex)	When lifted above the crib and suddenly lowered (or in response to a loud noise), the arms and legs symmetrically extend and then abduct while the fingers spread to form a "C."	4 to 6 months
Sucking	Sucking motion begins when a nipple is placed in the neonate's mouth.	6 months
Babinski's	When the sole on the side of the small toe is stroked, the neonate's toes fan upward.	2 years
Stepping	When held upright with the feet touching a flat surface, the neonate exhibits dancing or stepping movements.	Variable

Locating the fontanels

The locations of the anterior and posterior fontanels are depicted in this illustration of the top of a neonatal skull. The anterior fontanel typically closes by age 18 months; the posterior fontanel, by age 2 months.

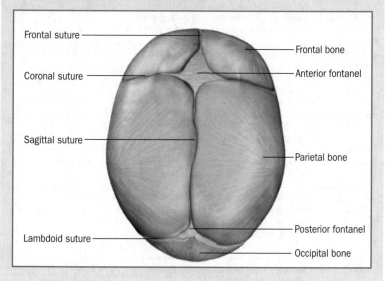

Frontal suture — Frontal bone

Coronal suture — Anterior fontanel

Sagittal suture — Parietal bone

Posterior fontanel

Lambdoid suture — Occipital bone

GI and GU systems

Findings for a GI and genitourinary (GU) assessment are described here.

Inspection
· GI: Abdomen symmetrical and fairly prominent when sitting or standing (flat when supine); no umbilical herniation
· GU: Urethra free from discharge or inflammation; no inguinal herniation; both testes descended
· Visible peristaltic waves may be a normal finding in infants and thin children; however, they may also indicate obstructive disorders such as pyloric stenosis.

Auscultation
· GI: Normal bowel sounds; possible borborygmi

· GU: No bruits over renal arteries
· Absent or hyperactive bowel sounds warrant further investigation because each usually indicates a GI disorder.

Percussion
· GI: Tympany over empty stomach or bowels; dullness over liver, full stomach, or stool in bowels
· GU: No tenderness or pain over kidneys

Palpation
· GI: No tenderness, masses, or pain; strong and equal femoral pulses
· GU: No tenderness or pain over kidneys

Tips for pediatric abdominal assessment

• Warm your hands before beginning the assessment.
• Note guarding of the abdomen and the child's ability to move around on the examination table.
• Flex the child's knees to decrease abdominal muscle tightening.
• Have the child use deep breathing or distraction during the examination; a parent can help divert the child's attention.
• Have the child "help" with the examination.
• Place your hand over the child's hand on the abdomen and extend your fingers beyond the child's fingers to decrease ticklishness when palpating the abdomen.
• Auscultate the abdomen before palpation (palpation can produce erratic bowel sounds); lightly palpate tender areas last.

Musculoskeletal assessment

Normal findings for a musculoskeletal assessment are described here.

Inspection
• Extremities are symmetrical in length and size.
• No gross deformities are present.
• Good body alignment is evident.
• The child's gait is smooth with no involuntary movements.
• The child can perform active range of motion with no pain in all muscles and joints.
• No swelling or inflammation is present in joints or muscles.
• A lateral curvature of the spine indicates scoliosis.

Palpation
• Muscle mass shape is normal, with no swelling or tenderness.
• Muscles are equal in tone, texture, and shape bilaterally.
• No involuntary contractions or twitching is evident.
• Bilateral pulses are equally strong.

Sequence of tooth eruption

A child's primary and secondary teeth will erupt in a predictable order, as shown in these illustrations.

Primary tooth eruption

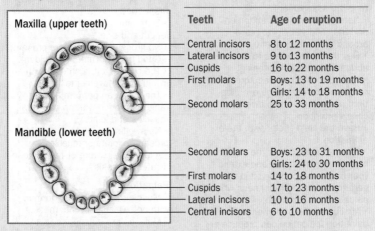

	Teeth	Age of eruption
Maxilla (upper teeth)		
	Central incisors	8 to 12 months
	Lateral incisors	9 to 13 months
	Cuspids	16 to 22 months
	First molars	Boys: 13 to 19 months
		Girls: 14 to 18 months
	Second molars	25 to 33 months
Mandible (lower teeth)		
	Second molars	Boys: 23 to 31 months
		Girls: 24 to 30 months
	First molars	14 to 18 months
	Cuspids	17 to 23 months
	Lateral incisors	10 to 16 months
	Central incisors	6 to 10 months

Secondary (or permanent) tooth eruption

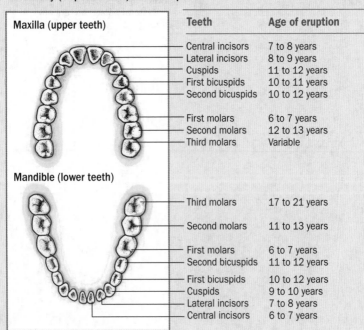

	Teeth	Age of eruption
Maxilla (upper teeth)		
	Central incisors	7 to 8 years
	Lateral incisors	8 to 9 years
	Cuspids	11 to 12 years
	First bicuspids	10 to 11 years
	Second bicuspids	10 to 12 years
	First molars	6 to 7 years
	Second molars	12 to 13 years
	Third molars	Variable
Mandible (lower teeth)		
	Third molars	17 to 21 years
	Second molars	11 to 13 years
	First molars	6 to 7 years
	Second bicuspids	11 to 12 years
	First bicuspids	10 to 12 years
	Cuspids	9 to 10 years
	Lateral incisors	7 to 8 years
	Central incisors	6 to 7 years

Pain assessment

Assessing pain in infants and young children requires the cooperation of the parents and the use of age-specific assessment tools. If the child can communicate verbally, he can also aid in the process.

History questions

To help you better understand the child's pain, ask the parents these questions:

· What kinds of pain has your child had in the past?
· How does your child usually respond to pain?
· How do you know your child is in pain?
· What do you do when he's hurting?
· What does your child do when he's hurting?
· What works best to relieve your child's pain?
· Is there anything special you would like me to know about your child and pain?

Behavioral responses to pain

Behavior is the language infants and children rely on to convey information about their pain. In an infant, facial expression is the most common and consistent behavioral response to all stimuli, painful or pleasurable, and may be the single best indicator of pain for the provider and the parent. Facial expressions that tend to indicate that the infant is in pain include:

· mouth stretched open
· eyes tightly shut
· brows and forehead knitted (as they are in a grimace)
· cheeks raised high enough to form a wrinkle on the nose.

In young children, facial expression is joined by other behaviors to convey pain. In these patients, look for such signs as:

· narrowing of the eyes
· grimace or fearful appearance
· frequent and longer-lasting bouts of crying, with a tone that's higher and louder than normal
· less receptiveness to comforting by parents or other caregivers
· holding or protecting the painful area.

FLACC Scale

The Face, Legs, Activity, Cry, Consolability (FLACC) Scale uses the characteristics listed here to measure pain in infants.

   The FLACC Scale is a behavioral pain assessment tool for use in nonverbal patients unable to provide reports of pain. Here's how to use it: 1. Rate the patient in each of the five measurement categories; 2. Add the scores together; 3. Document the total pain score.

Category	Score		
	0	1	2
Face	No particular expression or smile	Occasional grimace or frown, withdrawn, disinterested	Frequent to constant frown, clenched jaw, and quivering chin
Legs	Normal position or relaxed	Uneasy, restless, tense	Kicking or legs drawn up
Activity	Lying quietly, normal position, moves easily	Squirming, shifting back and forth, tense	Arched, rigid, or jerking
Cry	No cry (awake or asleep)	Moans or whimpers, occasional complaint	Crying steadily, screams or sobs, frequent complaints
Consolability	Content, relaxed	Reassured by occasional touching, hugging, or "talking to," distractible	Difficult to console or comfort

Adapted with permission from "The FLACC: A behavioral scale for scoring postoperative pain in young children," by S. Merkel, et al. *Pediatric Nursing,* 23(3), 1997, p. 293-297. © 2002, The Regents of the University of Michigan.

Chip tool

The chip tool uses four identical chips to signify levels of pain and can be used for the child who understands the basic concept of adding one thing to another to get more. If available, you can use poker chips. If not, simply cut four uniform circles from a sheet of paper. Here's how to present the chips:
· First say, "I want to talk with you about the hurt you might be having right now."
· Next, align the chips horizontally on the bedside table, a clipboard, or other firm surface where the child can easily see and reach them.
· Point to the chip at the child's far left and say, "This chip is just a little bit of hurt."
· Point to the second chip and say, "This next chip is a little more hurt."
· Point to the third chip and say, "This next chip is a lot of hurt."
· Point to the last chip and say, "This last chip is the most hurt you can have."
· Ask the child, "How many pieces of hurt do you have right now?" (You won't need to offer the option of "no hurt at all" because the child will tell you if he doesn't hurt.)
· Record the number of chips. If the child's answer isn't clear, talk to him about his answer and then record your findings.

Recognizing child abuse and neglect

If you suspect a child is being harmed, contact your local child protective services or the police. Contact the Childhelp USA National Child Abuse Hotline (1-800-4-A-CHILD) to find out where and how to file a report.

These signs may indicate child abuse or neglect.

Children
· Show sudden changes in behavior or school performance
· Haven't received help for physical or medical problems brought to the parent's attention
· Are always watchful, as if preparing for something bad to happen
· Lack adult supervision
· Are overly compliant, passive, or withdrawn
· Come to school or activities early, stay late, and don't want to go home

Parents
· Show little concern for the child
· Deny or blame the child for the child's problems in school or at home
· Request that teachers or caregivers use harsh physical discipline if the child misbehaves
· See the child as entirely bad, worthless, or burdensome
· Demand a level of physical or academic performance the child can't achieve
· Look primarily to the child for care, attention, and satisfaction of emotional needs

Parents and children
· Rarely look at each other
· Consider their relationship to be entirely negative
· State that they don't like each other

Signs of child abuse

Here are some signs associated with specific types of child abuse and neglect. These types of abuse are typically found in combination rather than alone.

Physical abuse
· Has unexplained burns, bites, bruises, broken bones, or black eyes
· Has fading bruises or marks after absence from school
· Cries when it's time to go home
· Shows fear at the approach of adults
· Reports injury by a parent or care-giver

Neglect
· Is frequently absent from school
· Begs or steals food or money
· Lacks needed medical or dental care, immunizations, or glasses
· Is consistently dirty and has se-vere body odor
· Lacks sufficient clothing for the weather

Sexual abuse
· Has difficulty walking or sitting
· Suddenly refuses to change for gym or join in physical activities
· Reports nightmares or bedwetting
· Demonstrates bizarre, sophisticat-ed, or unusual sexual knowledge or behavior
· Becomes pregnant or contracts a venereal disease when younger than age 14

Emotional maltreatment
· Shows extremes in behavior, such as overly compliant or demanding behavior, extreme passivity, or ag-gression
· Is inappropriately adult (parenting other children) or inappropriately in-fantile (frequent rocking or head banging)
· Shows delayed physical or emo-tional development
· Reports a lack of attachment to the parent
· Has attempted suicide

Suicide warning signs

Watch for these warning signs of impending suicide:
· withdrawal or social isolation
· signs of depression, which may in-clude crying, fatigue, helplessness, hopelessness, poor concentration, reduced interest in daily activities, sadness, constipation, and weight loss
· farewells to friends and family
· putting affairs in order
· giving away prized possessions
· expression of covert suicide mes-sages and death wishes
· obvious suicide messages such as, "I would be better off dead."

Answering a threat

If an adolescent shows signs of im-pending suicide, assess the seri-ousness of the intent and the im-mediacy of the risk. Consider an adolescent with a chosen method who plans to commit suicide in the next 48 to 72 hours a high risk.

Tell the adolescent that you're concerned. Urge him to avoid self-destructive behavior until the staff has an opportunity to help him. Consult with the treatment team about psychiatric hospitalization.

Initiate these safety precautions for those at high risk for suicide:
· Provide a safe environment.
· Remove dangerous objects, such as belts, razors, suspenders, elec-tric cords, glass, knives, nail files, and clippers.
· Make the adolescent's specific re-strictions clear to staff members, and plan for observation of the pa-tient.
· Stay alert when the adolescent is taking medication or using the bath-room.
· Encourage continuity of care and consistency of primary nurses.

Calculating pediatric medication dosage

Common calculations

$$\text{child's dose in mg} = \text{child's body surface area (BSA) in m}^2 \times \frac{\text{pediatric dose in mg}}{\text{mg}^2/\text{day}}$$

$$\text{child's dose in mg} = \frac{\text{child's BSA in m}^2}{\text{average adult BSA (1.73 m}^2)} \times \text{average adult dose}$$

$$\text{mcg/ml} = \text{mg/ml} \times 1{,}000$$

$$\text{ml/minute} = \frac{\text{ml/hour}}{60}$$

$$\text{mg/minute} = \frac{\text{mg in bag}}{\text{ml in bag}} \times \text{flow rate} \div 60$$

$$\text{mcg/minute} = \frac{\text{mg in bag}}{\text{ml in bag}} = 0.06 \times \text{flow rate}$$

$$\text{mcg/kg/minute} = \frac{\text{mcg/ml} \times \text{ml/minute}}{\text{weight in kg}}$$

Common conversions

1 kg	=	1,000 g
1 g	=	1,000 mg
1 mg	=	1,000 mcg
1″	=	2.54 cm
1 L	=	1,000 ml
1 ml	=	1,000 microliters
1 tsp	=	5 ml
1 tbs	=	15 ml
2 tbs	=	30 ml
8 oz	=	240 ml
1 oz	=	30 g
1 lb	=	454 g
2.2 lb	=	1 kg

Estimating BSA in children

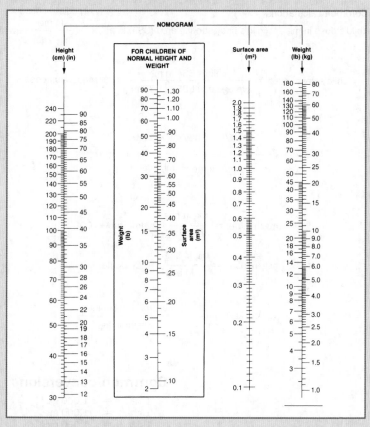

NOMOGRAM

Height (cm) (in)

FOR CHILDREN OF NORMAL HEIGHT AND WEIGHT

Surface area (m²)

Weight (lb) (kg)

Adapted with permission from Behrman, R.E., et al. *Nelson Textbook of Pediatrics,* 16th ed. Philadelphia: W.B. Saunders Co., 2000.

Preventing burns

Because children are tall enough to reach the stovetop, and can walk to and touch a fireplace or a wood stove, they can easily incur burns. Preventive measures to teach parents include:
· setting the hot water heater thermostat at a temperature less than 120° F (48.9° C)
· checking bath water temperature before a child enters the tub
· keeping pot handles turned inward and using the back burners on the stovetop
· keeping electrical appliances toward the backs of counters
· placing burning candles, incense, hot foods, and cigarettes out of reach
· avoiding the use of tablecloths so the curious child doesn't pull it to see

Preventing burns (continued)

what's on the table (possibly spilling hot foods or liquids on himself)
· teaching the child what "hot" means and stressing the danger of open flames
· storing matches and cigarette lighters in locked cabinets, out of reach
· burning fires in fireplaces or wood stoves with close supervision and using a fire screen when doing so

· securing safety plugs in all unused electrical outlets and keeping electrical cords tucked out of reach
· teaching preschoolers who can understand the hazards of fire to "stop, drop, and roll" if their clothes are on fire
· practicing escapes from home and school with preschoolers
· visiting a fire station to reinforce learning
· teaching preschoolers how to call 911 (for emergency use only).

Causes of burns

Type	Causes
Thermal	Flames, radiation, or excessive heat from fire, steam, or hot liquids or objects
Chemical	Various acids, bases, and caustics
Electrical	Electrical current and lightning
Light	Intense light sources or ultraviolet light, including sunlight
Radiation	Nuclear radiation and ultraviolet light

Classifying burns

Burns are classified according to the depth of the injury:

· **First-degree burns** are limited to the epidermis. Sunburn is a typical first-degree burn. These burns are painful but self-limiting. They don't lead to scarring and require only local wound care.
· **Second-degree burns** extend into the dermis but leave some residual dermis viable. These burns are painful, and the skin will appear swollen and red with blister formation.
· **Third-degree**, or full-thickness, burns involve the destruction of the entire

dermis, leaving only subcutaneous tissue exposed. These burns look dry and leathery and are painless because the nerve endings are destroyed.
· **Fourth-degree burns** are a rare type of burn usually associated with lethal injury. They extend beyond the subcutaneous tissue, involving the muscle, fasciae, and bone. Occasionally termed *transmural burns*, these injuries are commonly associated with complete transection of an extremity.

Estimating the extent of burns

Lund-Browder chart
Use to estimate the extent of an infant's or a child's (up to age 7) burns.

Rule of Nines
Use to estimate the extent of an older child's or a teenager's burns.

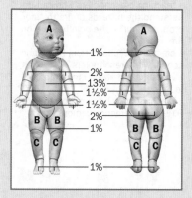

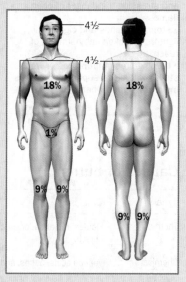

Relative percentage of burned body surface by age

At birth	0 to 1 year	1 to 4 years	5 to 9 years	10 to 15 years	16+ years
A: Half of head 9½%	8½%	6½%	5½%	4½%	3½%
B: Half of one thigh 2½%	3½%	4%	4½%	4½%	4½%
C: Half of one leg 2½%	2½%	2½%	3%	3½%	3½%

Calculating pediatric fluid needs

Determining and meeting the fluid needs of children are important nursing responsibilities. Keep in mind that fluid replacement can also be affected by clinical conditions that cause fluid retention or loss. Children with these conditions should receive fluids based on their individual needs.

Fluid needs based on weight

· Children weighing under 10 kg require 100 ml of fluid per kilogram of body weight per day:

$$\text{weight in kg} \times 100 \text{ ml/kg/day} = \text{fluid needs in ml/day}$$

· Children weighing 10 to 20 kg require 1,000 ml of fluid per day for the first 10 kg plus 50 ml for every kilogram over 10:

$$(\text{total kg} - 10 \text{ kg}) \times 50 \text{ ml/kg/day} = \text{additional fluid need in ml/day}$$

$$1{,}000 \text{ ml/day} + \text{additional fluid need} = \text{fluid needs in ml/day}$$

· Children weighing more than 20 kg require 1,500 ml of fluid for the first 20 kg plus 20 ml for each additional kilogram:

$$(\text{total kg} - 20 \text{ kg}) \times 20 \text{ ml/kg/day} = \text{additional fluid need in ml/day}$$

$$1{,}500 \text{ ml/day} + \text{additional fluid need} = \text{fluid needs in ml/day}$$

Fluid needs based on calories

A child should receive 120 ml of fluid for every 100 kilocalories of metabolism (calorie requirements can be found in a table of recommended dietary allowances for children, or calculated by a dietitian):

$$\text{fluid requirements in ml/day} = \frac{\text{calorie requirements}}{100 \text{ kcal}} \times 120 \text{ ml}$$

Fluid needs based on body surface area (BSA)

Multiply the child's BSA by 1,500 to calculate the daily fluid needs of a child who isn't dehydrated:

$$\text{fluid maintenance needs in ml/day} = \text{BSA in m}^2 \times 1{,}500 \text{ ml/day/m}^2$$

SIDS prevention

Sudden infant death syndrome (SIDS) is the sudden death of a previously healthy infant when the cause of death isn't confirmed by a postmortem examination. It's the most common cause of death between ages 1 month and 1 year, and the third leading cause of death in all infants from birth to age 1 year. Even so, the incidence of SIDS has declined dramatically by more than 40% since 1992, which is mostly attributed to the 1992 initiative to put babies on their backs for sleeping, called the "Back to Sleep" campaign.

Preventive strategies

Parents should be informed of simple measures that they can take to prevent SIDS, including:
· putting the infant on his back to sleep
· not smoking anywhere near the infant
· removing from the infant's crib or sleeping environment all pillows, quilts, stuffed toys, and other soft surfaces that may trap exhaled air
· using a firm mattress with a snug-fitting sheet
· making sure the infant's head remains uncovered while sleeping
· keeping the infant warm while sleeping but not overheated.

Handling temper tantrums

As they assert their independence, toddlers demonstrate "temper tantrums," or violent objections to rules or demands. These tantrums include such behaviors as lying on the floor and kicking their feet, screaming, or holding their breath.

How to handle them

Dealing with a child's temper tantrums can be a challenge for parents who may be frustrated, embarrassed, or exhausted by their child's behavior. Reassure the parents that temper tantrums are a normal occurrence in toddlers and that the child will outgrow them as he learns to express himself in more productive ways. This type of reassurance should be accompanied by some concrete suggestions for dealing effectively with temper tantrums.
· Provide a safe, childproof environment.
· Hold the child to keep him safe if his behavior is out of control.
· Give the toddler frequent opportunities to make developmentally appropriate choices.
· Give the child advance warning of a request to help prevent tantrums.
· Remain calm and be supportive of a child having a tantrum.
· Ignore tantrums when the toddler is seeking attention or trying to get something he wants.
· Help the toddler find acceptable ways to vent his anger and frustration.

When to get help

Parents should be advised to seek help from a health care provider when problematic tantrums:
· persist beyond age 5
· occur more than five times per day
· occur with a persistent negative mood
· cause property destruction
· cause harm to the child or others.

Choking hazards

Choking can easily occur in toddlers because they're still exploring their environments with their mouths. Toddlers may ingest small objects, and the small size of their oral cavities increases the risk of choking while eating. Foods that are round and less than 1″ (2.5 cm) in diameter can obstruct the airway of a child when swallowed whole.

Common items that may cause choking include:
· foods, such as popcorn, peanuts, whole grapes, cherry or grape tomatoes, chunks of hot dogs, raw carrots, hard candy, bubble gum, long noodles, dried beans, and marshmallows
· small toys, such as broken latex balloons, button eyes, beaded necklaces, and small wheels
· common household items, such as broken zippers, pills, bottle caps, and nails and screws.

Preventive strategies
· Cut food into small pieces to prevent airway obstruction. Slicing hot dogs into short, lengthwise pieces is a safe option.
· Avoid fruits with pits, fish with bones, hard candy, chewing gum, nuts, popcorn, whole grapes, and marshmallows.
· Encourage the child to sit whenever eating.
· Keep easily aspirated objects out of a toddler's environment.
· Be especially cautious about what toys the child plays with (choose sturdy toys without small, removable parts).
· Learn how to relieve airway obstruction in infants and children as part of a cardiopulmonary resuscitation course.

Toilet training

Physical readiness for toilet training occurs between ages 18 and 24 months; however, many children aren't cognitively ready to begin toilet training until they're between ages 36 and 42 months.

Signs of readiness
When physically and cognitively ready, the child can start toilet training. The process can take 2 weeks to 2 months to complete successfully. It's important to remember that there's considerable variation from one child to another. Other signs of readiness include:
· periods of dryness for 2 hours or more, indicating bladder control
· child's ability to walk well and remove clothing
· cognitive ability to understand the task
· facial expression or words suggesting that the child knows when he's about to defecate.

Step-by-step
Steps to toilet training include:
· teaching words for voiding and defecating
· teaching the purpose of the toilet or potty chair
· changing the toddler's diapers frequently to give him the experience of feeling dry and clean
· helping the toddler make the connection between dry pants and the toilet or potty chair
· placing the child on the potty chair or toilet for a few moments at regular intervals and rewarding successes
· helping the toddler understand the physiologic signals by pointing out behaviors he displays when he needs to void or defecate
· rewarding successes but not punishing failures.

Preventing poisoning

As a young child's gross motor skills improve and he becomes more curious, he's able to climb onto chairs and reach cabinets where medicines, cosmetics, cleaning products, and other poisonous substances are stored. Preventive measures to teach parents include:
· keeping medicines and other toxic materials locked away in high cupboards, boxes, or drawers
· using child-resistant containers and cupboard safety latches
· avoiding storage of a large supply of toxic agents
· teaching the child that medication isn't candy or a treat (even though it might taste good)
· teaching the child that plants inside or outside aren't edible and keeping houseplants out of reach
· promptly discarding empty poison containers and never reusing them to store a food item or other poison
· always keeping original labels on containers of toxic substances
· having the poison control center number (1-800-222-1222) prominently displayed on every telephone. (The American Academy of Pediatrics no longer recommends keeping syrup of ipecac in the home to treat poisoning; instead, parents should keep the poison control center number clearly posted.)

Preventing drowning

Toddlers and preschoolers are quite susceptible to drowning because they can walk onto docks or pool decks and stand or climb on seats in a boat. Drowning can also occur in mere inches of water, resulting from falls into buckets, bathtubs, hot tubs, toilets, and even fish tanks. Preventive strategies to teach parents include:
· instituting close adult supervision of any child near water
· teaching children never to go into water without an adult and never to horseplay near the water's edge
· using child-resistant pool covers and fences with self-closing gates around backyard pools
· emptying buckets when not in use and storing them upside-down
· using U.S. Coast Guard-approved child life jackets near water and on boats
· providing the child with swimming lessons.

Preventing falls

Young children can easily fall as their gross motor skills improve and they're able to move chairs to climb onto counters, climb ladders, and open windows. Preventive strategies to teach parents include:
· providing close supervision at all times during play
· keeping crib rails up and the mattress at the lowest position
· placing gates across the tops and bottoms of stairways
· installing window locks on all windows to keep them from opening more than 3″ (7.6 cm) without adult supervision
· keeping doors locked or using child-proof doorknob covers at entries to stairs, high porches or decks, and laundry chutes
· removing unsecured scatter rugs
· using a nonskid bath mat or decals in the bathtub or shower
· avoiding the use of walkers, especially near stairs
· always restraining children in shopping carts and never leaving them unattended
· providing safe climbing toys and choosing play areas with soft ground cover and safe equipment.

Motor vehicle and bicycle safety

Children can easily incur motor vehicle and bicycle injuries because they may be able to unbuckle seat belts, resist riding in a car seat, or refuse to wear a bicycle helmet.
   Preventive measures to teach parents include:
· learning about the proper fit and use of bicycle helmets and requiring the child to wear a helmet every time he rides a bicycle
· teaching the preschool-age child never to go into a road without an adult
· not allowing the child to play on a curb or behind a parked car
· checking the area behind vehicles before backing out of the driveway (small children may not be visible in rear-view mirrors because of blind spots, especially in larger vehicles)
· providing a safe, preferably enclosed, area for outdoor play for younger children (and keeping fences, gates, and doors locked)
· learning how to use child safety seats for all motor vehicle trips and ensuring proper use by having the seats inspected (many local fire departments offer free inspections)
· encouraging older children to wear brightly colored clothing whenever riding bicycles. (Discourage the child from riding his bicycle during dusk hours or after dark; if he must ride during these hours, affix reflective tape to his clothing to make him easily visible and make sure his bicycle has a light and reflectors.)

Car safety seat guidelines

Proper installation and use of a car safety seat are critical. In addition to the weight and age guidelines outlined in the chart below, these guidelines for booster seat use will help ensure a child's safety while riding in a vehicle.
· Always make sure belt-positioning booster seats are used with both lap and shoulder belts.
· Make sure the lap belt fits low and right across the lap/upper thigh area and the shoulder belt fits snug, crossing the chest and shoulder to avoid abdominal injuries.
· All children younger than age 12 should ride in the back seat.

Weight and age	Seat type	Seat position
Up to 1 year or 20 lb (9 kg)	Infant-only or rear-facing convertible	Rear-facing
Up to 1 year and over 20 lb	Rear-facing convertible	Rear-facing
Over 1 year and 20 to 40 lb (9 to 18 kg)	Rear-facing convertible (until meeting the seat manufacturer's limit for maximum weight and height), then forward-facing	Forward-facing
4 to 8 years and over 40 lb	Booster seat	Forward-facing

Nutritional guidelines for infants and toddlers

· Breast-feeding is recommended exclusively for the first 6 months of life and then should be continued in combination with infant foods until age 1 year.
· If breast-feeding isn't possible or desired, bottle-feeding with iron-fortified infant formula is an acceptable alternative for the first 12 months of life.
· After age 1, whole cow's milk can be used in place of breast milk or formula.
· New foods should be introduced to the infant's diet one at a time, waiting 5 to 7 days between them. If the infant rejects a food initially, the parents should offer it again later.
· Unpasteurized products, such as honey or corn syrup, should be avoided.
· Toddlers should be offered a variety of foods, including plenty of fruits, vegetables, and whole grains.
· Serving size should be approximately 1 tablespoon of solid food per year of age (or one-fourth to one-third the adult portion size) so as not to overwhelm the child with larger portions.

Solid foods and infant age

Age	Type of food	Rationale
4 months	Rice cereal mixed with breast milk or formula	Are less likely than wheat to cause an allergic reaction
5 to 6 months	Strained vegetables (offered first) and fruits	Offered first because they may be more readily accepted than if introduced after sweet fruits
7 to 8 months	Strained meats, cheese, yogurt, rice, noodles, pudding	Provide an important source of iron and add variety to the diet
8 to 9 months	Finger foods (bananas, crackers)	Promote self-feeding
10 months	Mashed egg yolk (no whites until age 1); bite-size cooked food (no foods that may cause choking)	Decrease the risk of choking (Avoiding foods that can cause choking is the safest option, even though the infant chews well.)
12 months	Foods from the adult table (chopped or mashed according to the infant's ability to chew foods)	Provide a nutritious and varied diet that should meet the infant's nutritional needs

Nutritional guidelines for children older than age 2 years

Key recommendations for children and adolescents from the Dietary Guidelines for Americans (2005) issued by the U.S. Department of Health and Human Services and the U.S. Department of Agriculture are listed here. All children should be encouraged to eat a variety of fruits, vegetables, and whole grains.

Weight management
· For overweight children and adolescents, reduce body weight gain while achieving normal growth and development. Consult with a health care practitioner before placing a child on a weight-reduction diet.
· For overweight children with chronic diseases or those on medication, consult with a health care practitioner before starting a weight-reduction program to ensure management of other health conditions.

Physical activity
· Children and adolescents should engage in at least 60 minutes of physical activity on most (preferably all) days.

Food groups to encourage
· At least one-half of grains consumed should be whole grains.

· Children ages 2 to 8 years should consume 2 cups of fat-free or low-fat milk (or equivalent milk product) per day.
· Children ages 9 years and older should consume 3 cups of fat-free or low-fat milk (or equivalent milk product) per day.

Fats
· For children ages 2 to 3 years, fat intake should be 30% to 35% of total daily calories consumed.
· For children ages 4 to 18 years, fat intake should be 25% to 35% of total daily calories consumed.
· Most fats should come from sources of polyunsaturated and monounsaturated fatty acids, such as fish, nuts, and vegetable oils.

Food safety
· Infants and young children shouldn't eat or drink raw (unpasteurized) milk or products made from unpasteurized milk, raw or partially cooked eggs or foods containing raw eggs, raw or undercooked meat or poultry, raw or uncooked fish or shellfish, unpasteurized juices, or raw sprouts.

Preventing obesity

Obesity and overweight have become serious health problems. An estimated 16% of children and adolescents are now overweight. Over the last two decades, this rate has skyrocketed in young Americans; it's doubled in children and tripled in adolescents. Excess body fat is problematic because it increases a person's risk of developing such serious health problems as type 2 diabetes, hypertension, dyslipidemia, certain types of cancers, and more. Additionally, overweight children have a high probability of becoming obese adults.

What to do

Weight-loss diets may not be the answer for children and adolescents because growth and development increase nutritional needs. However, some dietary changes can have significant results. Suggestions include:
- avoiding fast food
- eating low-fat after-school snacks
- switching from whole milk to 1% or skim milk
- substituting fresh vegetables for fried snack foods
- eating a variety of fresh and dried fruits.

Additionally, children who are overweight or even of normal weight should be encouraged to participate in some type of daily vigorous, aerobic activity to help reduce or prevent childhood obesity and promote a habit of daily exercise that will last a lifetime.

Healthy snacks for children

Encourage parents of your pediatric patients to begin good eating habits early by offering healthy snacks to their children. Here are some suggestions:
- peanut butter spread on apple slices or rice cakes
- frozen yogurt topped with berries or fruit slices
- raw or dried fruit served with a dip such as low-fat yogurt or pudding
- raw red and green peppers, carrots, and celery sticks served with low-fat salad dressing as a dip
- fruit smoothies made with blended low-fat milk or yogurt and fresh or frozen fruit
- applesauce.

Sleep guidelines

Age-group	Hours of sleep needed per day	Special considerations
Infant Birth to 6 months	15 to 16½	• To help prevent sudden infant death syndrome, all infants should be placed on their backs to sleep.
6 to 12 months	13¾ to 14½	• At ages 4 to 6 months, infants are physiologically capable of sleeping (without feeding) for 6 to 8 hours at night. • From birth to age 3 months, infants may take many naps per day; from ages 4 to 9 months, two naps per day; and by 9 to 12 months, only one nap per day.
Toddler 1 to 2 years	10 to 15	• Most toddlers sleep through the night without awakening.
2 to 3 years	10 to 12	• A consistent routine (set bedtime, reading, and a security object) helps toddlers prepare for sleep. • Up to age 3, toddlers take one nap per day; after age 3, many toddlers don't need a nap.
Preschool age	10 to 12	• If the preschooler no longer naps, a "quiet" or rest period may be useful. • Dreams or nightmares become more real as magical thinking increases and a vivid imagination develops. • Problems falling asleep may occur because of overstimulation, separation anxiety, or fear of the dark or monsters.
School age	9 to 10	• Compliance at bedtime becomes easier. • Nightmares are usually related to a real event in the child's life and can usually be eradicated by resolving any underlying fears the child might have. • Sleepwalking and sleeptalking may begin.
Adolescent	At least 8	• Sleep requirements increase because of physical growth spurts and high activity levels. • The hours needed for sleep can't be made up or stored ("catch-up" sleep on the weekends isn't effective in replenishing a teen's sleep store).

II

Disease profiles

9 Adult disorders 472

10 Maternal-neonatal disorders 519

11 Pediatric disorders 550

Adult disorders

Alzheimer's disease

DESCRIPTION

- *Alzheimer's disease* is an acquired syndrome of decline in short- and long-term memory and other cognitive functions.
- It's progressive and disabling, and there's no cure or definitive treatment.
- It accounts for 60% to 80% of all cases of dementia.
- It isn't an inherent aspect of aging.
- It causes memory loss that's associated with impairment in abstract thinking and judgment.
- It's also known as *AD*.

PATHOPHYSIOLOGY

- AD's findings are detected only on an autopsy.
- Neuropathologic findings include extracellular deposition of amyloid-beta protein, intracellular neurofibrillary tangles, and loss of neurons.
- Amyloid-beta protein is thought to interfere with neuronal function by stimulating free radical production, which can result in neuronal cell death.
- Hyperphosphorylated neurofibrillary tangles deposit in neurons, leading to cell death.
- Neuronal cell death and synapse loss affect neurotransmitter pathways; deficient production of acetylcholine, serotonin, and norepinephrine occurs.

CAUSES

- Unknown
- Familial early-onset AD: found with genetic mutations in chromosome 21, 14, and 1 (accounts for less than 5% of cases)

ASSESSMENT FINDINGS

- History obtained from a family member or caregiver
- Insidious onset
- Forgetfulness
- Memory loss
- Difficulty learning and remembering new information
- General deterioration in personal hygiene
- Inability to concentrate or handle complex tasks
- Tendency to perform repetitive actions and to be restless
- Personality changes (irritability, depression, paranoia, hostility)
- Nocturnal awakening
- Disorientation
- Disturbance symptoms that interfere with work, social activities, and relationships
- Language difficulties
- Mood swings, sudden angry outbursts, and sleep disturbances
- Impaired stereognosis
- Gait disorders
- Tremors (if Parkinson-related dementia)
- Positive snout reflex
- Urinary or fecal incontinence (end-stage)

TEST RESULTS

- Diagnosis is made by clinical evaluation.

- Positive diagnosis is made on an autopsy.
- Positron emission tomography reveals metabolic activity of the cerebral cortex. It's performed when there's alteration in brain metabolism.
- Computed tomography scan may reveal excessive and progressive brain atrophy; this rules out pressure hydrocephalus.
- Magnetic resonance imaging rules out intracranial lesions.
- Cerebral blood flow studies may reveal abnormalities in blood flow to the brain (rarely done).
- EEG shows slowing of the brain waves in late stages of the disease.
- Neuropsychologic test results show impaired cognitive ability and reasoning.

TREATMENT

- Well-balanced diet and exercise (may need to be monitored)
- Safe activities as tolerated (may need to be monitored)
- Antidepressants as needed
- Antipsychotics as needed
- Acetylcholinesterase inhibitors
- Individual or group therapy
- Family support group
- Experimental therapies: anti-inflammatory agents, vitamin E, ginkgo biloba, a diet rich in omega-3, statins (see *Managing Alzheimer's disease*)

KEY PATIENT OUTCOMES

The patient (or family) will:
- perform activities of daily living to maximum ability to enhance quality of life
- maintain daily caloric requirements
- remain free from signs and symptoms of infection and pain
- perform self-care needs to maximum ability
- attain adequate management of symptoms

Managing Alzheimer's disease

Neuropsychiatric evaluation and behavioral interventions, either patient-centered or involving caregiver training, along with dietary consultation and occupational therapy consultation, can enhance the patient's and family's quality of life throughout the stages of the disease. Focus on managing cognitive and behavioral changes in a structured environment.

- use support systems and develop adequate coping behaviors.

NURSING INTERVENTIONS

- Establish a daily routine for the patient.
- Provide an effective communication system.
- Use soft tones and a slow, calm manner when speaking to the patient.
- Allow the patient sufficient time to answer questions.
- Protect the patient from injury.
- Provide rest periods; minimize sleep disturbance.
- Provide an exercise program.
- Encourage independence.
- Offer frequent toileting.
- Assist with hygiene and dressing.
- Give prescribed medication.
- Provide familiar objects to help with orientation and behavior control.
- Manage hypersexuality, aggression, and agitation.
- Evaluate the patient's response to medications.
- Monitor fluid intake and nutrition status.
- Adjust the environment for safety.

PATIENT TEACHING

Be sure to cover (with the caregiver):
- the disease process

- the diet and exercise regimen
- the importance of cutting food and providing finger foods, if indicated
- the use of plates with rim guards, built-up utensils, and cups with lids
- the importance of maintaining as much independence as possible
- how to access the Alzheimer's Association
- location and contact information for a local support group and local services.

Asthma

DESCRIPTION

- *Asthma* is a chronic inflammatory disorder of the airways involving episodic, reversible airway obstruction resulting from bronchospasms, increased mucus secretions, and mucosal edema.
- It may begin dramatically, with simultaneous onset of severe, multiple symptoms, or insidiously, with gradually increasing respiratory distress.
- Its signs and symptoms range from mild wheezing and dyspnea to life-threatening respiratory failure.
- It's classified into types: allergic, nonallergic/intrinsic, exercise-induced, nocturnal, occupational, and steroid-resistant. (See *Cardiac asthma*.)

PATHOPHYSIOLOGY

- Tracheal and bronchial linings overreact to various stimuli, causing episodic smooth-muscle spasms that severely constrict the airways.
- Mucosal edema and thickened secretions further block the airways.
- Immunoglobulin (Ig) E antibodies, attached to histamine-containing mast cells and receptors on cell membranes, initiate intrinsic asthma attacks.

- When exposed to an antigen such as pollen, the IgE antibody combines with the antigen. On subsequent exposure to the antigen, mast cells degranulate and release mediators.
- The mediators cause the bronchoconstriction and edema of an asthma attack.
- During an asthma attack, expiratory airflow decreases, trapping gas in the airways and causing alveolar hyperinflation.
- Atelectasis may develop in some lung regions.
- The increased airway resistance initiates labored breathing.

CAUSES

Allergic asthma: triggered by allergens
- Animal dander
- Cockroaches
- Dust mites
- House dust or mold
- Pollen
- Pollutants
- Smoke
- Dramatic emotional response (crying or laughing)
- Drugs, such as aspirin, beta-adrenergic blockers, and nonsteroidal anti-inflammatory drugs
- Emotional stress
- Kapok or feather pillows
- Sensitivity to specific external allergens or from internal, nonallergenic factors
- Infection
- Food additives containing sulfites and any other sensitizing substance

Intrinsic asthma: triggered by respiratory irritants
- Cold air
- Perfume or scents
- Fumes
- Cleaning agents
- Upper respiratory infection
- Gastroesophageal reflux disease (GERD)

Exercise-induced asthma: triggered while exercising
- Strenuous exercise
- Cold, dry conditions while exercising

Nocturnal asthma: triggered while sleeping (day or night)
- Allergens in bedding or bedroom
- Low room temperature
- GERD

Occupational asthma: triggered by being exposed to irritants over an extended length of time
- Chemical fumes
- Wood dust

ASSESSMENT FINDINGS

- History of exposure to a particular trigger followed by the sudden onset of dyspnea and wheezing, and by tightness in the chest accompanied by a cough that produces thick, clear, or yellow sputum
- Visibly dyspneic
- Ability to speak only a few words before pausing for breath
- Use of accessory respiratory muscles
- Diaphoresis
- Increased anteroposterior thoracic diameter
- Hyperresonance
- Tachycardia; tachypnea; mild systolic hypertension
- Inspiratory and expiratory wheezes
- Prolonged expiratory phase of respiration
- Diminished breath sounds
- Cyanosis, confusion, and lethargy indicating the onset of life-threatening status asthmaticus and respiratory failure

TEST RESULTS

- Arterial blood gas (ABG) analysis reveals hypoxemia.
- Serum IgE level is increased from an allergic reaction.

Cardiac asthma

The term *cardiac asthma* doesn't refer to true asthma. Cardiac asthma does involve wheezing, but it's associated with the pulmonary congestion caused by heart failure, rather than inflammation of the airways. Other signs and symptoms that are similar to asthma include shortness of breath and coughing; however, heart and liver enlargement and fluid retention also occur. Cardiac asthma can develop at any age and, unlike true asthma, is treated with diuretics to increase fluid output and decrease lung congestion.

- Complete blood count with differential shows an increased eosinophil count.
- Chest X-rays may show hyperinflation with areas of focal atelectasis.
- Pulmonary function studies show decreased peak flows and forced expiratory volume in 1 second, low-normal or decreased vital capacity, and increased total lung and residual capacities.
- Skin testing identifies specific allergens.
- Bronchial challenge testing shows the clinical significance of allergens identified by skin testing.
- Pulse oximetry measurements show decreased oxygen saturation.

TREATMENT

- Identification and avoidance of precipitating factors
- Desensitization to specific antigens
- Establishment and maintenance of a patent airway
- Fluid replacement
- Activity as tolerated
- Bronchodilators
- Corticosteroids
- Histamine antagonists

- Leukotriene antagonists
- Antibiotics
- Low-flow oxygen
- Endotracheal (ET)intubation and ventilation (with status asthmaticus)
- Heliox trial (before intubation)

KEY PATIENT OUTCOMES

The patient will:
- maintain adequate ventilation
- maintain a patent airway
- use effective coping strategies
- report feelings of comfort.

NURSING INTERVENTIONS

- Give prescribed drugs, and evaluate their effects.
- Place the patient in high Fowler's position.
- Encourage pursed-lip and diaphragmatic breathing.
- Monitor ABG results, pulmonary function test results, and pulse oximetry.
- Administer prescribed oxygen; adjust according to ABG values.
- Assist with ET intubation and mechanical ventilation, if appropriate.
- Perform postural drainage and chest percussion, if tolerated.
- Perform tracheal suctioning as needed.
- Administer I.V. fluids as ordered.
- Anticipate bronchoscopy or bronchial lavage.
- Keep the room temperature comfortable.
- Monitor vital signs and intake and output.
- Monitor response to treatment.
- Auscultate breath sounds before and after treatments, and every 2 to 4 hours.
- Assess level of anxiety.

PATIENT TEACHING

Be sure to cover:
- the disorder, diagnosis, and treatment

- medications and potential adverse reactions
- when to notify the physician
- avoidance of known allergens and irritants
- metered-dose inhaler or dry powder inhaler use
- pursed-lip and diaphragmatic breathing
- the use of a peak flow meter
- effective coughing techniques
- maintaining adequate hydration
- how to access the American Lung Association or Asthma and Allergy Foundation of America
- location and contact information for a local support group and local services.

Breast cancer

DESCRIPTION

- Breast cancer involves cancerous cells affecting the breast.
- Early detection and treatment influence the prognosis considerably. (See *Discovering breast cancer.*)
- It's the second leading cause of cancer deaths in women.

PATHOPHYSIOLOGY

- It involves a malignant proliferation of epithelial cells lining the ducts or lobules of the breast.
- Breast cancer metastasizes by way of the lymphatic system or the bloodstream.

Classification

- Ductal carcinoma in situ: cancer cells limited to milk ducts and haven't spread to the fatty tissue of the breast
- Invasive ductal carcinoma: 70% to 80% of all breast cancers; malignant cells have infiltrated the fatty tissue of the breast; may metastasize
- Inflammatory: rare; growing rapidly and causing overlying skin to

become edematous, inflamed, and indurated
• Lobular carcinoma in situ: involving the lobes of glandular tissue
• Medullary or circumscribed: well-defined tumor boundary
• Mucinous: mucus-producing cancer cells that spread into surrounding tissue
• Paget's disease of the nipple: rare; initiates in the milk duct and spreads to the nipple
• Phyloddes tumor: rare; forms from the connective tissue of the breast

CAUSES

• No known cause

RISK FACTORS

• Gender: occurs in women more than men
• Aging: 77% of women with breast cancer age 50 or over
• Gene mutation: BRCA1 and BRCA2 genes, ataxia-telangiectasia gene, p53 tumor suppressor gene is present
• Family history of breast cancer: risk doubles with one first-degree relative
• Personal history of breast cancer: 3 to 4 times increased chance of developing breast cancer in the other breast or another part of the breast where breast cancer already occurred (not recurrence of the first cancer)
• Race: occurs more in white women but higher cause of death in African-American women
• Previous abnormal breast biopsy: 1.5 to 5 times increased chance
• Previous breast radiation (for another type of cancer): significantly increased risk (up to 12 times more likely)
• Menstruating before age 12 or menopause after age 55: slightly higher risk

Discovering breast cancer

Finding breast cancer early greatly improves the chances of successful treatment. Early detection of breast cancer can occur by breast self-examination, followed by an immediate professional evaluation of any abnormality. However, mammography is also a useful technique for the detection of early breast cancer. Both physical examination and mammography are necessary for early diagnosis. Between 30% and 50% of detection occurs from mammography (theoretically, slow-growing breast cancer may take up to 8 years to become palpable at 1 cm), and 47% is detected by palpation.

• No children or having children after age 30: slightly higher risk
• Hormone replacement therapy: long-term use increases risk
• Alcohol: increased risk with 2 to 5 drinks daily
• Obesity: higher risk with weight gain as an adult, rather than being overweight since childhood

ASSESSMENT FINDINGS

• Detection of a hard, painless lump or mass in the breast (see *Breast tumor sources and sites,* page 478)
• Change in breast tissue
• History of risk factors
• Clear, milky, or bloody nipple discharge, nipple retraction, scaly skin around the nipple, and skin changes, such as dimpling or inflammation
• Arm edema
• Lymphadenopathy

TEST RESULTS

• Alkaline phosphatase level and liver function test results reveal distant metastases.

Breast tumor sources and sites

About 90% of all breast tumors arise from the epithelial cells lining the ducts. About half of all breast cancers develop in the breast's upper outer quadrant—the section containing the most glandular tissue.

The second most common cancer site is the nipple, where all of the breast ducts converge.

The next most common site is the upper inner quadrant, followed by the lower outer quadrant and, finally, the lower inner quadrant.

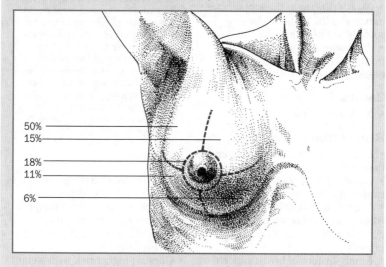

50%
15%
18%
11%
6%

• Hormonal receptor assay determines whether the tumor is estrogen- or progesterone-dependent; it also guides decisions to use therapy that blocks the action of the estrogen hormone that supports tumor growth.
• Mammography may show a mass.
• Ultrasonography distinguishes between a fluid-filled cyst and a solid mass.
• Chest X-ray may identify metastases in the chest.
• Scans of the bone, brain, liver, and other organs detect distant metastases.

TREATMENT

• Based on the stage, disease type, woman's age, and menopausal status, and any disfiguring effects of surgery
• With adjunctive therapy: survival of 10 or more years in 70% to 75% of women with negative lymph nodes (compared to 20% to 25% of women with positive lymph nodes)

Local (targeted treatment)
• Primary radiation therapy
• Preoperative breast irradiation
• Lumpectomy
• Partial, total, or modified radical mastectomy

Systemic (treats whole body)
• Chemotherapy used in combinations: doxorubicin (Adriamycin), cyclophosphamide (Cytoxan), fluorouracil (Efudex), methotrexate

- Hormonal (anti-estrogen) therapy: aromatase inhibitors (Arimidex), selective estrogen receptor modulators (Tamoxifen), estrogen-receptor downregulators, fulvestrant (Faslodex)
- Immune therapy (for stage II, III, or IV cancer): trastuzumab (Herceptin)
- Anti-angiogenesis therapy (in clinical trials): stops the growth of new blood vessels that supply the cancer cells

KEY PATIENT OUTCOMES

The patient will:
- recognize limitations imposed by the illness and express feelings about these limitations
- express positive feelings about herself
- report feelings of comfort
- express an increased sense of well-being
- use situational supports to reduce fear.

NURSING INTERVENTIONS

- Provide information about the disease process, diagnostic tests, and treatment.
- Give prescribed drugs, and evaluate their effects.
- Provide emotional support, and monitor psychological status.
- Observe the wound site for infection or bleeding, and change dressings as ordered.
- Monitor for postoperative complications.
- Check vital signs and intake and output.
- Track white blood cell count.
- Assess and help manage pain.

PATIENT TEACHING

Be sure to cover:
- disease process
- all procedures and treatments

- activities or exercises that promote healing
- breast self-examination
- risks and signs and symptoms of recurrence
- avoidance of venipuncture or blood pressure monitoring on the affected side
- how to access the American Cancer Society
- location and contact information for a local support group and local services.

Diabetes mellitus

DESCRIPTION

- *Diabetes mellitus* is a chronic disease in which high levels of blood glucose occur because of the body's inability to produce insulin, to produce enough insulin, or to properly utilize the insulin that's produced.
- It's characterized by disturbances in carbohydrate, protein, and fat metabolism.
- It has two primary forms.
  - Type 1 is an autoimmune disease that destroys pancreatic beta cells of the islets of Langerhans, which produce insulin.
  - Type 2 is a metabolic disease that results from insulin resistance with a defect in compensatory insulin production.
- It's also known as *DM*.

PATHOPHYSIOLOGY

- The effects result from insulin deficiency or resistance to endogenous insulin. (See *Understanding diabetes mellitus,* page 480.)
- Insulin allows glucose transport into the cells for use as energy or storage as glycogen.
- Insulin also stimulates protein synthesis and free fatty acid storage in the adipose tissues.

Understanding diabetes mellitus

Diabetes affects the way the body uses food to make energy.

Type 1 diabetes
· The pancreas makes little or no insulin.
· In genetically susceptible patients, a triggering event (possibly a viral infection) causes production of autoantibodies against the beta cells of the pancreas.
· The resultant destruction of beta cells leads to a decline in and ultimate lack of insulin secretion.
· Insulin deficiency leads to hyperglycemia, enhanced lipolysis, and protein catabolism. These occur when more than 90% of the beta cells have been destroyed.

Type 2 diabetes
· Genetic factors are significant, and onset is accelerated by obesity and a sedentary lifestyle. The pancreas produces some insulin, but it's either too little or ineffective.
· Factors that contribute to type 2 diabetes development include:
  – impaired insulin secretion
  – inappropriate hepatic glucose production
  – peripheral insulin insensitivity.

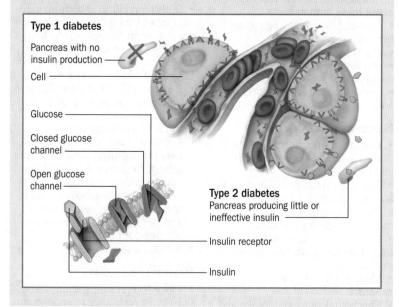

Type 1 diabetes
Pancreas with no insulin production
Cell
Glucose
Closed glucose channel
Open glucose channel
Type 2 diabetes
Pancreas producing little or ineffective insulin
Insulin receptor
Insulin

· Insulin deficiency compromises the body tissues' access to essential nutrients for fuel and storage.

CAUSES
· Autoimmune disease (type 1)
· Genetic factors (types 1 and 2)

Risk factors (type 2)
· Family history: increased risk if close relative has type 2 diabetes
· Age: more common after age 40—incidence in younger people increasing
· Race: higher incidence in African Americans, Latinos, Hispanics, Native Americans, Pacific Americans, and Asian Americans

- Child-bearing: increased risk of developing type 2 diabetes later in life in women with gestational diabetes or who deliver infants greater than 9 lb (4.1 kg)
- Overweight: increased risk with increased body fat
- Smoking: blood sugar harder to control
- High blood pressure and elevated cholesterol: associated with insulin resistance and heart disease
- Inactivity

ASSESSMENT FINDINGS

Type 1
- Rapidly developing symptoms
- Dehydration
- Weight loss and hunger; muscle wasting, and loss of subcutaneous fat
- Weakness, fatigue
- Frequent skin and urinary tract infections (UTIs)
- Sexual problems
- Numbness or pain in the hands or feet
- Postprandial feeling of nausea or fullness
- Nocturnal diarrhea

Type 2
- Vague, long-standing symptoms that develop gradually
- Family history of diabetes
- Pregnancy
- Fungal infection
- Other endocrine diseases
- Recent stress or trauma
- Use of drugs that increase blood glucose levels
- Slow-healing wounds
- Obesity, particularly in the abdominal area

Both types
- Polydipsia
- Polyuria
- Retinopathy or cataract formation
- Skin changes, especially on the legs and feet

- Dry mucous membranes
- Decreased peripheral pulses
- Cool skin temperature
- Diminished deep tendon reflexes
- Orthostatic hypotension
- Characteristic "fruity" breath odor in ketoacidosis
- Possible hypovolemia and shock in ketoacidosis and hyperosmolar hyperglycemic state

TEST RESULTS

- Fasting plasma glucose level is greater than or equal to 126 mg/dl on at least two occasions.
- Random blood glucose level is greater than or equal to 200 mg/dl.
- Two-hour postprandial blood glucose level is greater than or equal to 200 mg/dl.
- Glycosylated hemoglobin (HbA_{1c}) level is increased.
- Urinalysis may show acetone or glucose.
- Ophthalmologic examination may show diabetic retinopathy.

TREATMENT

- Tight glycemic control for prevention of complications
- Modest caloric restriction for weight loss or maintenance
- American Diabetes Association recommendations for reaching target glucose, HbA_{1c}, lipid, and blood pressure levels (see *Target numbers for diabetes mellitus,* page 482)
- Regular aerobic exercise
- Exogenous insulin (type 1 and possibly type 2)
- Oral antihyperglycemic drugs (type 2): sulfonylureas, biguanides, alpha-glucosidase inhibitors, thiazolidinediones, and meglitinides
- Pancreas transplantation (rare)
- Referral to a dietitian and a diabetes educator who can assist in teaching the patient ways to gain dietary control of blood glucose

Target numbers for diabetes mellitus

To help patients reduce their risk of complications from diabetes, the American Diabetes Association has recommended important target numbers. Teach your patient to monitor his target numbers for blood glucose, HbA$_{1c}$, blood lipids, and blood pressure.

• Blood glucose: Some meters and test strips report blood glucose as plasma glucose values, which are 10% to 15% higher than whole blood glucose values. Be sure to find out whether the meter and strips provide whole blood or plasma results.

– The target glucose range for most people using whole blood is 80 to 120 mg/dl before meals and 100 to 140 mg/dl at bedtime.

– The target glucose range for most people using plasma is 90 to 130 mg/dl before meals and 110 to 150 mg/dl at bedtime.

• HbA$_{1c}$: measures how well blood glucose has been controlled over the previous 3 months; it should be performed twice per year.

– The target: HbA$_{1c}$ for most people with diabetes is less than 7%.

• Blood lipids: low-density lipoprotein (LDL) is the cholesterol that causes the vessels to narrow and harden, which can lead to a heart attack.

– The target LDL cholesterol for most people with diabetes is less than 100 mg/dl.

• Blood pressure: high blood pressure makes the heart work harder and can lead to strokes and kidney disease. Blood pressure should be checked at every physician visit.

– The target blood pressure for most people with diabetes is less than 130/80 mm Hg.

From: National Institutes of Health, *www.ndep.nih.gov/diabetes/control/principles/html.*

KEY PATIENT OUTCOMES

The patient will:
• achieve and maintain optimal body weight
• maintain appropriate diet
• monitor capillary blood sugars
• verbalize an understanding of signs and symptoms of hypoglycemia and hyperglycemia and how to treat them
• remain free from infection
• avoid complications
• verbalize an understanding of the disorder and treatment
• demonstrate adaptive coping behaviors.

NURSING INTERVENTIONS

• Administer prescribed drugs, and evaluate their effects.
• Give rapidly absorbed carbohydrates for hypoglycemia or, if the patient is unconscious, glucagon or I.V. dextrose, as ordered.

• Administer I.V. fluids and insulin replacement for hyperglycemic crisis, as ordered.
• Provide meticulous skin care, especially to the feet and legs.
• Treat all injuries, cuts, and blisters immediately.
• Avoid constricting hose, slippers, or bed linens.
• Encourage adequate fluid intake.
• Encourage verbalization of feelings.
• Offer emotional support.
• Help to develop effective coping strategies.
• Monitor vital signs, intake and output, and daily weight.
• Monitor laboratory values, especially serum glucose and urine acetone.
• Assess renal and cardiovascular status as needed.
• Watch for signs and symptoms of hypoglycemia, hyperglycemia, hy-

perosmolar coma, UTIs, vaginal infections, and diabetic neuropathy.

PATIENT TEACHING

Be sure to cover:
- the disorder, diagnosis, and treatment
- medication and potential adverse reactions
- when to notify the physician
- the prescribed meal plan
- the prescribed exercise program
- signs and symptoms of infection, hypoglycemia, hyperglycemia, and diabetic neuropathy
- self-monitoring of blood glucose
- complications of hyperglycemia
- foot and wound care
- the importance of annual ophthalmologic examinations
- the importance of annual podiatry examination
- proper footwear
- the proper management of diabetes during illness
- contact information for diabetic teaching and nutritional counseling
- how to access the Juvenile Diabetes Research Foundation, the American Association of Diabetes Educators, and the American Diabetes Association to obtain additional information
- location and contact information for a local support group and local services.

Disseminated intravascular coagulation

DESCRIPTION

- *Disseminated intravascular coagulation* is a syndrome of activated coagulation characterized by bleeding or thrombosis.
- It complicates diseases and conditions that accelerate clotting, causing occlusion of small blood vessels, organ necrosis, depletion of circulating clotting factors and platelets, and activation of the fibrinolytic system.
- It's a life-threatening illness.
- It can be acute or chronic.
- It's also known as *DIC, consumption coagulopathy,* and *defibrination syndrome.*

PATHOPHYSIOLOGY

- Typical accelerated clotting results in generalized activation of prothrombin and a consequent excess of thrombin.
- Excess thrombin converts fibrinogen to fibrin, producing fibrin clots in the microcirculation.
- This process consumes exorbitant amounts of coagulation factors (especially platelets, factor V, prothrombin, fibrinogen, and factor VIII), causing thrombocytopenia, deficiencies in factors V and VIII, hypoprothrombinemia, and hypofibrinogenemia.
- Circulating thrombin activates the fibrinolytic system, which lyses fibrin clots into fibrinogen degradation products (FDPs).
- The hemorrhage that occurs may be caused by the anticoagulant activity of FDPs and depletion of plasma coagulation factors. (See *Understanding disseminated intravascular coagulation,* page 484.)
- Acute and chronic DIC differ; chronic DIC occurs at a more gradual pace, and some compensatory mechanisms decrease bleeding but cause a hypercoagulable state.

CAUSES

Acute DIC
- Infections from bacteria, fungi, viruses, and rickettsiae; sepsis
- Inflammatory bowel disease
- Obstetric complications from abruptio placentae, abortion (especially therapeutic), amniotic fluid embolism, and hemorrhagic shock

Understanding disseminated intravascular coagulation

This flowchart shows the pathophysiologic process of disseminated intravascular coagulation and points for treatment intervention.

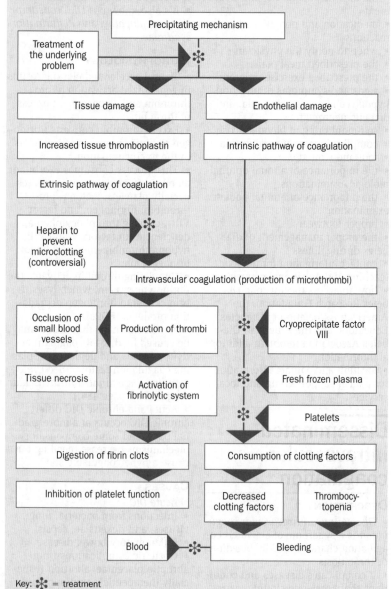

Key: ✱ = treatment

- Malignancies, such as acute leukemia or disseminated prostate cancer
- Brain infarction or hemorrhage
- Snake or spider venom
- Massive tissue destruction
- Heparin-induced thrombocytopenia thrombosis
- Purpura fulminans (in neonates)

Chronic DIC
- Chronic infection, such as tuberculosis or osteomyelitis
- Inflammatory bowel disease
- Dead fetus syndrome or retained products of conception
- Malignancies, such as lung, breast, or GI cancer
- Aortic aneurysm
- Giant hemangioma
- Chronic kidney disease

ASSESSMENT FINDINGS
Acute DIC
- Abnormal bleeding without a history of a serious hemorrhagic disorder, from at least three unrelated sites
- Signs of bleeding into the skin, such as cutaneous oozing, petechiae, ecchymoses, and hematomas
- Possible bleeding from surgical or invasive procedure sites, such as incisions or venipuncture sites
- Ischemic tissue
- Confusion, disorientation
- Dyspnea

Chronic DIC
- Signs and symptoms of deep vein or arterial thrombosis, possibly at multiple sites
- Superficial thrombosis
- Repeated episodes of thrombosis

TEST RESULTS
Acute DIC
- Prothrombin time (PT), partial thromboplastin time (PTT), and thrombin time are elevated.
- Fibrinogen levels are decreased.

- FDP levels are increased.
- Platelet count is decreased.
- D-dimer test is positive.
- Shistocytes appear on a peripheral smear.

Chronic DIC
- PT may be increased.
- PTT is decreased.
- Thrombin time is usually normal
- Platelet and fibrinogen levels may be increased, decreased, or normal.
- FDP is increased.
- Thrombin time is prolonged.

TREATMENT
Acute DIC
- Prompt recognition and adequate treatment of the underlying disorder
- Supportive care alone, if the patient isn't actively bleeding
- If bleeding, administration of fresh frozen plasma, platelets, packed red blood cells, and cryoprecipitate
- If ischemia occurs, anticoagulants possibly administered after correction of bleeding risk

Chronic DIC
- Long-term treatment with low-weight molecular heparin
- Possible treatment with warfarin (Coumadin)

KEY PATIENT OUTCOMES
The patient will:
- achieve resolution of the underlying disorder
- maintain balanced intake and output
- not show signs of bleeding
- have laboratory values return to normal
- verbalize an understanding of the disorder and treatment.

NURSING INTERVENTIONS
- Provide treatment for underlying disorder as directed.
- Provide emotional support.

- Reposition the patient every 2 hours.
- Perform range-of-motion exercises.
- Give prescribed oxygen therapy.
- Protect the patient from injury.
- Monitor for bleeding; if bleeding occurs, use pressure and topical hemostatic agents to control it.
- Watch for transfusion reactions and signs of fluid overload when administering blood products.
- Obtain daily weight.
- Monitor vital signs and intake and output.
- Monitor laboratory values.
- Monitor for signs of thrombosis.
- Provide supportive care as indicated.

PATIENT TEACHING
Be sure to cover:
- an explanation of the disorder and treatment
- the need for blood products and how they help the condition (with acute)
- the signs and symptoms of thrombosis and when to seek medical help (with chronic).

Emphysema

DESCRIPTION
- *Emphysema* is a chronic lung disease characterized by permanent enlargement of air spaces distal to the terminal bronchioles with destruction of their walls and with obvious fibrosis.
- It causes exertional dyspnea in early stages and, in later stages, respiratory difficulty, even at rest.
- It's one of several diseases usually labeled collectively as *chronic obstructive pulmonary disease* or *chronic obstructive lung disease*.

PATHOPHYSIOLOGY
- Recurrent inflammation associated with the release of proteolytic enzymes from lung cells causes abnormal, irreversible enlargement of the air spaces distal to the terminal bronchioles.
- Enlargement leads to the destruction of alveolar walls, which results in a breakdown of elasticity.
- Oxygen and carbon dioxide exchange becomes impaired.

CAUSES
- Damage to air sacs in lungs, usually by an irritant

Risk factors
- Cigarette smoking (greatest risk factor)
- Genetic deficiency of alpha$_1$-antitrypsin (A_1AT)
- Environmental pollution
- Frequent respiratory infections
- Immune deficiency disorder
- Connective tissue disorder
- I.V. drug user (caused by the insoluble filler used in drugs)

ASSESSMENT FINDINGS
- History of smoking
- Shortness of breath with exertion
- Chronic cough with small amounts of colorless sputum
- Anorexia and weight loss
- Barrel chest
- Pursed-lip breathing, use of accessory muscles
- Clubbed fingers and toes
- Tachypnea; decreased tactile fremitus and chest expansion
- Hyperresonance
- Diminished breath sounds, possible wheezing
- Distant heart sound

TEST RESULTS
- Pulmonary function tests reveal:
  – increased residual volume, functional residual capacity, and total lung capacity

- reduced diffusing capacity
- increased inspiratory flow.
• Chest X-ray may show:
  - hyperinflation of the lungs (flattened diaphragm, vertical heart, large retrosternal air space)
  - reduced vascular markings at the lung periphery
  - enlarged anteroposterior chest diameter.
• Computed tomography scan outlines bullae not seen on chest X-ray (this isn't routinely done for diagnosis).
• Arterial blood gas (ABG) analysis shows decreased partial pressure of oxygen and normal partial pressure of carbon dioxide (Pco_2) in the early stages of the disease. Later stages of the disease show increased Pco_2.
• Red blood cell count reveals an increased hematocrit late in the disease.
• Electrocardiography may show tall, symmetrical P waves in leads II, III, and aV_F; a vertical QRS axis; and signs of right ventricular hypertrophy (late in the disease).
• A_1AT concentration may be low (if inherited-type emphysema).

TREATMENT
• Smoking cessation
• Chest physiotherapy
• Supplemental oxygen therapy; endotracheal intubation and mechanical ventilation in severe exacerbation
• Adequate hydration
• High-protein, high-calorie diet
• Activity as tolerated
• Bronchodilators
• Mucolytics
• Corticosteroids
• Antibiotics as needed
• Surgery (bullectomy for giant bullae, lung volume reduction or lung transplantation)

KEY PATIENT OUTCOMES
The patient will:

• maintain a patent airway and adequate ventilation
• demonstrate energy conservation techniques
• express an understanding of the illness and treatment
• demonstrate effective coping strategies.

NURSING INTERVENTIONS
• Encourage smoking cessation.
• Monitor respiratory status.
• Provide supplemental oxygen.
• Administer prescribed medications.
• Provide supportive care.
• Help the patient adjust to lifestyle changes as needed.
• Encourage the patient to express his fears and concerns.
• Perform chest physiotherapy.
• Provide a high-calorie, protein-rich diet in small, frequent meals.
• Encourage daily activity and diversional activities.
• Provide frequent rest periods.
• Monitor vital signs, intake and output, and daily weight.
• Monitor ABG values.

PATIENT TEACHING
Be sure to cover:
• the disorder, diagnosis, and treatment
• the importance of smoking cessation
• medication and potential adverse reactions
• when to notify the physician
• avoidance of crowds and people with known infections
• avoidance of areas where smoking is permitted
• home oxygen therapy, if indicated
• coughing and deep-breathing exercises
• high-calorie, high-protein diet
• adequate oral fluid intake
• avoidance of respiratory irritants
• signs and symptoms of pneumothorax

• the need for influenza and pneumococcal pneumonia immunizations
• how to access the American Lung Association to obtain additional information.
• location and contact information for a local support group and local services.

Gastroesophageal reflux disease

DESCRIPTION

• *Gastroesophageal reflux disease* is a chronic condition in which backflow of gastric contents or duodenal contents, or both, causes inflammation or damage to the lining of the esophagus.
• Reflux of gastric acid results in acute epigastric pain, usually after a meal.
• It's popularly called *heartburn* or *GERD*.

PATHOPHYSIOLOGY

• Reflux occurs when lower esophageal sphincter (LES) pressure is deficient or when pressure in the stomach exceeds LES pressure. LES relaxes or has weak contractions, and gastric contents regurgitate into the esophagus.
• Acid in the esophagus causes nerve fibers to be stimulated, typically causing a burning pain.
• The degree of mucosal injury is based on the amount and concentration of refluxed gastric acid, proteolytic enzymes, and bile acids.

CAUSES

• Any condition or position that increases intra-abdominal pressure
• Hiatal hernia with incompetent sphincter
• Pyloric surgery (alteration or removal of the pylorus), which allows reflux of bile or pancreatic juice

ASSESSMENT FINDINGS

• Minimal or no symptoms in one-third of patients
• Heartburn that typically occurs $1\frac{1}{2}$ to 2 hours after eating
• Heartburn that worsens with vigorous exercise, bending, lying down, wearing tight clothing, coughing, constipation, and obesity
• Reported relief by using antacids or sitting upright
• Regurgitation
• Possible nausea or belching
• Feeling of fluid accumulation in the throat without a sour or bitter taste
• Chronic pain radiating to the neck, jaws, and arms that may mimic angina pectoris
• Nocturnal hypersalivation and wheezing
• Odynophagia (sharp substernal pain on swallowing), possibly followed by a dull substernal ache
• Bright red or dark brown blood in vomitus
• Laryngitis and morning hoarseness
• Chronic cough

TEST RESULTS

• Esophageal acid test reveals the degree of gastroesophageal reflux (considered the "gold standard").
• Barium swallow with fluoroscopy reveals evidence of recurrent reflux.
• Esophageal motility test evaluates function of the esophageal muscle.
• Esophageal manometry reveals abnormal LES pressure and sphincter incompetence.
• Gastric emptying studies determine the rate in which the stomach empties.
• An acid perfusion (Bernstein) test determines whether chest pain is caused by acid reflux (rarely used).
• Upper GI endoscopy (esophagogastroduodenoscopy) and biopsy confirm pathologic changes in the mucosa or identify complications.

TREATMENT

- Modification of lifestyle (smoking cessation)
- Positional therapy
- Weight reduction, if appropriate
- Dietary modifications (see *Factors affecting LES pressure*)
- Chewing gum after meals
- Small, frequent meals and avoidance of eating 2 hours before bedtime
- Antacids
- Histamine-2 receptor antagonists (ranitidine [Zantac] or famotidine [Pepcid])
- Proton pump inhibitors (omeprazole [Prilosec] or pantoprazole [Protonix])
- Foam barrier (Gaviscon) (combination of aluminum hydroxide gel, magnesium trisilicate, and alginate)
- Fundoplication
- Endoscopic surgery or treatment

KEY PATIENT OUTCOMES

The patient will:
- state and demonstrate an understanding of the disorder and its treatment
- express feelings of increased comfort and decreased episodes of heartburn
- have minimal or no complications
- demonstrate lifestyle modifications.

NURSING INTERVENTIONS

- Offer emotional and psychological support.
- Help the patient identify appropriate lifestyle changes.
- Assist with diet modification.
- Stress remaining upright for 2 hours after meals.
- Administer prescribed medications, and evaluate their effects.
- Ensure pain control.
- Monitor vital signs, intake and output, and bowel function.
- Provide postoperative care as appropriate.

Factors affecting LES pressure

Various dietary and lifestyle elements can increase or decrease lower esophageal sphincter (LES) pressure. Take these into account as you plan the patient's treatment program.

What increases LES pressure
- Carbohydrates
- Low-dose ethanol
- Nonfat milk
- Protein

What decreases LES pressure
- Antiflatulent (simethicone [Gas-X, Mylanta Gas, Phazyme])
- Chocolate
- Cigarette smoking
- Fatty foods
- High-dose ethanol
- Lying on the right or left side
- Citrus juices
- Tomato-based products
- Peppermint
- Caffeinated products

PATIENT TEACHING

Be sure to cover:
- the disorder, diagnosis, and treatment
- causes of gastroesophageal reflux
- prescribed antireflux regimen of medication, diet, and positional therapy
- how to develop a dietary plan
- the need to identify situations or activities that increase intra-abdominal pressure
- smoking cessation, if appropriate
- signs and symptoms to watch for and report
- how to access the American Gastroenterological Association to obtain additional information
- location and contact information for a local support group and local services.

Heart failure

DESCRIPTION

- *Heart failure* is a chronic, progressive cardiovascular disorder that causes fluid buildup in the heart from impaired myocardium contractility.
- It usually occurs from a damaged left ventricle, but it may also result from right ventricular damage.
- It's classified according to physical limitations. (See *Classifying heart failure.*)
- It's the fastest growing cardiac disorder in the United States.
- It's also known as *congestive heart failure.*

Classifying heart failure

The New York Heart Association classification is a universal gauge of heart failure severity based on physical limitations.

Class I: Minimal
· The patient has no limitations.
· Ordinary physical activity doesn't cause undue fatigue, dyspnea, palpitations, or angina.

Class II: Mild
· The patient has lightly limited physical activity.
· The patient is comfortable at rest.
· Ordinary physical activity results in fatigue, palpitations, dyspnea, or angina.

Class III: Moderate
· The patient has markedly limited physical activity.
· The patient is comfortable at rest.
· Less-than-ordinary activity produces symptoms.

Class IV: Severe
· The patient is unable to perform physical activity without discomfort.
· Angina or symptoms of cardiac inefficiency may develop at rest.

PATHOPHYSIOLOGY

Left-sided heart failure

- Ineffective left ventricle contractile function results in decreased cardiac output.
- Blood backs up into the left atrium and lungs, causing pulmonary congestion.
- If the condition persists, pulmonary edema and right-sided heart failure may occur.

Right-sided heart failure

- Ventricular injury that impedes contractile ability of cardiac cells of the right ventricle leads
- Ineffective pumping of the ventricle leads to blood backup in the right atrium and, eventually, in the peripheral circulation
- If condition persists, peripheral edema and engorgement of the kidneys and other organs possibly occurring

CAUSES

- Abnormal cardiac muscle function
- Abnormal left ventricle volume
- Abnormal left ventricle pressure
- Abnormal left ventricle filling (see *Causes of heart failure*)

ASSESSMENT FINDINGS

Left-sided heart failure (early stages)

- Dyspnea
- Orthopnea
- Paroxysmal nocturnal dyspnea
- Fatigue
- Nonproductive cough

Left-sided heart failure (late stages)

- Crackles on auscultation
- Hemoptysis
- Point of maximal impulse displaced toward the left anterior axillary line
- Tachycardia

Causes of heart failure

Cause	Examples
Abnormal cardiac muscle function	• Myocardial infarction • Cardiomyopathy
Abnormal left ventricular volume	• Valvular insufficiency • High-output states: – Chronic anemia – Arteriovenous fistula – Thyrotoxicosis – Pregnancy – Septicemia – Beriberi – Infusion of a large volume of I.V. fluids in a short period
Abnormal left ventricular pressure	• Hypertension • Pulmonary hypertension • Chronic obstructive pulmonary disease • Aortic or pulmonic valve stenosis
Abnormal left ventricular filling	• Mitral valve stenosis • Tricuspid valve stenosis • Atrial myxoma • Constrictive pericarditis • Atrial fibrillation • Impaired ventricular relaxation: – Hypertension – Myocardial hibernation – Myocardial stunning

• Third (S_3) and fourth (S_4) heart sounds on auscultation
• Cool, pale skin
• Restlessness and confusion

Right-sided heart failure
• Elevated jugular vein distention
• Positive hepatojugular reflux and hepatomegaly
• Right upper quadrant abdominal pain
• Anorexia; fullness and nausea
• Nocturia
• Weight gain
• Peripheral edema
• Ascites or anasarca

TEST RESULTS
• B-type natriuretic peptide immunoassay is elevated.
• Chest X-rays show increased pulmonary vascular markings, interstitial edema, or pleural effusion and cardiomegaly.
• Electrocardiography may indicate hypertrophy, ischemia or infarction, tachycardia, or extrasystole.
• Pulmonary artery pressure monitoring typically shows elevated pulmonary artery and pulmonary artery wedge pressures, left ventricular end-diastolic pressure in left-sided heart failure, and elevated right atrial or central venous pressure in right-sided heart failure.

• Echocardiography reveals wall motion abnormalities, decreased left ventricular function, valvular disease, cardiac tamponade, and constriction.
• Liver function tests may be abnormal, blood urea nitrogen and creatinine may be elevated, and prothrombin time may be prolonged.

TREATMENT

• Treatment of the underlying cause
• Supplemental oxygen
• Diuretics
• Nesiritide (Natrecor)
• Angiotensin-converting enzyme inhibitors (with left-ventricular dysfunction)
• Digoxin
• Beta-adrenergic blockers (with class II or III heart failure)
• Inotropic drugs
• Morphine sulfate
• Nitrates
• Lifestyle modifications: diet, weight reduction, exercise
• Surgery (coronary artery bypass, angioplasty, valvular repair, heart transplantation)
• Ventricular assist device or biventricular pacemaker

KEY PATIENT OUTCOMES

The patient will:
• maintain hemodynamic stability
• maintain adequate cardiac output
• carry out activities of daily living without excess fatigue or decreased energy
• maintain adequate ventilation
• maintain adequate fluid balance.

NURSING INTERVENTIONS

• Place in Fowler's position, and provide supplemental oxygen.
• Assess respiratory status.
• Monitor cardiac rhythm.
• Assist with range-of-motion exercises.

• Apply antiembolism or sequential compression stockings; check for calf pain and tenderness.
• Monitor weight and intake and output.
• Assess for peripheral edema.
• Administer prescribed medications, and evaluate their effects.
• Monitor vital signs, pulse oximetry, and hemodynamic parameters, if available.
• Monitor laboratory and arterial blood gas values.

PATIENT TEACHING

Be sure to cover:
• the disorder, diagnosis, and treatment
• signs and symptoms of worsening heart failure
• when to notify the physician
• the importance of follow-up care
• the need to avoid high-sodium foods
• instructions about fluid restrictions
• the importance of monitoring weight daily and reporting increases of 3 to 5 lb (1.5 to 2.5 kg) in 1 week
• the importance of smoking cessation, if appropriate
• weight reduction as needed
• medication dosage, administration, potential adverse effects, and monitoring needs
• how to access the American Heart Association to obtain additional information
• location and contact information for a local support group and local services.

Hip fracture

DESCRIPTION

• *Hip fracture* is a break in the head or neck of the femur (usually the head).
• It's the most common fall-related injury resulting in hospitalization.

- It's the leading cause of disability among older adults.
- It may permanently change a patient's level of functioning and independence.
- Almost 25% of patients die within 1 year.
- It affects more than 200,000 people each year.
- It occurs in one of five women by age 80 and is more common in females than in males.

PATHOPHYSIOLOGY

- With bone fracture, the periosteum and blood vessels in the marrow, cortex, and surrounding soft tissues are disrupted.
- Disruption of the periosteum and blood vessels results in bleeding from the damaged ends of the bone and from the neighboring soft tissue.
- Clot formation occurs within the medullary canal, between the fractured bone ends, and beneath the periosteum.
- Bone tissue immediately adjacent to the fracture dies, and the necrotic tissue causes an intense inflammatory response.
- Vascular tissue invades the fracture area from surrounding soft tissue and marrow cavity within 48 hours, increasing blood flow to the entire bone.
- Bone-forming cells in the periosteum, endosteum, and marrow are activated to produce subperiosteal procallus along the outer surface of the shaft and over the broken ends of the bone.
- Collagen and matrix, which become mineralized to form callus, are synthesized by osteoblasts within the procallus.
- During the repair process, remodeling occurs; unnecessary callus is resorbed, and trabeculae are formed along stress lines.

- New bone, not scar tissue, is formed over the healed fracture.

CAUSES

- Cancer metastasis
- Falls
- Osteoporosis
- Skeletal disease
- Trauma

ASSESSMENT FINDINGS

- Affected extremity possibly appearing shorter
- Edema and discoloration of the surrounding tissue
- Fall or trauma to the bones
- In an open fracture, bone protruding through the skin
- Limited or abnormal range of motion (ROM)
- Outward rotation of affected extremity
- Pain exacerbated by movement
- Pain in the affected hip and leg

TEST RESULTS

- X-rays show the fracture's location.
- Computed tomography scan shows abnormalities in complicated fractures.

TREATMENT

- Based on age, comorbidities, cognitive functioning, support systems, and functional ability
- Possible skin traction
- Total hip arthroplasty
- Hemiarthroplasty
- Percutaneous pinning
- Internal fixation using a compression screw and plate
- Analgesics and stool softeners
- Physical therapy
- Non-weight-bearing transfers
- Bed rest, initially
- Ambulation as soon as possible after surgery
- Well-balanced diet
- Foods rich in vitamin C and A, calcium, and protein

• Adequate vitamin D

KEY PATIENT OUTCOMES

The patient will:
• identify factors that increase the potential for injury
• maintain muscle strength and tone and joint ROM
• verbalize feelings of increased comfort
• attain the highest degree of mobility possible within the confines of the injury
• maintain skin integrity.

NURSING INTERVENTIONS

• Give prescribed medications.
• Give prescribed prophylactic anticoagulation medications after surgery.
• Maintain traction.
• Maintain proper body alignment.
• Use logrolling techniques to turn the patient in bed.
• Maintain non-weight-bearing status.
• Increase the patient's activity level as prescribed.
• Consult physical therapy as early as possible.
• Assist with active ROM exercises to unaffected limbs, and monitor mobility and ROM.
• Encourage coughing and deep-breathing exercises and the use of incentive spirometry.
• Prevent skin breakdown; keep the patient's skin clean and dry.
• Encourage good nutrition; offer high-protein, high-calorie snacks.
• Monitor vital signs.
• Measure and evaluate intake and output.
• Assess level of pain.
• Assess incision and dressings, and perform wound care.
• Apply a sequential compression stocking to prevent deep vein thrombosis.
• Observe for complications.
• Monitor coagulation study results.

• Observe for signs of bleeding.
• Assess neurovascular status.
• Assess skin integrity.
• Observe for signs and symptoms of infection.

PATIENT TEACHING

Be sure to cover:
• the disorder, diagnosis, and treatment
• prescribed medications and potential adverse effects
• ROM exercises
• meticulous skin care
• proper body alignment
• wound care
• signs of infection
• coughing and deep-breathing exercises and incentive spirometry
• assistive devices
• activity restrictions and lifestyle changes
• safe ambulation practices
• nutritious diet and adequate fluid intake.

Human immunodeficiency virus

DESCRIPTION

• *Human immunodeficiency virus (HIV) type I* is a retrovirus causing acquired immunodeficiency syndrome (AIDS).
• It causes patients to become susceptible to opportunistic infections, unusual cancers, and other abnormalities.
• It's marked by progressive failure of the immune system.
• It's transmitted by contact with infected blood or body fluids and associated with identifiable high-risk behaviors.

PATHOPHYSIOLOGY

• HIV strikes helper T cells bearing the CD4$^+$ antigen.

- The antigen serves as a receptor for the retrovirus and lets it enter the cell.
- After invading a cell, HIV replicates, leading to cell death, or becomes latent.
- HIV infection leads to profound pathology, either directly, through destruction of CD4$^+$ cells, other immune cells, and neuroglial cells, or indirectly, through the secondary effects of CD4$^+$ T-cell dysfunction and resultant immunosuppression.

CAUSES
- Infection with HIV, a retrovirus

Risk factors
- Unprotected sexual intercourse with an infected partner or multiple partners
- History of sharing needles with I.V. drug abusers
- History of sexually transmitted disease
- Received blood products before 1985
- Born to a mother who's HIV-infected and wasn't treated
- Use of nonsterile needles while acquiring a tattoo or piercing
- Exposure to infected blood or body fluid without recommended barriers

ASSESSMENT FINDINGS
- A high-risk exposure and inoculation, followed by a mononucleosis-like syndrome (patient then possibly asymptomatic for years)
- In the latent stage, laboratory evidence of seroconversion, the only sign of HIV infection
- Neurologic symptoms resulting from HIV encephalopathy
- Nonspecific symptoms (weight loss, fatigue, night sweats, fevers)
- Opportunistic infection or cancer (Kaposi's sarcoma)
- Persistent generalized adenopathy

TEST RESULTS
- CD4$^+$ T-cell count is at least 200 cells/ml.
- Screening test enzyme-linked immunosorbent assay and confirmatory test (Western blot) detect the presence of HIV antibodies.
- Direct testing detects HIV itself; these tests include antigen testing, HIV cultures, nucleic acid probes of peripheral blood lymphocytes, and polymerase chain reaction tests.

TREATMENT
- Various therapeutic options for opportunistic infections (the leading cause of morbidity and mortality in patients infected with HIV)
- Disease-specific therapy for a variety of neoplastic and premalignant diseases and organ-specific syndromes
- Symptom management (fatigue and anemia)
- Well-balanced diet
- Regular exercise, as tolerated, with adequate rest periods
- Immunomodulatory agents
- Anti-infective agents
- Antineoplastic agents
- Highly active antiretroviral therapy—three or more of the following:
  - Protease inhibitors
  - Nucleoside reverse transcriptase inhibitors
  - Nonnucleoside reverse transcriptase inhibitors
  - Fusion inhibitors

KEY PATIENT OUTCOMES
The patient will:
- achieve management of illness symptoms
- demonstrate the use of protective measures, including conservation of energy, maintenance of a well-balanced diet, and getting adequate rest
- follow safer sex practices
- use available support systems to assist with coping

• voice feelings about changes in sexual identity and social response to disease
• develop no complications of illness
• comply with the treatment regimen.

NURSING INTERVENTIONS

• Help the patient to cope with an altered body image, the emotional burden of serious illness, and the threat of death.
• Avoid glycerin swabs for mucous membranes. Use normal saline or bicarbonate mouthwash for daily oral rinsing.
• Ensure adequate fluid intake during episodes of diarrhea.
• Encourage the patient to maintain as much physical activity as he can tolerate. Make sure his schedule includes time for exercise and rest.
• Monitor vital signs, especially temperature, noting any pattern.
• Assess skin integrity and provide skin care.
• Observe for signs of illness, such as cough, sore throat, or diarrhea.
• Assess for swollen, tender lymph nodes.
• Monitor laboratory values, including complete blood count; electrolyte, blood urea nitrogen, and creatinine levels; and chest X-rays.
• Record calorie intake.
• Monitor progression of lesions in Kaposi's sarcoma.
• Observe for opportunistic infections or signs of disease progression.
• Discuss and monitor compliance with medication regimen.

PATIENT TEACHING

Be sure to cover:
• the disorder, diagnosis, and treatment
• medication regimens
• the importance of informing potential sexual partners, caregivers, and health care workers of HIV infection, and the need to practice barrier precautions to prevent contracting HIV
• the need for the caregiver to properly dispose of items contaminated with body fluids
• signs of impending infection and the importance of seeking immediate medical attention
• symptoms of AIDS dementia and its stages and progression
• how to access the Centers for Disease Control and Prevention to obtain additional information
• location and contact information for a local support group and local services.

Intestinal obstruction

DESCRIPTION

• *Intestinal obstruction* is a partial or complete blockage of the lumen of the small or large bowel.
• It's commonly a medical emergency.
• It's the leading cause of small-bowel obstruction in postoperative adhesions followed by malignancy, Crohn's disease, and hernias.
• Without treatment, a complete obstruction in any part of the bowel can cause death within hours from shock and vascular collapse.

PATHOPHYSIOLOGY

• Mechanical or nonmechanical (neurogenic) blockage of the lumen occurs.
• Fluid, air, or gas collects near the site.
• Peristalsis increases temporarily in an attempt to break through the blockage.
• Intestinal mucosa is injured, and distention at and above the site of obstruction occurs.

• Venous blood flow is impaired, and normal absorptive processes cease.
• Water, sodium, and potassium are secreted by the bowel into the fluid pooled in the lumen.
• Increased bowel mucosal permeability can lead to bacterial leakage and systemic toxicity.
• Bowel ischemia can lead to partial or complete perforation and fecal soilage of the peritoneum.

CAUSES

Mechanical obstruction
• Adhesions
• Carcinomas
• Compression of the bowel wall from stenosis, intussusception, volvulus of the sigmoid or cecum, tumors, and atresia
• Foreign bodies
• Strangulated hernias

Nonmechanical obstruction
• Electrolyte imbalances
• Neurogenic abnormalities
• Paralytic ileus
• Thrombosis or embolism of mesenteric vessels
• Toxicity such as that associated with uremia or generalized infection

ASSESSMENT FINDINGS
• Recent change in bowel habits
• Hiccups

Mechanical obstruction
• History of abdominal surgery, pelvic surgery, or radiation therapy
• Colicky pain
• Nausea, vomiting
• Constipation
• Distended abdomen
• Borborygmi and rushes (occasionally loud enough to be heard without a stethoscope)
• Abdominal tenderness
• Rebound tenderness
• Hyperresonance on percussion
• Fever and tachycardia

Nonmechanical obstruction
• Diffuse abdominal discomfort
• Frequent vomiting
• Severe abdominal pain (if obstruction results from vascular insufficiency or infarction)
• Abdominal distention
• Decreased bowel sounds (early), then absent bowel sounds

TEST RESULTS
• Serum sodium, chloride, and potassium levels are decreased.
• White blood cell count is elevated.
• Serum amylase level is increased if pancreas is irritated by a bowel loop.
• Blood urea nitrogen and creatinine are increased with dehydration.
• Abdominal X-rays reveal the presence and location of intestinal gas or fluid; in small-bowel obstruction, a typical "stepladder" pattern emerges, with alternating fluid and gas levels apparent in 3 to 4 hours.
• Barium enema reveals a distended, air-filled colon or a closed loop of sigmoid with extreme distention (in sigmoid volvulus).

TREATMENT
• Nasogastric (NG) tube insertion for decompression of the bowel and relief of vomiting and distention
• Surgery usually the treatment of choice (exception is paralytic ileus, in which nonoperative therapy is usually attempted first)
• Correction of fluid and electrolyte imbalances
• Treatment of shock and peritonitis
• Nothing by mouth if surgery is planned
• Parenteral nutrition until the bowel is functioning
• High-fiber diet when obstruction is relieved and peristalsis returns
• Bed rest during acute phase
• Postoperatively, avoidance of lifting and contact sports

- Broad-spectrum antibiotics
- Analgesics
- Blood replacement
- Type of surgery dependent on the cause of blockage

KEY PATIENT OUTCOMES

The patient will:
- maintain stable vital signs
- express feelings of increased comfort
- maintain normal fluid volume
- return to normal bowel function
- maintain caloric requirement.

NURSING INTERVENTIONS

- Insert an NG tube, and attach to low-pressure, intermittent suction.
- Maintain the patient in semi-Fowler's position.
- Provide mouth and nose care.
- Begin and maintain I.V. therapy as ordered.
- Administer prescribed medications.
- Monitor vital signs.
- Assess for signs and symptoms of shock.
- Assess bowel sounds and signs of returning peristalsis.
- Monitor NG tube function and drainage.
- Assess pain control, and provide comfort measures.
- Monitor the abdominal girth measurement to detect progressive distention.
- Assess hydration and nutritional status.
- Monitor electrolytes and signs and symptoms of metabolic derangements.
- Assess the wound site (postoperatively), and provide wound care.

PATIENT TEACHING

Be sure to cover:
- the disorder (focusing on the patient's type of intestinal obstruction), diagnosis, and treatment

- techniques for coughing and deep breathing, and the use of incentive spirometry
- colostomy or ileostomy care, if appropriate
- incision care
- postoperative activity limitations and why these restrictions are necessary
- the proper use of prescribed medications, focusing on correct administration, desired effects, and possible adverse reactions
- the importance of following a structured bowel regimen, particularly if the patient had a mechanical obstruction from fecal impaction
- referral information to an enterostomal specialist, if appropriate.

Leukemia, acute

DESCRIPTION

- *Acute leukemia* is the malignant proliferation of white blood cell (WBC) precursors, or *blasts*, in bone marrow or lymph tissue. Blasts accumulate in peripheral blood, bone marrow, and body tissues.
- It's the most common form of cancer among children.
- It has several common forms.
  – *Acute lymphoblastic (lymphocytic) leukemia (ALL)* is characterized by abnormal growth of lymphocyte precursors (lymphoblasts). It's the most common form of leukemia in children.
  – *Acute myeloblastic (myelogenous) leukemia (AML)* causes rapid accumulation of myeloid precursors (myeloblasts).
  – Acute monoblastic (monocytic) leukemia, or *Schilling's type*, results in a marked increase in monocyte precursors (monoblasts).

Understanding leukemia

Leukemias cause an abnormal proliferation of white blood cells (WBCs) and suppression of other blood components. A rapidly progressing disease, acute leukemia is characterized by the malignant proliferation of WBC precursors (blasts) in bone marrow or lymph tissue and by their accumulation in peripheral blood, bone marrow, and body tissues. In chronic forms of leukemia, disease onset occurs more insidiously, commonly with no symptoms.

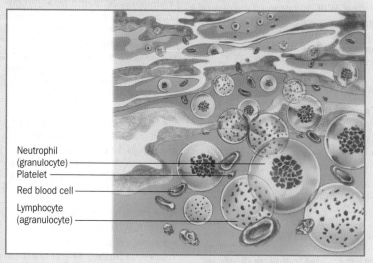

Neutrophil
(granulocyte)
Platelet
Red blood cell
Lymphocyte
(agranulocyte)

PATHOPHYSIOLOGY

• Immature, nonfunctioning WBCs appear to accumulate first in the tissue where they originate, such as lymphocytes in lymph tissue and granulocytes in bone marrow.
• The immature, nonfunctioning WBCs spill into the bloodstream and overwhelm red blood cells (RBCs) and platelets; from there, they infiltrate other tissues. (See *Understanding leukemia*.)

CAUSES

• Unknown

Risk factors
• Radiation exposure
• Drugs
• Genetic abnormalities
• Toxins

• Viruses
• Myelodysplastic syndrome

ASSESSMENT FINDINGS

• Sudden onset of high fever
• Abnormal bleeding or bruising; petechiae
• Fatigue and night sweats
• Weakness, lassitude, frequent and recurrent infections, and chills
• Abdominal or bone pain in patients with ALL, AML, or acute monoblastic leukemia
• Tachycardia, palpitations, and a systolic ejection murmur
• Pallor
• Decreased ventilation
• Liver or spleen enlargement
• Lymph node enlargement
• Headaches
• Weight loss

Test results

- Blood counts show low, normal, or elevated WBC count, and WBC differential shows the cell type. Hemoglobin is low.
- Computed tomography scan shows the affected organs, and cerebrospinal fluid analysis showing abnormal WBC invasion of the central nervous system.
- Bone marrow aspiration shows a proliferation of immature WBCs (confirming acute leukemia).
- Lumbar puncture detects meningeal involvement.

Treatment

- Transfusions of platelets to prevent bleeding
- Transfusions of RBCs to prevent anemia
- Bone marrow transplantation in some patients
- Stem cell transplantation
- Radiation therapy in case of brain or testicular infiltration
- Chemotherapeutic and radiation treatment, depending on diagnosis
- Well-balanced diet
- Frequent rest periods

For meningeal infiltration

- Intrathecal instillation of methotrexate (Rheumatrex) or cytarabine (Tarabine PFS) with cranial radiation

For ALL

- Vincristine (Oncovin), prednisone (Orasone), high-dose cytarabine, and daunorubicin
- Intrathecal methotrexate or cytarabine because ALL carries a 40% risk of meningeal infiltration
- Induces remission in 90% of children (with best survival rate among children ages 2 to 8) and in 65% of adults

For AML

- A combination of I.V. daunorubicin and cytarabine
- If combination of I.V. daunorubicin and cytarabine fails to induce remission, some or all of the following medications: a combination of cyclophosphamide, vincristine, prednisone, or methotrexate; high-dose cytarabine alone or with other drugs; amsacrine; etoposide; and 5-azacytidine and mitoxantrone
- Average survival time of 1 year after diagnosis, even with aggressive treatment (remissions lasting 2 to 10 months in 50% of children)

For acute monoblastic leukemia

- Cytarabine and thioguanine with daunorubicin or doxorubicin
- Anti-infective agents, such as antibiotics, antifungals, and antiviral drugs and granulocyte injections

Key patient outcomes

The patient will:
- be free from infection
- have no further weight loss
- exhibit intact mucous membranes
- express feelings of increased comfort.

Nursing interventions

- Encourage verbalization, and provide comfort.
- Provide adequate hydration.
- After bone marrow or stem cell transplantation, keep the patient in a sterile room, administer antibiotics, and transfuse packed RBCs as necessary.
- Administer prescribed medications.
- Control mouth ulceration by checking often for obvious ulcers and gum swelling and by providing frequent mouth care and saline rinses.
- Observe for complications from treatment, especially signs and symptoms of infection.

- Assess the patient's hydration and nutritional status.
- Test urine pH (should be above 7.5).
- Monitor vital signs.
- Observe for signs and symptoms of bleeding.

PATIENT TEACHING

Be sure to cover:
- the disorder, diagnosis, and treatment
- medication, including administration, dosage, and possible adverse effects
- use of a soft toothbrush and avoidance of hot, spicy foods and commercial mouthwashes
- signs and symptoms of infection
- signs and symptoms of abnormal bleeding
- the importance of planned rest periods during the day
- how to access the American Cancer Society or the Leukemia and Lymphoma Society to obtain additional information
- location and contact information for a local support group and local services.

Lung cancer

DESCRIPTION

- *Lung cancer* involves malignant tumors arising from the respiratory epithelium.
- It's the most common fatal cancer in the United States.
- Its most common types are epidermoid (squamous cell), adenocarcinoma, small-cell (oat cell), and large-cell (anaplastic).
- Its most common site is the wall or epithelium of the bronchial tree.

PATHOPHYSIOLOGY

- It involves bronchial epithelial changes progressing from squamous cell alteration or metaplasia to carcinoma in situ.
- Tumors originating in the bronchi are thought to be more mucus-producing.
- Partial or complete obstruction of the airway occurs with tumor growth, resulting in lobar collapse distal to the tumor.
- Early metastasis occurs in other thoracic structures, such as hilar lymph nodes or the mediastinum.
- Distant metastasis occurs in the brain, liver, bone, and adrenal glands. (See *How lung cancer develops,* page 502.)

CAUSES

- Exact cause unknown

Risk factors

- Tobacco smoking (in 90% of patients)
- Exposure to carcinogens
- Chronic interstitial pneumonitis
- Genetic predisposition

ASSESSMENT FINDINGS

- Possibly no symptoms; history of tobacco use
- Coughing
- Decreased breath sounds
- Dilated chest and abdominal veins (superior vena cava syndrome)
- Dyspnea on exertion
- Edema of the face, neck, and upper torso
- Enlarged liver and lymph nodes
- Exposure to carcinogens
- Fatigue
- Finger clubbing
- Hemoptysis
- Hoarseness
- Orthopnea
- Persistent low-grade fever
- Pleural friction rub
- Recurrent bronchitis or pneumonia
- Weight loss; cachexia
- Wheezing

How lung cancer develops

Lung cancer usually begins with the transformation of one epithelial cell within the patient's airway. Although the exact cause of such change remains unclear, some lung cancers originating in the bronchi may be more vulnerable to injuries from carcinogens.

As the tumor grows, it can partially or completely obstruct the airway, resulting in lobar collapse distal to the tumor. Early metastasis may occur to other thoracic structures as well.

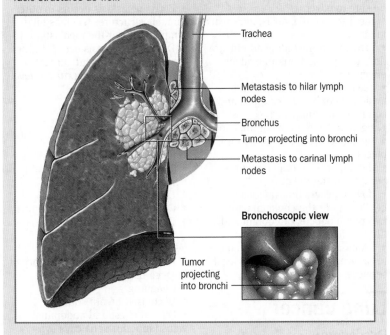

Trachea

Metastasis to hilar lymph nodes

Bronchus

Tumor projecting into bronchi

Metastasis to carinal lymph nodes

Bronchoscopic view

Tumor projecting into bronchi

TEST RESULTS

- Cytologic sputum analysis shows diagnostic evidence of pulmonary malignancy.
- Liver function test results are abnormal, especially with metastasis.
- Chest X-rays may show the size and location of advanced lesions (possibly as old as 2 years).
- Contrast studies of the bronchial tree (chest tomography, bronchography) demonstrate size, location, and spread of the lesion.
- Bone scan detects metastasis.

- Computed tomography (CT) of the chest detects malignant pleural effusion.
- CT of the brain detects metastasis.
- Positron emission tomography aids in the diagnosis of primary and metastatic sites.
- Bronchoscopy identifies the tumor site (bronchoscopic washings provide material for cytologic and histologic study).
- Needle biopsy of the lungs (which relies on biplanar fluoroscopic visual control to locate peripheral tumors before withdrawing a tissue

specimen for analysis) allows firm diagnosis in 80% of patients.
- Tissue biopsy of metastatic sites, including supraclavicular and mediastinal nodes and pleura, determines the stage of disease.
- Thoracentesis allows chemical and cytologic examination of pleural fluid.
- Gallium scans of the liver and spleen detect metastasis.
- Exploratory thoracotomy is used to obtain a biopsy specimen.

TREATMENT

- Various combinations of surgery, radiation therapy, and chemotherapy to improve prognosis
- Palliative (most treatments)
- Preoperative and postoperative radiation therapy
- Laser therapy (experimental)
- Well-balanced diet
- Activity, as tolerated per breathing capacity
- Chemotherapy drug combinations
- Immunotherapy (investigational)
- Partial removal of the lung (wedge resection, segmental resection, lobectomy, radical lobectomy)
- Total removal of the lung (pneumonectomy, radical pneumonectomy)

KEY PATIENT OUTCOMES

The patient will:
- maintain normal fluid volume
- maintain adequate ventilation
- maintain a patent airway
- express feelings of increased comfort and decreased pain.

NURSING INTERVENTIONS

- Provide supportive care.
- Administer supplemental oxygen; monitor oxygenation.
- Encourage verbalization.
- Assess pain control and provide comfort measures.
- Administer prescribed medications.

- Assess chest tube function and drainage.
- Observe for postoperative complications.
- Assess the wound site, and provide wound care.
- Monitor all vital signs.
- Assess sputum production.
- Monitor and record hydration and nutrition.

PATIENT TEACHING

Be sure to cover:
- the disorder, diagnosis, and treatment
- preoperative and postoperative procedures and equipment
- chest physiotherapy
- exercises to prevent shoulder stiffness
- medications, including dosage, administration, and possible adverse effects
- risk factors for recurrent cancer
- information about and referral to a smoking-cessation program
- referral for home care or hospice care
- how to access the American Cancer Society or the American Lung Association to obtain additional information
- location and contact information for a local support group and local services.

Multiple sclerosis

DESCRIPTION

- *Multiple sclerosis* is a progressive inflammatory demyelination of the white matter of the brain and spinal cord.
- It's characterized by exacerbations and remissions.
- Four types of the disease are recognized by the National Multiple Sclerosis Society.

How myelin breaks down

Myelin speeds electrical impulses to the brain for interpretation. This lipoprotein complex (formed of glial cells or oligodendrocytes) protects the neuron's axon, much like the insulation on an electrical wire. Its high electrical resistance and low capacitance allow the myelin to conduct nerve impulses from one node of Ranvier to the next.

Myelin is susceptible to injury (for example, by hypoxemia, toxic chemicals, vascular insufficiencies, or autoimmune responses). The sheath becomes inflamed, and the membrane layers break down into smaller components that become well-circumscribed plaques (filled with microglial elements, macroglia, and lymphocytes). This process is called *demyelination*.

The damaged myelin sheath can't conduct normally. The partial loss or dispersion of the action potential causes neurologic dysfunction.

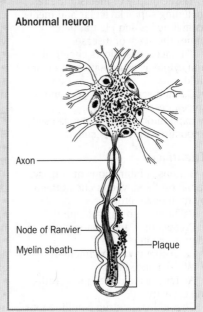

Abnormal neuron

Axon

Node of Ranvier

Myelin sheath

Plaque

– *Relapsing remitting* is the most common and involves partial or total recovery after each attack.
– *Primary progressive* is a continuous worsening disability without remission.
– *Secondary progressive* is a relapsing remitting course that becomes progressive with increasing disability.
– *Progressive relapsing* is a progressively worsening disability with acute exacerbations. It's rare.
• It's also known as *MS*.

PATHOPHYSIOLOGY

• MS is characterized by lymphocyte and macrophage infiltration of parenchyma of the brain, brain stem, spinal cord, and optic nerve that appears as plaques.
• Demyelination and destruction of neuron axons occurs, resulting in widespread and varied neurologic dysfunction. (See *How myelin breaks down*.)

CAUSES

• Exact cause unknown

Possible contributing factors

• Allergic response
• Autoimmune response of the nervous system
• Events that precede the onset:
  – Acute respiratory tract infections
  – Emotional stress
  – Fatigue
  – Overwork
  – Postpartum pregnancy
• Geographic factors (decreased incidence in northernmost and southernmost regions)
• Genetic factors
• Slow-acting viral infection

Assessment findings

- Symptoms related to the extent and site of myelin destruction, extent of remyelination, and adequacy of subsequent restored synaptic transmission
- Symptoms possibly transient or last for hours or weeks
- Symptoms unpredictable and difficult to describe
- Blurred vision or diplopia
- Bowel disturbances (involuntary evacuation or constipation)
- Dysphagia
- Emotional lability
- Fatigue (typically the most disabling symptom)
- Gait ataxia
- Intention tremor
- Muscle weakness of the involved area
- Nystagmus; scotoma
- Ophthalmoplegia
- Optic neuritis
- Paralysis, ranging from monoplegia to quadriplegia
- Poor articulation
- Spasticity; hyperreflexia
- Urinary problems
- Vision problems and sensory impairment (the first signs)

Test results

- Cerebrospinal fluid analysis shows mononuclear cell pleocytosis, an elevation in the level of total immunoglobulin (Ig) G, and the presence of oligoclonal Ig.
- Magnetic resonance imaging detects multiple sclerosis focal lesions.
- EEG abnormalities occur in one-third of patients with MS.
- Evoked potential studies show slowed conduction of nerve impulses.

Treatment

- Symptomatic treatment for acute exacerbations and related signs and symptoms
- Immunosuppressants

- Antimetabolites
- Alkylating drugs
- Biological response modifiers
- I.V. steroids followed by oral steroids
- High-fluid and high-fiber diet
- Frequent rest periods
- Physical therapy
- Supportive care

Key patient outcomes

The patient will:
- perform activities of daily living independently
- remain free from infection
- maintain mobility and range of motion
- express feelings of increased energy and decreased fatigue
- develop regular bowel and bladder habits
- use available support systems and coping mechanisms.

Nursing interventions

- Provide emotional and psychological support.
- Administer prescribed medications.
- Monitor the patient for response to medications and adverse drug reactions.
- Assist with the physical therapy program.
- Provide adequate rest periods.
- Keep the bedpan or urinal readily available because the need to void is immediate.
- Provide bowel and bladder training, if indicated.
- Assess the patient for sensory impairment, muscle dysfunction, and energy level.
- Observe for signs and symptoms of infection.
- Monitor the patient for speech and vision changes.
- Monitor appropriate laboratory values.

PATIENT TEACHING

Be sure to cover:
• the disease process
• the medication and adverse effects
• the avoidance of stress, infections, and fatigue
• maintaining independence
• avoiding exposure to bacterial and viral infections
• nutritional management
• adequate fluid intake and regular urination
• how to access the National Multiple Sclerosis Society to obtain additional information
• location and contact information for a local support group and local services.

Myocardial infarction

DESCRIPTION

• *Myocardial infarction* involves reduced blood flow through one or more coronary arteries, causing myocardial ischemia and necrosis.
• The infarction site depends on the vessels involved.
• Symptoms may differ between women and men.
• It's also called *MI* and *heart attack*.

PATHOPHYSIOLOGY

• At least one coronary artery becomes occluded.
• If coronary occlusion causes ischemia lasting longer than 30 to 45 minutes, irreversible myocardial cell damage and muscle death occur.
• Every MI has a central area of necrosis surrounded by an area of hypoxic injury; this injured tissue is potentially viable and may be salvaged if circulation is restored, or it may progress to necrosis.

CAUSES

• Atherosclerosis
• Coronary artery stenosis or spasm
• Platelet aggregation
• Thrombosis

ASSESSMENT FINDINGS

• Cardinal symptom in men: persistent, crushing substernal pain or pressure possibly radiating to the left arm, jaw, neck, and shoulder blades
• Women: commonly initially experience unusual fatigue and shortness of breath with complaint of upper back discomfort
• Shortness of breath
• A feeling of impending doom
• Diaphoresis
• Fatigue
• Nausea and vomiting
• Indigestion
• A fourth heart sound (S_4), a third heart sound (S_3), and paradoxical splitting of a second heart sound (S_2) with ventricular dysfunction
• Bradycardia and hypotension, in inferior MI
• Dyspnea
• Extreme anxiety and restlessness
• Hypertension
• In an elderly patient or a patient with diabetes, pain possibly absent; in others, pain possibly mild and confused with indigestion
• Low-grade fever during the next few days
• Pericardial friction rub with transmural MI or pericarditis
• Possible coronary artery disease with increasing anginal frequency, severity, or duration
• Sudden death (may be the first and only indication of MI)
• Systolic murmur of mitral insufficiency
• Tachycardia; palpitations (in women)

Test results

• Serum creatine kinase (CK) level, especially the CK-MB isoenzyme, the cardiac muscle fraction of CK, is elevated.

• Troponin I, a structural protein found in cardiac muscle, is elevated only in cardiac muscle damage. It's more specific than the CK-MB level. (Troponin levels increase within 4 to 6 hours of myocardial injury and may remain elevated for 5 to 11 days.)

• Characteristic electrocardiogram (ECG) abnormalities include ST-segment elevations and T-wave changes; leads with abnormalities identify the location of the MI.

• Serum lactate dehydrogenase (LD) level is elevated. LD_1 isoenzyme (found in cardiac tissue) is higher than LD_2 isoenzyme (found in serum).

• Myoglobin, the hemoprotein in cardiac and skeletal muscle that's released with muscle damage, is detected as soon as 2 hours after MI.

• Echocardiography shows ventricular wall dyskinesia with a transmural MI and helps to evaluate the ejection fraction.

• Nuclear medicine scans, using I.V. technetium 99m pertechnetate, identify acutely damaged muscle by picking up accumulations of radioactive nucleotide, which appear as a "hot spot" on the film.

• Myocardial perfusion imaging with thallium 201 reveals a "cold spot" in most patients during the first few hours after a transmural MI.

Treatment

• Aspirin
• Oxygen
• Nitroglycerin
• Morphine I.V.
• Pacemaker, electrical cardioversion or defibrillation, based on arrhythmia

• I.V. thrombolytic therapy started within 3 hours of the onset of symptoms
• Antiarrhythmics, antianginals
• Heparin I.V.
• Inotropic drugs
• Beta-adrenergic blockers
• Angiotensin-converting inhibitors
• Stool softeners
• Low-fat, low-cholesterol diet
• Calorie restriction, if indicated
• Bed rest with a bedside commode
• Gradual increase in activity as tolerated
• Calcium channel blockers
• Percutaneous revascularization
• Intra-aortic balloon pump for cardiogenic shock
• Surgical revascularization

Key patient outcomes

The patient will:
• maintain adequate cardiac output
• maintain hemodynamic stability
• demonstrate a normal perfusing rhythm without arrhythmias
• develop no complications of fluid volume excess
• express feelings of increased comfort and decreased pain
• exhibit adequate coping skills.

Nursing interventions

• Assess pain and give prescribed analgesics. Record the severity, location, type, and duration of the pain. Avoid I.M. injections.

• Check the patient's blood pressure before and after giving nitroglycerin or morphine.

• Obtain serial cardiac markers every 8 hours, then daily.

• Obtain an ECG every 8 hours in the first 24 hours, then daily and with episodes of chest pain.

• Monitor vital signs and heart and breath sounds.

• If the patient has undergone percutaneous transluminal coronary angioplasty, provide sheath care per facility protocol. Monitor distal

peripheral pulses for strength, and catheter site for signs of bleeding.
• Organize patient care and activities to provide periods of uninterrupted rest.
• Provide a low-cholesterol, low-sodium diet with caffeine-free beverages.
• Allow the patient to use a bedside commode.
• Provide emotional support, and help reduce stress and anxiety.
• Monitor the appropriate coagulation studies.
• Monitor daily weight and intake and output.
• Monitor cardiac rhythm for reperfusion arrhythmias (treat according to facility protocol).
• Encourage lifestyle changes, such as smoking cessation and weight loss, if appropriate.

PATIENT TEACHING

Be sure to cover:
• the disorder, diagnostic procedures, and treatment
• medication dosages, adverse reactions, and signs of toxicity to watch for and report
• dietary restrictions
• progressive resumption of sexual activity
• appropriate responses to new or recurrent symptoms
• typical or atypical chest pain to report
• how to access the American Heart Association to obtain additional information
• location and contact information for a local support group and local services.

Obesity

DESCRIPTION

• *Obesity* is an excess of body fat, generally 20% above ideal body weight.

• It involves a body mass index (BMI) of 30 or greater. (See *BMI measurements*.)
• It's the second leading cause of preventable deaths in the U.S.
• It affects more than one-third of U.S. residents, and one in five children.

PATHOPHYSIOLOGY

• Fat cells increase in size in response to dietary intake.
• When the cells can no longer expand, they increase in number.
• With weight loss, the size of the fat cells decreases but the number of cells doesn't.

CAUSES

• Excessive caloric intake combined with inadequate energy expenditure
• Possible contributing factors:
  – Abnormal absorption of nutrients
  – Environmental factors
  – Genetic predisposition
  – Hypothalamic dysfunction of hunger and satiety centers
  – Impaired action of GI and growth hormones and of hormonal regulators such as insulin
  – Psychological factors
  – Socioeconomic status

ASSESSMENT FINDINGS

• BMI of 30 or greater
• Complications of obesity, including type 2 diabetes, hypertension, osteoarthritis, sleep apnea, gallbladder disease, and liver disease
• Increasing weight

TEST RESULTS

• BMI of 30 or greater.
• Waist measurement is more than 35″ in women or 40″ in men.
• Anthropometric arm measurement over the 95th percentile may indicate overweight or obesity.

TREATMENT

- Behavior modification techniques
- Nutritional counseling
- Psychological counseling
- Reduction in daily caloric intake
- Increase in daily activity level
- Vertical-banded gastroplasty
- Gastric bypass surgery

KEY PATIENT OUTCOMES

The patient will:
- reduce BMI to normal level
- safely reduce weight to within normal limits for height, weight, and age
- demonstrate effective coping mechanisms to deal with long-term compliance.

NURSING INTERVENTIONS

- Obtain weight and BMI.
- Obtain an accurate diet history to identify eating patterns, dietary choices, and the importance of food to the patient's lifestyle.
- Note cultural or religious dietary guides.
- Promote increased physical activity as appropriate.
- Monitor dietary intake and compliance with dietary restrictions.
- Record and evaluate intake and output.
- Monitor vital signs.

PATIENT TEACHING

Be sure to cover:
- dietary guidelines that fit with the patient's lifestyle and cultural beliefs
- safe weight-loss practices
- physical activity guidelines
- the need for long-term maintenance after desired weight is achieved
- how to access the National Institutes of Health to obtain additional information
- location and contact information for a local support group and local services.

BMI measurements

Use these steps to calculate body mass index (BMI).
· Multiply the weight in pounds by 705.
· Divide this number by the height in inches.
· Divide this number by the height in inches again.
· Compare the results to these standards:
  – 18.5 to 24.9: normal
  – 25.0 to 29.9: overweight
  – 30 to 39.9: obese
  – 40 or greater: morbidly obese.

Parkinson's disease

DESCRIPTION

- *Parkinson's disease* is a chronic, progressive neurologic disease causing deterioration of muscle movement and control.
- Its usual cause of death is aspiration pneumonia.
- It's one of the most common crippling diseases in the United States.

PATHOPHYSIOLOGY

- Dopaminergic neurons degenerate, causing a loss of available dopamine.
- Dopamine deficiency prevents affected brain cells from performing their normal inhibitory function.
- Excess excitatory acetylcholine occurs at synapses.
- Nondopaminergic receptors may contribute to depression and other nonmotor symptoms.
- Motor neurons are depressed.
(See *Neurotransmitter action in Parkinson's disease,* page 510.)

CAUSES

- Usually unknown
- Possible contributing factors:

Neurotransmitter action in Parkinson's disease

Parkinson's disease is a degenerative process involving the dopaminergic neurons in the substantia nigra (the area of the basal ganglia that produces and stores the neurotransmitter dopamine). Dopamine deficiency prevents affected brain cells from performing their normal inhibitory function. Other nondopaminergic receptors may be affected, possibly contributing to depression and other nonmotor symptoms.

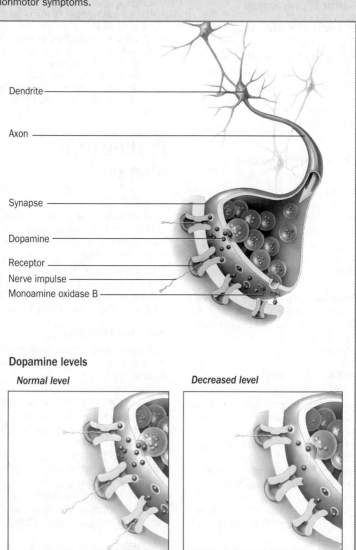

Dendrite

Axon

Synapse

Dopamine

Receptor

Nerve impulse

Monoamine oxidase B

Dopamine levels

Normal level

Decreased level

– Drug-induced (haloperidol [Haldol], methyldopa [Aldomet], reserpine [Serpalan])
– Exposure to such toxins as manganese dust and carbon monoxide
– Genetic factors
– Type A encephalitis

ASSESSMENT FINDINGS

- Tremor of hand or eye
- Slow, shuffling gait
- Muscle rigidity
- Loss of balance
- Dysarthria
- Dysphagia
- Fatigue with activities of daily living (ADLs)
- High-pitched, monotonous voice
- Increased perspiration
- Insidious (unilateral pill-roll) tremor; increases during stress or anxiety, decreases with purposeful movement and sleep
- Insomnia
- Masklike facial expression
- Mood changes
- Muscle cramps of legs, neck, and trunk
- Oculogyric crises (eyes fixed upward, with involuntary tonic movements)
- Oily skin

TEST RESULTS

- There's no definitive test.
- Diagnosis based on clinical findings
- Computed tomography scan or magnetic resonance imaging rules out other disorders such as intracranial tumors.

TREATMENT

- Levodopa, carbidopa
- Dopamine agonists
- Selegiline
- Catechol-O-methyltransferase inhibitors
- Anticholinergics
- Amantadine

- Coenzyme Q10
- Tricyclic antidepressants
- Small, frequent meals
- High-bulk foods
- Physical and occupational therapy
- Assistive devices to aid ambulation
- Surgery; thalamotomy, pallidotomy, deep brain stimulation

KEY PATIENT OUTCOMES

The patient will:
- perform ADLs independently
- participate in an exercise program
- avoid injury
- maintain an adequate caloric intake
- express positive feelings about himself
- develop adequate coping behaviors
- seek support resources.

NURSING INTERVENTIONS

- Provide emotional and psychological support.
- Encourage the patient to be independent.
- Monitor the response to drug therapy.
- Ensure adequate nutrition.
- Take measures to prevent aspiration.
- Protect the patient from injury.
- Stress the importance of rest periods between activities.
- Encourage the patient to enroll in a physical therapy program.
- Assist with ambulation and range-of-motion exercises.
- Monitor vital signs.
- Measure and evaluate intake and output.
- Postoperatively observe for signs of hemorrhage and increased intracranial pressure.

PATIENT TEACHING

Be sure to cover:
- the disorder, diagnosis, and treatment

- drug administration, dosage, and possible adverse effects
- the appropriate exercise program
- household safety measures
- the swallowing therapy regimen (aspiration precautions)
- how to access the National Parkinson Foundation or the National Institute of Neurological Disorders and Stroke to obtain additional information
- location and contact information for a local support group and local services.

Renal failure, acute

DESCRIPTION

- *Acute renal failure* results from a sudden interruption of renal function resulting from obstruction, reduced circulation, or renal parenchymal disease.
- It's classified as prerenal failure, intrarenal failure (also called *intrinsic* or *parenchymal failure*), or postrenal failure.
- It's usually reversible with medical treatment.
- If not treated, it may progress to end-stage renal disease, uremia, and death.
- It's seen in 5% of hospitalized patients.
- It normally occurs in three distinct phases: oliguric, diuretic, and recovery.

Oliguric phase

- This phase may last a few days to several weeks.
- A patient's urine output may drop below 400 ml/day.
- Fluid volume excess, azotemia, and electrolyte imbalance occur.
- Local mediators are released, causing intrarenal vasoconstriction.
- Medullary hypoxia causes cellular swelling and adherence of neutrophils to capillaries and venules.

- Hypoperfusion occurs in this phase.
- Cellular injury and necrosis occur.
- Reperfusion causes reactive oxygen species to form, leading to further cellular injury.

Diuretic phase

- Renal function is recovered.
- Urine output gradually increases.
- Glomerular filtration rate improves, although tubular transport systems remain abnormal.

Recovery phase

- This phase may last 3 to 12 months, or longer.
- The patient gradually returns to normal or near-normal renal function.

PATHOPHYSIOLOGY

Prerenal failure

- Prerenal failure is caused by impaired blood flow.
- Decrease in filtration pressure causes a decline in glomerular filtration rate (GFR).
- Failure to restore blood volume or blood pressure may cause acute tubular necrosis (ATN) or acute cortical necrosis.

Intrarenal failure

- A severe episode of hypotension, commonly associated with hypovolemia, is typically a significant contributing event.
- Cell swelling, injury, and necrosis—a form of reperfusion injury that may also be caused by nephrotoxins—results from ischemia-generated, toxic oxygen-free radicals and anti-inflammatory mediators.

Postrenal failure

- Postrenal failure usually occurs with urinary tract obstruction, such as prostatic hyperplasia, that affects the kidneys bilaterally.

Causes

Prerenal failure

- Hemorrhagic blood loss
- Hypotension or hypoperfusion
- Hypovolemia
- Loss of plasma volume
- Water and electrolyte losses

Intrarenal failure

- ATN
- Coagulation defects
- Glomerulopathies
- Malignant hypertension

Postrenal failure

- Bladder neck obstruction
- Obstructive uropathies, usually bilateral
- Ureteral destruction

Assessment findings

- Oliguria or anuria, depending on the renal failure phase
- Altered level of consciousness
- Bibasilar crackles
- Bleeding abnormalities
- Dry mucous membranes
- Dry, pruritic skin
- Elevated blood pressure
- Fatigue
- Irritability, drowsiness, or confusion
- Nausea, vomiting
- Peripheral or generalized edema
- Seizure
- Tachycardia
- Uremic breath odor

Test results

- Blood urea nitrogen, serum creatinine, and potassium levels are elevated.
- Hematocrit, blood pH, bicarbonate, and hemoglobin levels are decreased.
- Urine casts and cellular debris are present, and specific gravity is decreased.
- In glomerular disease, proteinuria and urine osmolality are close to serum osmolality level.

- Urine sodium level is normal, decreased (below 20 mEq/L, caused by decreased perfusion in oliguria), or increased (above 40 mEq/L, caused by an intrarenal problem during the oliguric phase).
- Urine creatinine clearance measures GFR and estimates the number of remaining functioning nephrons.
- Kidney ultrasonography, kidney-ureter-bladder radiography, excretory urography renal scan, retrograde pyelography, computed tomography scan, and nephrotomography may reveal obstruction.
- Renal angiography reveals abnormality of blood vessels, if that's the cause.
- Electrocardiography reveals tall, peaked T waves; a widening QRS complex; and disappearing P waves if hyperkalemia is present.

Treatment

- Treatment of the underlying cause
- Hemodialysis or peritoneal dialysis (if appropriate)
- High-calorie, low-protein, low-sodium, and low-potassium diet
- Fluid restriction
- Rest periods when fatigued
- Antibiotics, diuretics
- In hyperkalemia, hypertonic glucose-and-insulin infusions, sodium bicarbonate, sodium polystyrene sulfonate

Key patient outcomes

The patient will:

- regain normal kidney function
- avoid complications
- maintain fluid balance
- maintain hemodynamic stability
- verbalize diet and medication rationales and regimen.

Nursing interventions

- Provide treatment for underlying cause.
- Measure and evaluate intake and output.

- Monitor appropriate renal function studies.
- Administer prescribed medications.
- Encourage the patient to express his feelings.
- Provide emotional support.
- Monitor daily weight.
- Assess the patient's vital signs.
- Monitor the effects of excess fluid volume.
- Assess the dialysis access site for bruit and thrill.

PATIENT TEACHING

Be sure to cover:
- the disorder, diagnosis, and treatment
- administration, dosages, and possible adverse reactions to the medications
- recommended fluid allowance
- compliance with diet and drug regimen
- signs and symptoms of edema and the importance of reporting them to the physician
- how to access the National Kidney Foundation to obtain additional information
- location and contact information for a local support group and local services.

Stroke

DESCRIPTION

- *Stroke* is a sudden impairment of blood circulation to the brain.
- It's the third most common cause of death in the United States.
- It affects 700,000 people each year, causing 158,000 deaths.
- It's the most common cause of neurologic disability.
- About 15% to 30% of stroke survivors are permanently disabled.
- Recurrences are possible within weeks, months, or years.

- It's also known as *cerebrovascular accident* or *brain attack*.

PATHOPHYSIOLOGY

- The blood and oxygen supply to the brain is interrupted or diminished.
- In ischemic (thrombotic or embolic) stroke, neurons die from lack of oxygen.
- In hemorrhagic stroke, impaired cerebral perfusion causes infarction.

CAUSES

- Cerebral embolism
- Cerebral hemorrhage
- Cerebral thrombosis

Risk factors (controllable)
- High blood pressure
- Smoking
- Diabetes mellitus
- Carotid artery or peripheral artery disease
- Atrial fibrillation
- Heart disease
- Blood disorders that increase red blood cell count; sickle cell anemia
- Elevated cholesterol and triglyceride levels
- Obesity
- Minimal physical activity
- Alcohol or illegal drug use
- Use of hormonal contraceptives, especially in those who smoke and have hypertension

Risk factors (uncontrollable)
- Increasing age
- Family history of stroke
- Gender
- Prior history of stroke or transient ischemic attack

ASSESSMENT FINDINGS

- Presence of one or more risk factors for stroke
- Sudden onset of hemiparesis or hemiplegia
- Sudden severe headache (not always present)

- Sudden confusion, cognitive impairment, or difficulty speaking
- Sudden visual disturbance
- Sudden difficulty with motor coordination or dizziness
- Dysphagia
- Urinary incontinence
- Decreased deep tendon reflexes
- Hemianopsia on the affected side of the body
- Sensory losses

TEST RESULTS

- Computed tomography scan detects structural abnormalities.
- Magnetic resonance imaging and magnetic resonance angiography show the location and size of the lesion.
- Cerebral or magnetic resonance angiography details the disruption of cerebral circulation and is the test of choice for examining the entire cerebral blood flow.
- Positron emission tomography provides data on cerebral metabolism and cerebral blood flow changes.
- Laboratory tests—including anticardiolipin antibodies, antiphospholipid, factor V (Leiden) mutation (the most common hereditary contributor to hypercoagulability), antithrombin III, protein S, and protein C, factor VIII, and erythrocyte sedimentation rate—show increased thrombotic risk; prothrombin time or International Normalized Ratio may be increased if the patient was on anticoagulant therapy.
- Other tests include:
  - transcranial Doppler studies to evaluate the velocity of blood flow
  - carotid Doppler to measure blood flow through the carotid arteries
  - two-dimensional echocardiogram to evaluate the heart for dysfunction

- cerebral blood flow studies to measure blood flow to the brain
  - electrocardiogram to evaluate electrical activity in an area of cortical infarction.

TREATMENT

- Airway management
- Thrombolytics when the cause isn't hemorrhagic (with administration within 3 hours of onset of the symptoms)
- Blood pressure management
- Anticonvulsants
- Stool softeners
- Anticoagulants
- Analgesics
- Antidepressants
- Antiplatelets
- Antilipemics
- Pureed dysphagia diet or tube feedings, if indicated
- Physical, speech, and occupational rehabilitation
- Surgery, if indicated, which may include craniotomy, carotid endarterectomy, extracranial-intracranial bypass, ventricular shunts

KEY PATIENT OUTCOMES

The patient will:
- maintain adequate ventilation
- remain free from injury
- achieve maximal independence
- maintain joint mobility and range of motion
- verbalize risk factors for stroke and modify lifestyle appropriately.

NURSING INTERVENTIONS

- Maintain a patent airway and oxygenation.
- Administer medications as ordered.
- Monitor vital signs and cardiac rhythm.
- Insert an indwelling urinary catheter, if necessary.
- Ensure adequate fluid, electrolyte, and nutritional intake.

Preventing stroke

To decrease the risk of another stroke, teach the patient and family members about the need to correct risk factors. For example, if the patient smokes, refer him to a smoking-cessation program. Teach the importance of maintaining an ideal weight and controlling diabetes and hypertension. Teach all patients to follow a low-cholesterol, low-sodium diet; perform regular physical exercise; avoid prolonged bed rest; and minimize stress. Early recognition of signs and symptoms of complications or impending stroke is imperative, as is seeking prompt treatment.

• Follow the physical therapy program, and assist the patient with exercise.
• Turn the patient every 2 hours, and provide skin care.
• Establish and maintain effective communication.
• Provide psychological support for patient and family members.
• Set realistic short-term goals.
• Protect the patient from injury and complications.
• Provide careful positioning to prevent aspiration and contractures.
• Monitor the patient for complications.

PATIENT TEACHING

Be sure to cover:
• the disorder, diagnosis, and treatment
• occupational and speech therapy programs
• dietary and drug regimens
• adverse drug reactions
• stroke prevention (see *Preventing stroke*)
• how to access the American Stroke Association to obtain additional information

• location and contact information for local support group and local services.

Tuberculosis

DESCRIPTION

• *Tuberculosis* is an acute or chronic lung infection characterized by pulmonary infiltrates and the formation of granulomas with caseation, fibrosis, and cavitation.
• Its prognosis is excellent with proper treatment and compliance.
• It's also known as *TB.*

PATHOPHYSIOLOGY

• Multiplication of the bacillus *Mycobacterium tuberculosis* causes an inflammatory process where deposited.
• A cell-mediated immune response follows, usually containing the infection within 4 to 6 weeks.
• The T-cell response causes granulomas to form around the bacilli, making them go dormant. This confers immunity to subsequent infection.
• Bacilli within granulomas may remain viable for many years, causing a positive result for the purified protein derivative or other skin test for TB.
• Active disease develops in 5% to 15% of those infected.
• Transmission occurs when an infected person coughs or sneezes.

CAUSES

• Exposure to *M. tuberculosis*
• Exposure to other strains of mycobacteria (sometimes)

Risk factors
• Close contact with a newly diagnosed TB patient
• A history of TB exposure
• Multiple sexual partners

- Being a recent immigrant from Africa, Asia, Mexico, or South America
- History of gastrectomy
- A history of silicosis, diabetes, malnutrition, cancer, Hodgkin's disease, or leukemia
- Drug or alcohol abuse problems
- Being a resident in a nursing home, mental health facility, or prison
- Immunosuppressed patients and those who use corticosteroids
- Homeless patients
- Crowded, poorly ventilated, unsanitary living conditions

Assessment findings

- History of one or more risk factors
- Signs and symptoms of primary infection:
  - May be asymptomatic after a 4- to 8-week incubation period
  - Weakness and fatigue
  - Anorexia, weight loss
  - Low-grade fever
  - Night sweats
- Signs and symptoms of reactivated infection:
  - Chest pain
  - Productive cough for blood, or mucopurulent or blood-tinged sputum
  - Low-grade fever
- Other possible signs and symptoms:
  - Dullness over the affected area
  - Crepitant crackles
  - Bronchial breath sounds
  - Wheezes
  - Whispered pectoriloquy

Test results

- Tuberculin skin test result is positive in both active and inactive tuberculosis.
- Stains and cultures of sputum, cerebrospinal fluid, urine, abscess drainage, or pleural fluid show heat-sensitive, nonmotile, aerobic, and acid-fast bacilli.
- Chest X-rays show nodular lesions, patchy infiltrates, cavity formation, scar tissue, and calcium deposits.
- Computed tomography or magnetic resonance imaging shows presence and extent of lung damage.
- Bronchoscopy specimens show heat-sensitive, nonmotile, aerobic, acid-fast bacilli in specimens.

Treatment

- Antitubercular therapy for at least 6 months, with daily oral doses of:
  - Ethambutol (Myambutol), in some cases
  - Isoniazid (INH)
  - Pyrazinamide
  - Rifampin (Rifadin)
- Second-line drugs:
  - Amikacin (Amikin)
  - Capreomycin (Capastat)
  - Ethionamide (Trecator)
  - Gatifloxacin (Tequin)
  - Levofloxacin (Levaquin)
  - Moxifloxacin (Avelox)
  - Para-aminosalicylic acid
- Well-balanced, high-calorie diet
- Rest initially; then activity as tolerated
- Possible surgery for certain complications

Key patient outcomes

The patient will:
- express an understanding of the illness
- maintain adequate ventilation
- use support systems to assist with coping
- identify measures to prevent or reduce fatigue
- comply with the treatment regimen
- resume normal activities after 2- to 4-week infectious period, while continuing to take medication.

Preventing tuberculosis

Explain respiratory and standard precautions to a hospitalized patient with tuberculosis (TB). Before discharge, tell him that he must take precautions to prevent spreading the disease, such as wearing a mask around others, until his physician tells him he's no longer contagious. He should tell all health care providers he sees, including his dentist and optometrist, that he has TB so that they can institute infection-control precautions.

Teach the patient other specific precautions to avoid spreading the infection. Tell him to cough and sneeze into tissues and to dispose of the tissues properly. Stress the importance of washing his hands thoroughly in hot, soapy water after handling his own secretions. Also, instruct him to wash his eating utensils separately in hot, soapy water.

Nursing interventions

- Isolate the patient in a quiet, properly ventilated room, and maintain tuberculosis precautions. (See *Preventing tuberculosis.*)
- Administer drug therapy.
- Properly dispose of secretions.
- Provide supportive care.
- Provide diversional activities.
- Provide adequate rest periods.
- Provide well-balanced, high-calorie foods.
- Provide small, frequent meals.
- Consult with a dietitian if oral supplements are needed.
- Perform chest physiotherapy.
- Monitor the patient's vital signs, intake and output, and daily weight.
- Monitor the patient for potential complications, including massive pulmonary tissue damage, respiratory failure, bronchopleural fistulas, pneumothorax, pleural effusion, pneumonia infection of other body organs by small mycobacterial foci, liver involvement, and disease caused by drug therapy.
- Observe for adverse reactions to drugs; monitor the patient's visual acuity if he's taking ethambutol.
- Monitor the results of liver and kidney function tests.

Patient teaching

Be sure to cover:
- the disorder, diagnosis, and treatment
- the medication and potential adverse effects
- when to notify the physician
- the need for isolation
- postural drainage and chest percussion
- coughing and deep-breathing exercises
- the importance of regular follow-up examinations
- signs and symptoms of recurring TB
- possible decreased hormonal contraceptive effectiveness during rifampin therapy
- the need for a high-calorie, high-protein, balanced diet
- how to access the American Lung Association to obtain additional information
- location and contact information for a local support group and local services.

10 Maternal-neonatal disorders

Maternal disorders

Dysfunctional labor

DESCRIPTION
- *Dysfunctional labor* is abnormal or difficult labor.
- It may determine the need for cesarean delivery.
- It's also called *inertia.*
- Uterine contractions don't progress in a normal fashion, causing unacceptable cervical effacement and dilation.
- Fetal position or presentation disrupts the normal progression of labor.
- It's also characterized by an insufficient pelvic structure or birth canal.

PATHOPHYSIOLOGY
- Dysfunctional labor can occur during the first or second stage of labor. Contractions may be hypertonic, hypotonic, or uncoordinated.
- *Hypertonic* contractions have an increased resting tone, occur in the latent phase of labor, and have incomplete relaxation with no effacement or dilation of the cervix.
- *Hypotonic* contractions usually occur during the active phase of labor. Contractions begin normally but diminish in frequency and strength. Cervical changes may cease.
- *Uncoordinated* contractions are contractions that prevent normal progress of cervical effacement and dilation and descent of the fetus.

CAUSES
- Fetal malposition or malpresentation, or an unusually large fetus
- Abnormal contractions (see *Types of contractions,* page 520)
- Abnormality of birth canal or pelvis, including pelvic contractures
- Medications, such as analgesics or anesthetics, given too early during labor
- Other conditions, such as a distended bladder or bowel

ASSESSMENT FINDINGS
Hypotonic contractions
- Most common during the active phase and result in protraction of this phase
- Number usually low, or occur infrequently
- Commonly limited to two or three in a 10-minute period
- Highly irregular pattern; typically doesn't cause pain
- Resting tone of the uterus: remains below 10 mm Hg
- Strength of contractions: doesn't rise above 25 mm Hg

Hypertonic contractions
- Most common during the latent phase and results in protraction of this phase
- Intensity of contractions possibly similar to hypotonic contractions
- Tend to occur frequently
- Resting tone of the uterus: increases to more than 15 mm Hg
- Patient: complains of pain

Uncoordinated contractions
- Occur erratically

Types of contractions

Here are illustrations of the different uterine activity types. Depending on your assessment, you may need to intervene to promote adequate labor contractions.

Typical contractions

Typical uterine contractions occur every 2 to 5 minutes during active labor and typically last 30 to 90 seconds.

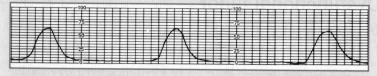

Hypotonic contractions

Hypotonic contractions are accompanied by a rise in pressure of no more than 10 mm Hg during each contraction.

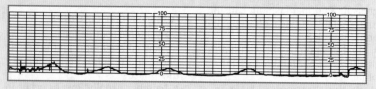

Hypertonic contractions

Hypertonic contractions don't allow the uterus to rest between contractions, as shown by a resting pressure of 40 to 50 mm Hg.

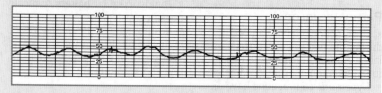

• Lack of regular pattern: interferes with the patient's ability to rest or use breathing techniques between contractions

TEST RESULTS

• Ultrasonography reveals fetal malposition, an unusually large fetus, or pelvic contractures.
• Uterine monitoring reveals hypotonic, hypertonic, or uncoordinated contractions.

TREATMENT

Hypotonic contractions

• Inducement or augmentation of labor, if contractions are too weak or infrequent to be effective
• Inducement of labor if the cervix is deemed ready for dilation, as evidenced by a score of 8 on the cervical readiness scale (see *Evaluating cervical readiness*)
• Inducement of labor if the fetus is in danger or if labor doesn't occur spontaneously and the fetus appears to be at term

Evaluating cervical readiness

Bishop's score is a tool you can use to assess whether a woman is ready for labor. A score ranging from 0 to 3 is given for each of five factors: cervical dilation, length (effacement), station, consistency, and position. If the woman's score exceeds 8, the cervix is considered suitable for induction.

Scoring factor	Score			
	0	**1**	**2**	**3**
Dilation (cm)	0	1 to 2	3 to 4	3 to 4
Effacement (%)	0 to 30	40 to 50	60 to 70	80
Station	−3	−2	−1 to 0	+1 to +2
Consistency	Firm	Medium	Soft	—
Position	Posterior	Mild position	Anterior	—

Adapted with permission from Bishop, E.H. "Pelvic Scoring for Elective Induction," *Obstetrics and Gynecology* 24:266, 1964.

- Cervical ripening via stripping of membranes or application of prostaglandin gel or laminaria may be done to prepare for the induction of labor
- Oxytocin administration

Hypertonic contractions
- Rest with analgesia (such as morphine sulfate) and possible inducement of sedation
- Comfort measures (changing the linens and the mother's gown, darkening room lights, and decreasing noise and stimulation)
- Cesarean delivery if late decelerations of fetal heart rate (FHR), first stage of labor is abnormally long, or progress isn't made with pushing (second-stage arrest)

Uncoordinated contractions
- Oxytocin administration
- Discontinuation of oxytocin if hypertension occurs

Problems with birth canal or fetus
- If the pelvic measurements (especially the inlet measurement) are borderline or just adequate and the fetal lie and position are good: possible trial labor
- If descent of the presenting part and dilation of the cervix are occurring: possible continuation of labor
- If labor doesn't progress or if complications develop: cesarean delivery

KEY PATIENT OUTCOMES
The patient will:
- exhibit a more coordinated uterine contraction pattern
- progress through labor without complications or evidence of fetal distress
- give birth to a viable neonate vaginally or by cesarean delivery.

NURSING INTERVENTIONS
- Explain the events to the patient and her family; explain the treatment plan.

- Provide comfort measures, including nonpharmacologic pain relief.
- Continuously monitor uterine contractions and FHR patterns.
- Offer oral fluids as appropriate; institute I.V. therapy.
- Assist with measures to induce or augment labor; monitor oxytocin infusion, if used.
- Encourage frequent voiding.

PATIENT TEACHING

Be sure to cover:
- the disorder, diagnosis, and treatment
- necessary monitoring techniques
- pain relief measures
- medications for augmenting labor, including possible adverse effects
- steps involved in a trial labor, if appropriate
- cesarean delivery, including indications
- postcesarean delivery care, if applicable.

Ectopic pregnancy

DESCRIPTION

- *Ectopic pregnancy* is the implantation of a fertilized ovum outside the uterine cavity, most commonly in the fallopian tube. (See *Implantation sites of ectopic pregnancy*.)
- It has a good maternal prognosis with prompt diagnosis, appropriate surgical intervention, and control of bleeding.
- It has poor fetal prognosis; there is a rare incidence of survival to term with abdominal implantation.
- Patients have about a 50% chance of giving birth to a live neonate in a subsequent pregnancy.
- Complications include rupture of the fallopian tube, hemorrhage, shock, peritonitis, infertility, disseminated intravascular coagulation, and death.

PATHOPHYSIOLOGY

- Transport of a blastocyst to the uterus is delayed.
- The blastocyst implants at another available vascularized site, usually the fallopian tube lining.
- Normal signs of pregnancy are initially present.
- Uterine enlargement occurs in about 25% of cases.
- Human chorionic gonadotropin (HCG) hormonal levels are lower than in uterine pregnancies.
- If not interrupted, internal hemorrhage occurs with rupture of the fallopian tube.

CAUSES

- May be idiopathic
- Congenital defects in the reproductive tract
- Diverticula
- Ectopic endometrial implants in the tubal mucosa
- Endosalpingitis
- Intrauterine device
- Previous surgery, such as tubal ligation or resection
- Sexually transmitted tubal infection
- Transmigration of the ovum
- Tumors pressing against the tube

ASSESSMENT FINDINGS

- Amenorrhea
- Abnormal menses (after fallopian tube implantation)
- Slight vaginal bleeding
- Unilateral pelvic pain over the mass
- If fallopian tube ruptures: sharp lower abdominal pain, possibly radiating to the shoulders and neck
- Possible extreme pain when the cervix is moved and the adnexa palpated
- Boggy and tender uterus
- Possible enlargement of the adnexa

Implantation sites of ectopic pregnancy

In about 95% of patients with ectopic pregnancy, the ovum implants in part of the fallopian tube: the fimbria, ampulla, or isthmus. Other possible abnormal sites of implantation include the interstitium, ovarian ligament, ovary, abdominal viscera, and internal cervical os.

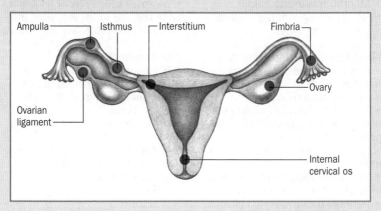

TEST RESULTS

• Serum HCG level is abnormally low; when repeated in 48 hours, the level remains lower than the levels found in a normal intrauterine pregnancy.
• Real-time ultrasonography may show an intrauterine pregnancy or ovarian cyst.
• Culdocentesis shows free blood in the peritoneum.
• Laparoscopy may reveal a pregnancy outside the uterus.

TREATMENT

• Oophorectomy for ovarian pregnancy
• Laparoscopy, laparotomy, or hysterectomy depending on location of ectopic pregnancy and stability of the patient
• Methotrexate (Rheumatrex) for chemical-induced abortion
• In the event of pelvic-organ rupture, management of shock
  – Transfusion with whole blood or packed red blood cells
  – Laparotomy and salpingectomy if culdocentesis shows blood in the peritoneum; possibly performed after laparoscopy to remove the affected fallopian tube and control bleeding
  – Microsurgical repair of the fallopian tube if possible to maintain fertility
• Activity determined by clinical status
• Diet determined by clinical status
• Broad-spectrum I.V. antibiotics
• Supplemental iron

KEY PATIENT OUTCOMES

The patient will:
• have stable vital signs
• express her feelings about her current situation
• use available support systems to aid in coping.

NURSING INTERVENTIONS

• Determine the date and description of the patient's last menstrual period.

- Monitor vital signs for changes.
- Assess vaginal bleeding, including amount and characteristics.
- Assess pain level; provide analgesia as ordered and evaluate its effect.
- Monitor intake and output.
- Assess for signs of hypovolemia and impending shock.
- Prepare the patient with excessive blood loss for emergency surgery.
- Administer prescribed blood transfusions.
- Provide emotional support.
- Administer $Rh_o(D)$ immune globulin (RhoGAM), as ordered, if the patient is Rh-negative.
- Provide a quiet, relaxing environment.
- Encourage the patient to express feelings of fear, loss, and grief.
- Help the patient develop effective coping strategies.
- Refer the patient to a mental health professional for additional counseling, if necessary, before discharge.

PATIENT TEACHING

Be sure to cover:
- the disorder, diagnosis, and treatment
- risk factors, including surgery involving the fallopian tubes and pelvic inflammatory disease
- postoperative care
- prompt treatment of pelvic infections
- how to contact the American Society for Reproductive Medicine
- location and contact information for local support groups and services.

Gestational hypertension

DESCRIPTION

- *Gestational hypertension* is high blood pressure (greater than 140 mm Hg systolic or 90 mm Hg diastolic) not accompanied by proteinuria, most commonly occurring after the 20th week of gestation in a nulliparous patient. It may be transient.
- It carries a high risk of fetal mortality because of the increased incidence of premature delivery, placental abruption, and intrauterine growth restriction.
- It's among the most common causes of maternal death in developed countries (especially with complications).
- It has several possible complications.
  - Abruptio placentae (premature detachment of the placenta)
  - Coagulopathy
  - Stillbirth
  - Seizures
  - Coma
  - Premature labor
  - Renal failure
  - Maternal hepatic damage
  - Hemolysis, elevated liver enzyme levels, and low platelet count (HELLP syndrome)
- There are several other types of hypertension in pregnancy.
  - *Chronic hypertension* is blood pressure greater than 140/90 mm Hg before the 20th week of gestation. It's a primary disorder in 90% to 95% of cases.
  - *Preeclampsia* is elevated blood pressure with proteinuria, and it occurs after the 20th week of gestation. It may be mild or severe. It occurs in approximately 5% of all pregnancies and 10% of first pregnancies.
  - *Eclampsia,* which is preeclampsia with seizures, occurs between the 24th week of gestation and the end of the first postpartum week.
- Formerly called *pregnancy-induced hypertension*

What happens in gestational hypertension

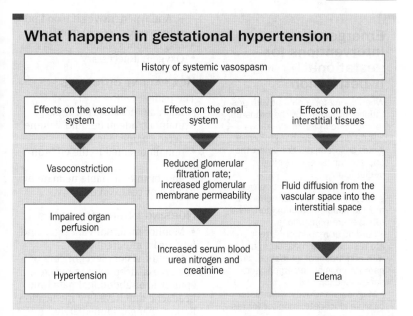

History of systemic vasospasm

Effects on the vascular system	Effects on the renal system	Effects on the interstitial tissues
Vasoconstriction	Reduced glomerular filtration rate; increased glomerular membrane permeability	Fluid diffusion from the vascular space into the interstitial space
Impaired organ perfusion	Increased serum blood urea nitrogen and creatinine	
Hypertension		Edema

PATHOPHYSIOLOGY

• Exact pathophysiology is unknown.
• Generalized arteriolar vasospasm is thought to cause decreased blood flow through the placenta and maternal organs, leading to intrauterine growth restriction, placental infarcts, and abruptio placentae. (See *What happens in gestational hypertension.*)

CAUSES

• Exact cause unknown

   Risk factors
   – First–time pregnancy
   – Multiple fetuses
   – Obesity
   – History of vascular disease
• Contributing factors
   – Autoimmune disease
   – Autointoxication
   – Autolysis of placental infarcts
   – Chronic hypertension
   – Diabetes
   – Geographic, ethnic, racial, nutritional, immunologic, and familial factors
   – Maternal age (younger than age 19 or older than age 35)
   – Maternal sensitization to total proteins
   – Preexisting vascular disease
   – Pyelonephritis
   – Uremia

ASSESSMENT FINDINGS

• Sudden weight gain
• Irritability
• Emotional tension
• Severe frontal headache
• Blurred vision, scotomata
• Epigastric pain or heartburn
• Generalized edema, especially of the face
• Pitting edema of the legs and feet
• Hyperreflexia
• Oliguria
• Vascular spasm, papilledema, retinal edema or detachment, and arteriovenous nicking or hemorrhage (seen on ophthalmoscopy)

Emergency interventions for gestational hypertension

When caring for a patient with gestational hypertension, be prepared to intervene in these situations.

· Fetal distress: prepare for emergency cesarean section; alert the obstetrician, anesthesiologist, and pediatrician

· Seizure: administer anticonvulsants; maintain a patent airway; provide supplemental oxygen; institute seizure precautions

· Cardiac or respiratory arrest: initiate resuscitative measures; assist with endotracheal intubation; prepare for possible emergency cesarean section

· Magnesium toxicity: administer calcium gluconate; monitor for respiratory arrest

TEST RESULTS

• Proteinuria of more than 300 mg/ 24 hours (1+ on dipstick) reveals preeclampsia.

• Proteinuria of 5 g/24 hours (3+) or more reveals severe eclampsia.

• Hemolysis, elevated liver enzymes, and a decreased platelet count reveals HELLP syndrome.

• Serial ultrasonography evaluates fetal well-being and the amniotic fluid volume.

• Nonstress tests and biophysical profiles evaluate fetal well-being.

TREATMENT

• Delivery of fetus is definitive treatment, especially if the patient is near term (38 weeks' gestation; advocated by some clinicians)

• Complete bed rest, preferably in the left lateral supine position

• Adequate nutrition
  – Limited caffeine and low-sodium diet if indicated

– Antihypertensives if blood pressure exceeds 160/90 mm Hg
• Magnesium sulfate
• Oxygen, if necessary

KEY PATIENT OUTCOMES

The patient will:
• maintain normal vital signs
• maintain adequate fluid volume
• avoid complications
• remain oriented to the environment
• give birth to a viable neonate by vaginal or cesarean delivery.

NURSING INTERVENTIONS

• Monitor maternal vital signs and fetal heart rate frequently.
• Monitor vision, level of consciousness, deep tendon reflexes, epigastric or abdominal pain, and headache unrelieved by medication. Report changes immediately.
• Give prescribed medications. (See *Emergency interventions for gestational hypertension.*)
• Monitor the extent of edema and the degree of pitting.
• Encourage elevation of edematous arms or legs.
• Eliminate constricting clothing, pantyhose, slippers, and bed linens.
• Monitor daily weight and intake and output.
• Assist with or insert an indwelling urinary catheter, if necessary.
• Provide a quiet, darkened room.
• Encourage compliance with bed rest.
• Provide emotional support, encouraging the patient to express her feelings.
• Help the patient develop effective coping strategies.
• Involve a significant other in daily care.

PATIENT TEACHING

Be sure to cover:
• the disorder, diagnosis, and treatment

- signs and symptoms of pre-eclampsia and eclampsia
- the importance of bed rest in the left lateral position, as ordered
- adequate nutrition and a low-sodium diet
- good prenatal care
- control of preexisting hypertension
- early recognition and prompt treatment of preeclampsia.

Isoimmunization

DESCRIPTION

- *Isoimmunization* is the development of Rh antibodies when a woman with Rh-negative blood is exposed to Rh-positive blood.
- It can occur from blood transfusion with Rh-positive blood, or pregnancy with the fetus having Rh-positive blood (most common).
- It carries a risk of hemolytic disease in the neonate, if untreated.
- It was formerly a major cause of kernicterus and neonatal death (prognosis improved with use of $Rh_o(D)$ immune globulin [Rho-GAM]).
- It's also known as *Rh incompatibility*.

PATHOPHYSIOLOGY

- An antigen-antibody immunologic reaction within the body occurs when an Rh-negative woman is exposed to Rh-positive blood.
- The Rh-negative woman is sensitized by exposure to Rh-positive fetal blood antigens during her first pregnancy, or she may also become sensitized through blood transfusions with alien Rh antigens, from inadequate doses of $Rh_o(D)$, or from failure to receive $Rh_o(D)$ after significant fetal-maternal leakage from abruptio placentae (premature detachment of the placenta).

- Subsequent pregnancy with an Rh-positive fetus provokes increasing amounts of maternal agglutinating antibodies to cross the placental barrier, attach to Rh-positive cells in the fetus, and cause hemolysis and anemia.
- To compensate for this, the fetus steps up the production of red blood cells (RBCs), and erythroblasts (immature RBCs) appear in the fetal circulation.
- Extensive hemolysis results in the release of large amounts of unconjugated bilirubin, which the liver can't conjugate and excrete, thereby causing hyperbilirubinemia and hemolytic anemia. (See *Pathogenesis of Rh isoimmunization,* page 528.)

CAUSES

- Rh-negative woman exposed to Rh-positive blood that may result from several factors
  - Pregnancy
  - Abdominal or pelvic trauma
  - Abortion
  - Blood transfusion
  - Ectopic pregnancy
  - In utero fetal death
  - Invasive obstetrical procedure
  - Placenta previa
  - Abruptio placentae

ASSESSMENT FINDINGS

- Known Rh negative blood type in mother; known Rh positive blood type in father
- No physical symptoms

TEST RESULTS

- Blood type reveals Rh negative blood.
- Increased concentration (optical density) of bilirubin and RBC breakdown products in the amniotic fluid may reveal isoimmunization.
- Anti-D antibody titer of 1:16 or greater may reveal isoimmunization.
- Radiologic studies may reveal edema and, in those with hydrops

Pathogenesis of Rh isoimmunization

Rh isoimmunization spans pregnancies in Rh-negative mothers who give birth to Rh-positive neonates. These illustrations outline the process of isoimmunization.

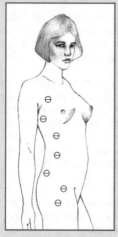

1. Before pregnancy, the woman has Rh-negative blood.

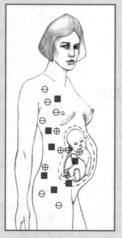

2. She becomes pregnant with an Rh-positive fetus. Normal antibodies appear.

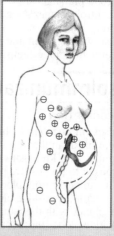

3. Placental separation occurs.

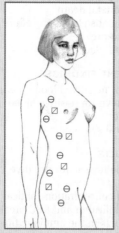

4. After delivery, the mother develops anti–Rh-positive antibodies.

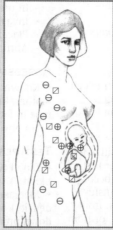

5. With the next Rh-positive fetus, anti-Rh antibodies enter fetal circulation, causing hemolysis.

KEY:
Rh − blood ⊕
Rh + blood ⊖
Normal antibodies ■
Anti-Rh antibodies ☑

fetalis, the halo sign (edematous, elevated, subcutaneous fat layers) and the Buddha position (fetus's legs crossed).

TREATMENT

• Monitoring of the indirect Coombs' test (measures level of antibodies in maternal blood)
• Delta optical density analysis of the amniotic fluid at 26 weeks' gestation
• Antibody titers
• Intrauterine (IU) fetal transfusion
• Possible early delivery
• Administration of RhoGAM at 28 weeks' gestation and within 72 hours after delivery of Rh-positive neonate to attain passive antibody protection for future pregnancies

KEY PATIENT OUTCOMES

The patient will:
• verbalize an understanding of the disorder and its treatment
• demonstrate adequate coping measures
• give birth to a viable neonate.

NURSING INTERVENTIONS

• Assess all pregnant women for possible Rh incompatibility.
• Administer RhoGAM as ordered.
• Assist with IU fetal transfusion as indicated.
• Before IU transfusion, obtain a baseline fetal heart rate (FHR) by electronic monitoring; explain the procedure and its purpose to the patient.
• Posttransfusion, carefully monitor the patient for uterine contractions, amniotic fluid leaking from the vagina, and fluid leakage from the puncture site.
• Monitor FHR for tachycardia, bradycardia, or variable decelerations.
• Prepare the patient for a planned delivery, usually 2 to 4 weeks before term date, depending on maternal

history, serologic tests, and amniocentesis results.
• Assist with induction of labor, if indicated.
• During labor, monitor the fetus electronically for oxygen saturation.
• Indication of fetal distress necessitates immediate cesarean delivery.
• Provide emotional support to the patient and her family.

PATIENT TEACHING

Be sure to cover:
• the disorder, diagnosis, and treatment
• procedures used to determine sensitization, including preprocedure and postprocedure care
• the need for follow-up
• RhoGAM administration
• plans for delivery, possibly before term due date.

Placenta previa

DESCRIPTION

• *Placenta previa* is abnormal placental implantation in the lower uterine segment, encroaching on the internal cervical os.
• It's the leading cause of third-trimester hemorrhage and a common cause of bleeding during the second half of pregnancy. (Among patients who develop placenta previa during the second trimester, less than 15% have persistent previa at term.)
• Preterm delivery occurs in 50% of women with placenta previa.
• Fetal prognosis varies by gestational age and amount of blood loss. Risk of death is greatly reduced by frequent monitoring and prompt management.

PATHOPHYSIOLOGY

• The placenta covers all or part of the internal cervical os. (See *Three types of placenta previa,* page 530.)

Three types of placenta previa

The degree of placenta previa depends largely on the extent of cervical dilation at the time of examination because the dilating cervix gradually uncovers the placenta, as shown here.

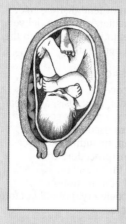 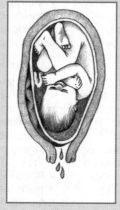 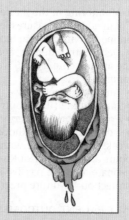

Marginal placenta previa
If the placenta covers just a fraction of the internal cervical os, the patient has marginal, or low-lying, placenta previa.

Partial placenta previa
The patient has the partial, or incomplete, form of the disorder if the placenta caps a larger part of the internal os.

Total placenta previa
If the placenta covers all of the internal os, the patient has total, complete, or central placenta previa. This type is associated with greater blood loss.

• Painless bleeding occurs, usually in the third trimester as placental attachment is disrupted by thinning of the lower uterine segment in preparation for labor.

Causes
• Exact cause unknown
• Several contributing factors
  – Advanced maternal age (older than age 35)
  – Defective vascularization of the decidua
  – Endometriosis
• Factors that may affect the site of placental attachment to the uterine wall:
  – Multiparity
  – Multiple gestation

  – Previous uterine surgery or cesarean section
  – Smoking

Assessment findings
• Onset of painless, bright red vaginal bleeding after 20 weeks' gestation
• Vaginal bleeding before onset of labor, typically episodic and stopping spontaneously
• May be asymptomatic
• Soft, nontender uterus
• Fetal malpresentation
• Minimal descent of fetal presenting part
• Good fetal heart tones

Test results

- Transvaginal ultrasonography determines placental position.
- Maternal hemoglobin level is decreased.
- Kleihauer-Betke testing in an Rh-negative mother may indicate the presence of fetal blood cells from fetomaternal hemorrhage greater than 30 ml.
- Pelvic examination is contraindicated.

Treatment

- Maternal stabilization and fetal monitoring
- Hospitalization with complete bed rest until 36 weeks' gestation with complete placenta previa
- Magnesium sulfate if preterm labor occurs
- Control of blood loss; blood replacement
- Delivery of viable neonate as close to term as possible
- Prevention of coagulation disorders
- Monitoring fetus of less than 36 weeks' gestation to determine the need for preterm delivery
- Possible vaginal delivery, with minimal bleeding or rapidly progressing labor; possible cesarean section with complete placenta previa
- Nothing by mouth initially, then as guided by clinical status
- I.V. fluids, using a large-bore catheter
- Immediate cesarean delivery in severe hemorrhage or at 36 weeks' gestation

Key patient outcomes

The patient will:
- maintain stable vital signs
- maintain normal fluid volume
- express her feelings of increased comfort
- verbalize her feelings and concerns about her condition

- use available support systems to aid in coping
- give birth to a viable neonate as close to term as possible.

Nursing interventions

- Institute complete bed rest.
- If the patient is experiencing active bleeding, continuously monitor her blood pressure, pulse rate, respirations, central venous pressure, intake and output, and amount of vaginal bleeding, as well as the fetal heart rate and rhythm.
- If continuation of the pregnancy is deemed safe for the patient and the fetus, administer magnesium sulfate as ordered for premature labor.
- Obtain blood samples for complete blood count and blood type and crossmatching.
- Administer prescribed I.V. fluids and blood products.
- Assist with application of electronic fetal monitoring as indicated by maternal and fetal status.
- Administer oxygen if fetal distress occurs, as indicated by bradycardia, tachycardia, late or variable decelerations, pathologic sinusoidal pattern, unstable baseline, or loss of variability.
- If the patient is Rh-negative and not sensitized, administer $Rh_o(D)$ immune globulin after every bleeding episode.
- Provide information about labor progress and the condition of the fetus.
- Prepare the patient and her family for a possible cesarean delivery and the birth of a preterm neonate, and provide thorough instructions for postpartum care.
- If the fetus is less than 36 weeks' gestation, expect to administer an initial dose of betamethasone to help mature the neonate's lungs; explain that additional doses may be

given again in 24 hours and, possibly, for the next 2 weeks.
• If necessary, request consultation with a neonatologist or pediatrician to discuss a treatment plan for the neonate after birth with the patient and her family.
• Encourage the patient and her family to verbalize their feelings, help them to develop effective coping strategies, and refer them for counseling, if necessary.
• Anticipate the need for a referral for home care if the patient's bleeding ceases and she returns home on bed rest.
• During the postpartum period, monitor the patient for signs of early and late postpartum hemorrhage and shock.

PATIENT TEACHING

Be sure to cover:
• the disorder, diagnosis, and treatment
• signs and symptoms of placenta previa
• the possibility of emergency cesarean delivery
• the possibility of the birth of a premature neonate or of fetal or neonatal demise
• postpartum physical and emotional changes.

Postpartum hemorrhage

DESCRIPTION

• *Postpartum hemorrhage* involves uterine blood loss greater than 500 ml with a vaginal birth, and greater than 1,000 ml with a cesarean delivery.
• In early postpartum hemorrhage, blood is lost during the first 24 hours after delivery.
• In late postpartum hemorrhage, blood is lost after the first postpartum day, anytime during the re-

maining 6-week postpartum period (most commonly 7 to 14 days after delivery).
• Predisposing factors include delivery of a large neonate, multiple gestation, hydramnios, dystocia, grand multiparity, trauma during delivery, and medications used during labor or surgery.
• It's also known as *PPH*.

PATHOPHYSIOLOGY

• Normally, after a vaginal delivery, a blood loss of up to 500 ml is considered acceptable; for a cesarean delivery, the acceptable range for blood loss is typically 1,000 ml.
• After delivery and placental detachment, the highly vascular yet denuded uterus is widely exposed.
• Interference with the ability of the uterus to contract leads to uterine atony.
• Subsequently, the opened vessels at the site of placental attachment continue to bleed.
• Any condition that interferes with the ability of the uterus to contract can lead to uterine atony and, subsequently, to PPH.
• Tearing of the uterine artery, such as with cervical lacerations or lacerations of the birth canal, can lead to hemorrhage.
• Abnormal placental implantation that leaves an area of separation between the placenta and decidua can lead to hemorrhage.

CAUSES

• Amnionitis
• Disseminated intravascular coagulation (DIC)
• Incomplete placental separation
• Lacerations of the birth canal
• Rapid fetal descent
• Retained placental fragments
• Trauma to the lower genital tract
• Uterine atony
• Uterine inversion
• Uterine overdistention

- Uterine rupture

Risk factors
- PPH after a previous pregnancy
- Chorioamnionitis
- Labor induction and augmentation
- High birth weight
- Use of magnesium sulfate

ASSESSMENT FINDINGS

- Bleeding that can occur suddenly in large amounts or gradually as seeping or oozing of blood
- Frequent saturation of perineal pads
- In uterine atony: soft, relaxed uterus on palpation to the right or left of midline with distended bladder
- With retained placental fragments: soft, noncontracting uterus on palpation and slow trickle, oozing, or frank hemorrhage
- With genital tract lacerations or trauma: continuous, bright red vaginal bleeding and firm uterus
- With continuous or copious bleeding: signs and symptoms of hypovolemic shock
  - Hypotension with mean arterial blood pressure below 60 mm Hg
  - Pallor
  - Decreased sensorium
  - Rapid, shallow respirations
  - Urine output less than 25 ml/hour
  - Rapid, thready peripheral pulses
  - Cold, clammy skin
  - Narrowing pulse pressure

TEST RESULTS

- Hemoglobin and hematocrit levels are decreased (a drop of 1 to 1.5 g/dl in hemoglobin level and approximately 2% to 4% drop in hematocrit from the baseline).
- Urine specific gravity and osmolality (if shock ensues) are increased.

- Arterial blood pH and partial pressure of arterial oxygen are decreased; partial pressure of arterial carbon dioxide (if shock occurs) is increased.
- Platelet and fibrinogen levels, coagulation factors, and antithrombin III levels are decreased; prolonged clotting times are prolonged; and the D-dimer test (if DIC is the cause) is increased.

TREATMENT

- Correcting the underlying cause
- Controlling blood loss and minimizing the extent of hypovolemic shock
- Blood and fluid replacement
- Monitoring of vital signs
- Intermittent uterine massage, if uterine atony is the cause
  - Oxytocin, if massage is ineffective or if the uterus can't be maintained in a contracted state
  - Possible bimanual massage, if other measures prove ineffective
  - Methylergonovine (Methergine), prostaglandins, or other agents to promote strong, sustained uterine contractions
  - Arterial embolization, if other therapies are ineffective
  - Hysterectomy (last resort)
- Surgical repair of lacerations
- Removal of retained placental fragments by dilatation and curettage
- Treatment of the underlying cause of DIC

KEY PATIENT OUTCOMES

The patient will:
- maintain adequate cardiac output and tissue perfusion
- maintain adequate fluid volume and urine output
- exhibit hemodynamic stability
- communicate feelings about her condition
- use available support systems to aid in coping

Emergency interventions for hypovolemic shock

Be prepared to perform these interventions if the patient develops signs and symptoms of hypovolemic shock.

• Begin an I.V. infusion with normal saline solution or lactated Ringer's solution delivered through a large-bore (14G to 18G) catheter; administer blood products as ordered.
• Assist with insertion of a central venous line or pulmonary artery catheter for hemodynamic monitoring; monitor cardiac output and central venous, right atrial, pulmonary artery, and pulmonary artery wedge pressures hourly or as ordered.
• Monitor and record blood pressure, heart rate, respiratory rate, and pulse oximetry every 15 minutes until stable.
• Continuously monitor heart rhythm and neurologic status.
• Assess the patient's skin color and temperature, noting any changes.
• Watch for signs of impending coagulopathy, such as petechiae, bruising, bleeding, or oozing from gums or venipuncture sites.
• Obtain arterial blood samples to measure arterial blood gas (ABG) levels.

• Administer oxygen by nasal cannula, face mask, or airway to ensure adequate tissue oxygenation, adjusting the oxygen flow rate as ABG results and pulse oximetry levels indicate.
• Assess respiratory status for signs of respiratory distress.
• Obtain venous blood samples, as ordered, for a complete blood count, electrolyte levels, typing and cross-matching, and coagulation studies.
• If the physician orders prostaglandin therapy, be alert for possible adverse effects, such as nausea, diarrhea, tachycardia, and hypertension. Inform the patient about these effects to alleviate her fear and anxiety should they occur.
• Monitor the fundus, and provide massage as often as necessary; monitor vaginal blood loss.
• Prepare the patient for possible treatments, such as bimanual massage, surgical repair of lacerations, or dilatation and curettage, as indicated.
• Provide emotional support to the patient; explain all events and treatments to help alleviate her anxiety and fear.

• remain free from complications associated with hemorrhage.

NURSING INTERVENTIONS

• Assess the patient's fundus frequently, and perform fundal massage to assist with uterine involution; notify the physician if the fundus doesn't remain contracted.
• Monitor lochia; note if the amount increases or becomes watery with a change in color.
• Weigh perineal pads, and monitor pad count.
• Inspect the sheet beneath the patient for pooling of blood; if necessary, weigh disposable bed linen pads.

• Inspect the perineal area closely for oozing from any lacerations.
• Monitor vital signs frequently for changes, noting any trends such as a continuously rising pulse rate; report any changes immediately. (See *Emergency interventions for hypovolemic shock.*)
• Assess intake and output; report urine output of less than 30 ml/hour.
• Encourage the patient to void frequently to prevent bladder distention.
• Insert an indwelling urinary catheter if the patient can't void.

PATIENT TEACHING

Be sure to cover:

- the disorder, diagnosis, and treatment
- assessing lochia flow
- measures to control bleeding
- medications being administered
- signs and symptoms of hemorrhage and the need to inform the obstetrician.

Neonatal disorders

Fetal alcohol syndrome

DESCRIPTION

- *Fetal alcohol syndrome* (FAS) is a cluster of birth defects resulting from in utero exposure to alcohol. (See *Terminology associated with FAS*.)
- It includes at least one abnormality in each of the following categories: growth retardation, central nervous system (CNS) abnormalities, and facial malformations.
- It's commonly found in neonates of women who ingested varying amounts of alcohol during pregnancy.
- It can develop in the first 3 to 8 weeks of pregnancy, before a patient even knows she's pregnant.

PATHOPHYSIOLOGY

- Alcohol is a teratogenic substance that's particularly dangerous during critical periods of organogenesis.
- Alcohol interferes with the passage of amino acids across the placental barrier.
- Alcohol consumed by the pregnant patient crosses through the placenta and enters the blood supply of the fetus.
- Variables that affect the extent of damage caused to the fetus by alcohol include the amount of alcohol consumed, timing of consumption, and pattern of alcohol use.

■
Terminology associated with FAS

Fetal alcohol syndrome (FAS) is characterized by physical and mental disorders apparent at birth and problematic throughout the child's life. A distinctive pattern of three specific findings characterizes FAS: growth restriction (prenatal and postnatal), craniofacial structural anomalies, and central nervous system dysfunction. However, because effects other than those typically associated with FAS also occur, additional terminology has been developed to address these concerns.

· *Fetal alcohol effects* is used to describe children with a variety of problems thought to be associated with alcohol consumption by the mother during pregnancy. These problems may include low birth weight, developmental delays, and hyperactivity.

· *Alcohol-related birth defects* is used to describe neonates with some but not all of the symptoms of FAS.

· *Alcohol-related neurologic defects* is used to describe neonates with neurologic symptoms associated with FAS, such as cognitive difficulties, hyperactivity problems, and mental impairments.

When the effects of prenatal exposure to alcohol are viewed on a continuum, FAS is considered severe.

CAUSES

- Intrauterine exposure to alcohol ingested by the mother during pregnancy

Risk factors

- Occurs with even moderate alcohol consumption (1 to 2 oz [30 to 59 ml] of alcohol daily)
- Increases proportionally with increased daily alcohol intake

Common facial characteristics of neonates with FAS

Eyes	• Short palpebral fissures • Strabismus • Ptosis • Myopia
Nose	• Short • Upturned • Flat or absent groove above upper lip
Mouth	• Thin upper lip • Receding jaw

ASSESSMENT FINDINGS

• History of alcohol ingestion by the mother
• Prenatal and postnatal growth retardation
• Several characteristic findings within the first 24 hours of life
  – Difficulty establishing respirations
  – Irritability
  – Lethargy
  – Seizure activity
  – Tremulousness
  – Opisthotonos
  – Poor sucking reflex
  – Abdominal distention
• Facial anomalies, such as microcephaly, microophthalmia, maxillary hypoplasia, and short palpebral fissures (see *Common facial characteristics of neonates with FAS*)
• CNS dysfunction, including decreased IQ, developmental delays, and such neurologic abnormalities as decreased muscle tone, poor coordination, and small brain

TEST RESULTS

• No specific test confirms the diagnosis.
• Radiography may reveal associated renal or cardiac defects.

TREATMENT

• Careful prenatal history and education
• Identification of women at risk, with referral to alcohol treatment centers, if necessary
• Prompt identification of neonates with FAS to ensure early intervention and appropriate referrals
• Heart defects may require surgery
• Later, learning disorder may need specialized education

KEY PATIENT OUTCOMES

The patient will:
• maintain a patent airway and adequate ventilation
• remain free from injury
• remain free from overstimulation
• ingest adequate nutrients to foster growth
• exhibit weight gain within acceptable parameters
• reach maximum potential for growth and development
• demonstrate bonding and attachment behaviors with the caregiver.

NURSING INTERVENTIONS

• Closely assess any neonate born to a mother who has used alcohol.
• Prevent and treat respiratory distress, including assessing breath sounds frequently, being alert for signs of distress, and suctioning as needed.
• Encourage successful feeding; assist with developing measures to enhance the neonate's intake.
• Monitor weight, and measure intake and output.
• Promote parent-neonate attachment; encourage frequent visiting and rooming in, if possible, with physical contact between the parent and the neonate.
• Provide emotional support and anticipatory guidance related to the neonate's condition.
• Refer to social services to evaluate the home situation and assess the

neonate's home health needs, if indicated.

PATIENT TEACHING

Be sure to cover with the parents:
- the disorder, diagnosis, and treatment
- measures to facilitate bonding
- nutritional needs and strategies
- possible complications
- danger signs and symptoms to report to primary care provider
- the need for long-term follow-up
- how to contact the National Organization on Fetal Alcohol Syndrome
- location and contact information for local support groups and services.

Hemolytic disease of the newborn

DESCRIPTION

- *Hemolytic disease of the newborn* is defined as hemolytic disease of the fetus and neonate that results from an incompatibility of fetal and maternal blood.
- Potential complications include fetal death in utero, severe fetal anemia, fetal edema (fetal hydrops), heart failure, and kernicterus.
- It's also called *erythroblastosis fetalis* and *alloimmunization*.

PATHOPHYSIOLOGY

ABO incompatibility
- Each blood group has specific antigens on red blood cells (RBCs) and specific antibodies in the serum.
- The maternal immune system forms antibodies against fetal cells when blood groups differ.
- This can cause hemolytic disease even if fetal erythrocytes don't escape into the maternal circulation during pregnancy.

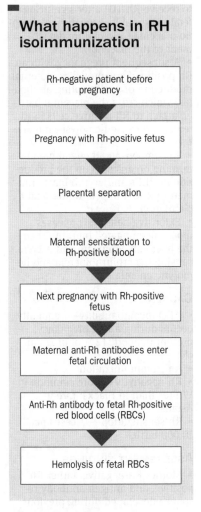

What happens in RH isoimmunization

Rh-negative patient before pregnancy

↓

Pregnancy with Rh-positive fetus

↓

Placental separation

↓

Maternal sensitization to Rh-positive blood

↓

Next pregnancy with Rh-positive fetus

↓

Maternal anti-Rh antibodies enter fetal circulation

↓

Anti-Rh antibody to fetal Rh-positive red blood cells (RBCs)

↓

Hemolysis of fetal RBCs

Rh incompatibility
- During her first pregnancy, an Rh-negative female becomes sensitized (during delivery or abortion) by exposure to Rh-positive fetal blood antigens inherited from the father. (See *What happens in Rh isoimmunization*.)
- A female may also become sensitized from receiving blood transfusions with alien Rh antigens; from inadequate doses of $Rh_o(D)$ immune globulin (RhoGAM), or from failure

to receive $Rh_o(D)$ after significant fetal-maternal leakage during abruptio placentae (premature detachment of the placenta).

• A subsequent pregnancy with an Rh-positive fetus provokes maternal production of agglutinating antibodies, which cross the placental barrier, attach to Rh-positive cells in the fetus, and cause hemolysis and anemia.

• To compensate, the fetal blood-forming organs step up the production of RBCs and erythroblasts (immature RBCs) appear in the fetal circulation.

• Extensive hemolysis releases more unconjugated bilirubin than the liver can conjugate and excrete, causing hyperbilirubinemia and hemolytic anemia.

CAUSES

• ABO incompatibility—frequently occurs during a first pregnancy; present in about 12% of pregnancies

• Rh isoimmunization

• Rh negativity—more common in Whites than in Blacks; rare in Asians

• Rh sensitization—11 cases per 10,000 births

ASSESSMENT FINDINGS

• Mother Rh-negative, father Rh-positive, and antigen-antibody response developed during previous pregnancy

• History of blood transfusion in the mother

• Maternal history of erythroblastotic stillbirths, abortions, previously affected children, or previous anti-Rh titers

• Bile-stained umbilical cord

• Edema

• Heart murmur

• Jaundice

• Mild to moderate hepatosplenomegaly

• Pallor

• Petechiae

• Pulmonary crackles

• Yellow- or meconium-stained amniotic fluid

TEST RESULTS

• Maternal blood type and Rh is necessary.

• Amniotic fluid analysis shows increased bilirubin and anti-Rh antibody titers.

• Direct Coombs' test of the umbilical cord is positive and documents presence of anti-A or anti-B antibodies.

• Direct antibodies test is positive in the mother and neonate.

• Cord hemoglobin level in the neonate is less than 10 g, indicating severe hemolytic disease and anemia.

• Many nucleated peripheral RBCs are present.

• Decreased blood glucose is common.

• Radiologic studies show edema and, in hydrops fetalis, the halo sign (edematous, elevated, subcutaneous fat layers) and the Buddha position (the fetus's legs are crossed).

TREATMENT

• Phototherapy (exposure to ultraviolet light to reduce bilirubin levels)

• Intubation of the neonate

• Removal of excess fluid

• Maintenance of body temperature

• Intrauterine-intraperitoneal transfusion (if amniotic fluid analysis suggests the fetus is severely affected and isn't mature enough to deliver)

• Exchange transfusion

• Albumin infusion

• Gamma globulin containing anti-Rh antibody $(Rh_o[D])$

• Planned delivery (usually 2 to 4 weeks before term date, depending on maternal history, serologic test results, and amniocentesis)

KEY PATIENT OUTCOMES

The patient will:
• exhibit adequate ventilation and tissue perfusion
• remain hemodynamically stable
• maintain fluid balance within normal limits
• maintain normal temperature.

NURSING INTERVENTIONS

• Encourage expression of fears by the family concerning possible complications of treatment.
• Prepare the neonate for treatment procedures, such as phototherapy or exchange transfusion.
• Promote parental bonding.
• Administer $Rh_o(D)$ immune globulin I.M. as ordered.
• Monitor cardiac rhythm and rate, airway and ventilation, and vital signs closely.
• Assist with transfusions, as ordered, and monitor for transfusion complications.
• Assess intake and output frequently.
• Encourage adherence to follow-up appointments.

PATIENT TEACHING

Be sure to cover with the parents:
• the disorder, diagnosis, and treatment
• medications, drug routes, and administration
• preventive measures for reoccurrence.

Hyperbilirubinemia, unconjugated

DESCRIPTION

• *Unconjugated hyperbilirubinemia* involves excessive serum bilirubin levels and mild jaundice resulting from hemolytic processes in the neonate.

• It can be physiologic (with jaundice the only symptom) or pathologic (resulting from an underlying disease).
• It's common in neonates, more common in males than in females, and more common in White infants than in Black infants.
• Potential complications include kernicterus, cerebral palsy, epilepsy, and mental retardation.
• It's also called *neonatal jaundice* or *physiologic jaundice of the newborn.*

PATHOPHYSIOLOGY

• As erythrocytes break down at the end of their neonatal life cycle, hemoglobin separates into globin (protein) and heme (iron) fragments.
• Heme fragments form unconjugated (indirect) bilirubin, which binds with albumin for transport to liver cells to conjugate with glucuronide, forming direct bilirubin.
• Unconjugated bilirubin, which is fat-soluble and can't be excreted in the urine or bile, may escape to extravascular tissue, especially fatty tissue and the brain, resulting in hyperbilirubinemia.
• Hyperbilirubinemia may develop when:
  – certain factors disrupt conjugation and usurp albumin–binding sites, including drugs (such as aspirin, tranquilizers, and sulfonamides) and conditions (such as hypothermia, anoxia, hypoglycemia, and hypoalbuminemia)
  – decreased hepatic function results in reduced bilirubin conjugation
  – increased erythrocyte production or breakdown results from hemolytic disorders or Rh or ABO incompatibility
  – biliary obstruction or hepatitis results in blockage of normal bile flow

Onset-related causes of hyperbilirubinemia

The neonate's age at onset of hyperbilirubinemia may provide clues as to the sources of this jaundice-causing disorder.

Day 1
• Blood type incompatibility (Rh, ABO, other minor blood groups)
• Intrauterine infection (rubella, cytomegalic inclusion body disease, toxoplasmosis, syphilis and, occasionally, such bacteria as *Escherichia coli, Staphylococcus, Pseudomonas, Klebsiella, Proteus,* and *Streptococcus*)

Day 2 or 3
• Abnormal red blood cell morphology
• Blood group incompatibilities
• Enclosed hemorrhage (skin bruises, subdural hematoma)
• Heinz body anemia from drugs and toxins (vitamin K_3, sodium nitrate)
• Infection (usually from gram-negative bacteria)
• Physiologic jaundice
• Polycythemia

• Red cell enzyme deficiencies (glucose-6-phosphate dehydrogenase, hexokinase)
• Respiratory distress syndrome (hyaline membrane disease)
• Transient neonatal hyperbilirubinemia

Day 4 and 5
• Breast-feeding, respiratory distress syndrome, and maternal diabetes
• Crigler-Najjar syndrome (congenital nonhemolytic icterus)
• Gilbert syndrome

Day 7 and later
• Bile duct atresia
• Choledochal cysts
• Galactosemia
• Infection (usually acquired in the neonatal period)
• Herpes simplex
• Hypothyroidism
• Neonatal giant cell hepatitis
• Pyloric stenosis

– maternal enzymes present in breast milk inhibit the infant's glucuronyl–transferase conjugating activity.

CAUSES
• Increased bilirubin production secondary to accelerated erythrocyte destruction, decreased levels of ligandin, and low activity of the bilirubin-conjugating enzyme (see *Onset-related causes of hyperbilirubinemia*)

ASSESSMENT FINDINGS
• Previous sibling with neonatal jaundice
• Familial history of anemia, bile stones, splenectomy, or liver disease
• Maternal illness suggestive of viral or other infection
• Maternal drug intake
• Delayed cord clamping

• Birth trauma with bruising
• Jaundice, icterus

TEST RESULTS
• Serum bilirubin levels are elevated.

TREATMENT
• Phototherapy
• Exchange transfusions
• Albumin
• Phenobarbital (rarely used)
• $Rh_0(D)$ immune globulin (RhoGAM) (to Rh-negative mother)

KEY PATIENT OUTCOMES
The patient will:
• exhibit normal body temperature
• maintain normal fluid balance
• maintain skin integrity
• have a reduced bilirubin level.

NURSING INTERVENTIONS

- Provide phototherapy as ordered; provide eye protection.
- Monitor skin integrity.
- Reassure the family that most neonates experience some degree of jaundice.
- Keep emergency equipment available when transfusing blood.
- Administer RhoGAM to an Rh-negative mother after amniocentesis or, to prevent hemolytic disease in subsequent infants, to an Rh-negative mother during the third trimester, after the birth of an Rh-positive infant, or after spontaneous or elective abortion.
- Monitor the neonate for jaundice.
- Assess serum bilirubin levels as ordered.
- Monitor vital signs closely.
- Assess intake and output, especially during treatment.
- Assess for signs and symptoms of bleeding and associated complications.

PATIENT TEACHING

Be sure to cover with the parents:
- the disorder, diagnosis, and treatment
- that the infant's stool contains some bile and may be greenish
- home phototherapy, if ordered.

Neonatal abstinence syndrome

DESCRIPTION

- *Neonatal abstinence syndrome* is a constellation of neurologic and physical behaviors exhibited by drug-exposed neonates.
- It has two types.
  - *Prenatal* refers to fetal exposure to drugs from maternal drug use during pregnancy.

- *Postnatal* results from abrupt discontinuation of drugs after prolonged administration to the neonate.
- Associated risks include congenital malformations, cerebrovascular complications, low birth weight, decreased head circumference, respiratory problems, drug withdrawal, and death.
- It's also known as *NAS*.

PATHOPHYSIOLOGY

- This is a neonatal addiction resulting from intrauterine exposure.
- Pathophysiology depends on which drug the fetus is exposed to; it's usually a multisystem disorder mainly affecting the neurovascular and GI systems.
- The drug acts as a teratogen, causing abnormalities in embryonic or fetal development.

CAUSES

- Intrauterine exposure to addictive substances
  - Barbiturates
  - Cocaine
  - Opiates and narcotics
  - Marijuana
  - Diazepam and lorazepam
  - Diphenhydramine
  - Selective serotonin reuptake inhibitors
  - Ethanol
  - Caffeine
  - Nicotine

ASSESSMENT FINDINGS

- Signs and symptoms of withdrawal dependent on the length of maternal addiction, the substance ingested, and the time of last ingestion before delivery (usually within 24 to 48 hours of delivery) (see *Signs and symptoms of opioid drug withdrawal,* page 542, and *Signs and symptoms of nonopioid drug withdrawal,* page 543)

■

Signs and symptoms of opioid drug withdrawal

Central nervous system signs and symptoms	GI signs and symptoms	Autonomic signs and symptoms
• Seizures • Tremors • Irritability • Increased wakefulness • High-pitched cry • Increased muscle tone • Increased deep tendon reflexes • Increased Moro reflex • Increased yawning • Increased sneezing • Rapid changes in mood • Hypersensitivity to noise and external stimuli	• Poor feeding • Uncoordinated and constant sucking • Vomiting • Diarrhea • Dehydration • Poor weight gain	• Increased sweating • Nasal stuffiness • Fever • Mottling • Temperature instability • Increased respiratory rate • Increased heart rate

TEST RESULTS
• Toxicology screen of urine or meconium is positive for drug use.
• Cultures are negative for an infectious agent.
• NAS scoring system measures the degree the neonate is experiencing withdrawal. (*See Neonatal drug withdrawal scoring system,* pages 544 and 545.)

TREATMENT
• Tight swaddling for comfort
• Increased caloric intake
• I.V. fluid with electrolytes
• A quiet, dark environment to decrease environmental stimuli
• A pacifier to meet sucking needs (for heroin withdrawal)
• Gavage feeding for poor sucking reflex (for methadone withdrawal)
• Maintenance of fluid and electrolyte balance
• Evaluate the appropriateness of breast-feeding for the specific mother and child
• Assessment for jaundice (methadone withdrawal)
• Medication to treat withdrawal manifestations, such as methadone (for heroin withdrawal), benzodiazepines (for alcohol withdrawal), or tincture of opium (for opioid withdrawal)
• Promotion of mother-infant bonding
• Evaluation for referral to child protective services, if warranted

KEY PATIENT OUTCOMES
The patient will:
• maintain a patent airway and adequate ventilation
• remain free from injury
• exhibit comfort
• ingest adequate nutrition
• demonstrate appropriate weight gain
• demonstrate positive bonding behaviors.

NURSING INTERVENTIONS
• Provide supportive care.
• Maintain a patent airway; have resuscitative equipment readily available.
• Elevate the neonate's head during feeding; offer a pacifier if the neonate demonstrates vigorous sucking

Signs and symptoms of nonopioid drug withdrawal

Substance	Signs and symptoms
Alcohol	Begin at birth and may last 18 months: crying, excessive eating, hyperactivity, irritability, poor sleeping pattern, poor sucking, seizures, tremors, sweating
Barbiturates	Begin in first 24 hours after birth or as late as 10 to 14 days old and may last 4 to 6 months with treatment: diarrhea, disturbed sleep, excessive crying, excessive eating, increased tone, irritability, noise intolerance, restlessness, severe tremors, vasomotor instability, vomiting
Caffeine	Begin after 24 hours and may last 7 days: bradycardia, jitteriness, tachypnea, vomiting
Chlordiazepoxide (Librium)	Begin at 21 days and may last 1½ months (with treatment) or 9 months (without treatment): irritability, tremors
Clomipramine (Anafranil)	Begin in first 12 hours after birth and may last 4 days (with treatment): cyanosis, hypothermia, tremors
Diazepam (Valium)	Begin at birth and may last 10 to 66 days (with treatment) or 8 months (without treatment): apnea, hyperactivity, hyperreflexia, hypertonia, hypothermia, hypotonia, poor sucking, tachypnea, tremors, vomiting
Ethchlorvynol (Placidyl)	Begin at birth and may last 10 days (with treatment): excessive eating, hypotonia, irritability, jitteriness, lethargy, poor sucking
Hydroxyzine (Vistaril)	Begin at birth and may last 5 weeks (with treatment): clonic movements, feeding problems, hyperactivity, hypotonia, irritability, jitteriness, myoclonic jerks, shrill cry, tachycardia, tachypnea, tremors
Meprobamate (Miltown)	Begin at birth and may last 3 months (with treatment) or 9 months (without treatment): abdominal pain, irritability, poor sleep pattern, tremors

(common in neonates of heroin-addicted mothers).
• Provide small, frequent feedings, positioning the nipple to ensure effective sucking.
• Monitor weight daily.
• Assess intake and output frequently, and monitor fluid and electrolyte balance.

• Administer medications as ordered, and evaluate their effect.
• Administer supplemental I.V. fluids as ordered.
• Assess the neonate for signs and symptoms of respiratory distress, and report them immediately if present.
• Assess breath sounds frequently for changes.

Neonatal drug withdrawal scoring system

Utilizing a scoring system, such as the Neonatal Drug Withdrawal Scoring System of Lipsitz, helps evaluate to what degree a neonate is experiencing drug withdrawal. The higher the score, the more severe is the withdrawal.

Signs	Score "0"	Score "1"
Tremors (muscle activity of limbs)	Normal	Minimally increased when hungry or disturbed
Irritability (excessive crying)	None	Slightly increased
Reflexes	Normal	Increased
Stools	Normal	Explosive, but normal frequency
Muscle tone	Normal	Increased
Skin abrasions	No	Redness of knees and elbows
Respiratory rate/minute	< 55	55 to 75
Repetitive sneezing	No	Yes
Repetitive yawning	No	Yes
Vomiting	No	Yes
Fever	No	Yes

Reproduced with permission from *Pediatrics*, vol. 17, pages 1-10, copyright © 1956 by the AAP.

• Administer supplemental oxygen as ordered, and assist with ventilatory support.
• Monitor arterial blood gas values and transcutaneous oxygen levels.
• Cluster care to prevent overstimulation, and allow for adequate rest.
• Firmly swaddle the neonate to promote comfort.
• Protect the neonate from injury during seizures.
• Maintain skin integrity, provide meticulous skin care, and frequently change the neonate's position.

PATIENT TEACHING

Be sure to cover with the parents:
• the disorder, diagnosis, and treatment

• nutrition and feeding
• comfort measures
• signs and symptoms of withdrawal
• methods to promote bonding and attachment
• location and contact information for local support groups and services.

Preterm neonate

DESCRIPTION

• *Preterm neonate* refers to the delivery of a neonate before the end of the 37th week of gestation.

Score "2"	Score "3"
Moderate or marked increase when disturbed; subside when fed or held snugly	Marked increase or continuous even when undisturbed, going on to seizurelike movements
Moderate to severe when disturbed or hungry	Marked even when undisturbed
Markedly increased	—
Explosive, more than eight per day	—
Rigidity	—
Breaking of skin	—
76 to 95	—
—	—
—	—
—	—

• It's associated with numerous problems because all body systems are immature.

• Preterm neonates between 28 and 37 weeks' gestation demonstrate the best chance of survival.

PATHOPHYSIOLOGY

• Preterm delivery may occur because of maternal disease that necessitates delivery of the neonate for the health of the mother—for example, preeclampsia.

• Preterm delivery may also be a direct result of preterm labor.

CAUSES

• Associated with maternal risk factors

– Adolescent pregnancy
– Cervical insufficiency
– Gestational hypertension
– High, unexplained alpha fetoprotein level in the second trimester
– Lack of prenatal care
– Multiple pregnancy
– Placenta previa
– Premature rupture of membranes
– Previous preterm delivery
– Substance abuse
– Uterine abnormalities

• Underlying condition that results in the delivery of the neonate before term

Assessment findings

- Low birth weight
- Minimal subcutaneous fat deposits
- Proportionally large head in relation to the body
- Prominent sucking pads in the cheeks
- Wrinkled features
- Thin, smooth, shiny skin that's almost translucent
- Veins clearly visible under the epidermis
- Lanugo hair over the body
- Sparse, fine, fuzzy hair on the head
- Soft, pliable ear cartilage (the ear may fold easily)
- Minimal creases in the soles and palms
- Prominent eyes, possibly closed
- Few scrotal rugae (males)
- Undescended testes (males)
- Prominent labia and clitoris (females)
- Inactivity (although may be unusually active immediately after birth)
- Extension of extremities
- Absence of suck reflex
- Weak swallow, gag, and cough reflexes
- Weak grasp reflex
- Ability to bring the neonate's elbow across the chest when eliciting the scarf sign
- Ability to easily bring the neonate's heel to the ear
- Inability to maintain body temperature
- Limited ability to excrete solutes in the urine
- Increased susceptibility to infection, hyperbilirubinemia, and hypoglycemia
- Periodic breathing, hypoventilation, and periods of apnea

Test results

- Chest X-rays may reveal underlying pulmonary problems.
- Echocardiography may reveal cardiac dysfunction.
- Arterial blood gas analysis reveals possible hypoxemia and acid-base abnormalities.
- Serum electrolytes reveal possible imbalances.
- Serum glucose levels may be decreased, indicating hypoglycemia.

Treatment

- Cardiac and respiratory assessment and assistance
- Resuscitation, if needed
- Maintenance of fluid and electrolyte balance
- Nutritional support
- Prevention of infection
- Assessment of neurologic status
- Maintenance of body temperature and a neutral thermal environment
- Monitoring of renal function
- Emotional support to the family
- Assessment of glucose and bilirubin levels

Key patient outcomes

The patient will:
- maintain thermoregulation
- maintain adequate ventilation, perfusion, and cardiac output
- remain free from injury
- demonstrate intake of adequate nutrients to support metabolic demands and growth
- demonstrate an increase in weight
- exhibit appropriate behavioral responses.

Nursing interventions

- Closely assess all body systems.
- Anticipate the need for endotracheal intubation and mechanical ventilation.
- Administer oxygen as ordered, avoiding concentrations that are too high.
- Monitor transcutaneous oxygen levels or pulse oximetry readings.
- Have emergency resuscitation equipment readily available.

- Administer medications to support cardiac and respiratory function.
- Institute measures to maintain a neutral thermal environment; anticipate the need for an incubator or a radiant warmer.
- Avoid vigorous stroking and rubbing; use a firm but gentle touch when handling the neonate.
- Support the head and maintain the extremities close to the body during position changes.
- Monitor fluid and electrolyte balance, assess intake and output, and administer I.V. fluid therapy, as ordered.
- Administer nutritional therapy as ordered.
- Provide emotional support and guidance to the family members; allow them to verbalize their concerns; and correct any misconceptions or erroneous information.
- Assist with referrals for supportive services.

PATIENT TEACHING

Be sure to cover with the parents:
- the disorder, diagnosis, and treatment
- procedures, equipment, and medications being used
- possible complications and risks
- nutritional needs
- methods to promote bonding and attachment
- expectations for growth and development
- necessary follow-up.

Respiratory distress syndrome

DESCRIPTION

- *Respiratory distress syndrome* is a respiratory disorder related to a developmental delay in lung maturity, involving widespread alveolar collapse.
- It's the most common cause of neonatal death.
- It affects approximately 10% of all premature neonates.
- It almost exclusively affects neonates born before the 27th gestational week and occurs in about 45% to 80% of those born before the 28th week if untreated antenatally.
- It most commonly occurs in neonates of mothers with diabetes, neonates delivered by cesarean birth, and neonates with perinatal asphyxia.
- If mild, it subsides slowly after about 3 days.
- It's also called *RDS* or *hyaline membrane disease.*

PATHOPHYSIOLOGY

- In premature neonates, immaturity of alveoli and capillary blood supply leads to alveolar collapse from lack of surfactant (a lipoprotein normally present in alveoli and respiratory bronchioles that lowers surface tension and helps maintain alveolar patency).
- Surfactant deficiency causes alveolar collapse, resulting in inadequate alveolar ventilation and shunting of blood through collapsed lung areas (atelectasis).
- Inadequate ventilation leads to hypoxia and acidosis.
- Compensatory grunting occurs, producing positive end-expiratory pressure (PEEP), which helps to prevent further alveolar collapse.

CAUSES

- Surfactant deficiency stemming from preterm birth

ASSESSMENT FINDINGS

- History of preterm birth, cesarean birth, or other stress during delivery

- Maternal history of diabetes or antepartum hemorrhage
- Rapid, shallow respirations
- Intercostal, subcostal, or sternal retractions
- Nasal flaring
- Audible expiratory grunting
- Pallor
- Frothy sputum
- Low body temperature
- Diminished gas exchange and crackles
- Possible hypotension, peripheral edema, and oliguria
- Possible apnea, bradycardia, and cyanosis

TEST RESULTS

- Partial pressure of arterial oxygen (Pao_2) is decreased; partial pressure of arterial carbon dioxide may be normal, decreased, or increased; and arterial pH is decreased (from respiratory or metabolic acidosis or both).
- Lecithin/sphingomyelin ratio shows prenatal lung development and RDS risk.
- Chest X-rays may show a fine reticulogranular pattern with a "ground glass" appearance.

TREATMENT

- Mechanical ventilation with PEEP or continuous positive airway pressure (CPAP) administered by a tight-fitting face mask or, when necessary, an endotracheal tube
- For a neonate who can't maintain adequate gas exchange, high-frequency oscillation ventilation
- Radiant warmer or Isolette
- Warm, humidified, oxygen-enriched gases given by oxygen hood or mechanical ventilation
- Tube feedings or total parenteral nutrition
- I.V. fluids and sodium bicarbonate
- Pancuronium bromide
- Prophylactic antibiotics

- Diuretics
- Surfactant replacement therapy
- Vitamin E
- Antenatal corticosteroids
- Possible tracheostomy

KEY PATIENT OUTCOMES

The patient (or family) will:
- maintain adequate ventilation
- maintain a patent airway
- remain free from infection
- maintain intact skin integrity
- identify factors that increase the risk of neonatal injury.

NURSING INTERVENTIONS

- Monitor vital signs, arterial blood gas (ABG) values, intake and output, central venous pressure, pulse oximetry, daily weight, skin color, respiratory status, and skin integrity.
- Give prescribed drugs.
- Check the umbilical catheter for arterial or venous hypotension, as appropriate.
- Suction as necessary.
- Change the transcutaneous Pao_2 monitor lead placement site every 2 to 4 hours.
- Adjust PEEP or CPAP settings as indicated by ABG values; monitor for signs of complications of PEEP or CPAP therapy, such as decreased cardiac output, pneumothorax, and pneumomediastinum.
- Monitor for signs and symptoms of infection, thrombosis, and decreased peripheral circulation.
- Implement measures to prevent infection.
- Provide mouth care every 2 hours.
- Encourage the parents to participate in the infant's care.
- Encourage the parents to ask questions and to express their fears and concerns.
- Advise the parents that full recovery may take up to 12 months.
- Offer emotional support.

PATIENT TEACHING

Be sure to cover with the parents:
• the disorder, diagnosis, and treatment
• drugs and possible adverse effects
• explanations of respiratory equipment, alarm sounds, and mechanical noise
• potential complications
• when to notify the physician
• how to contact the American Lung Association
• location and contact information for local support groups and services.

11 Pediatric disorders

Attention deficit hyperactivity disorder

DESCRIPTION

- *Attention deficit hyperactivity disorder* is a neurobehavioral disorder characterized by difficulty with inattention, impulsivity, hyperactivity, and boredom.
- It's difficult to diagnose before age 4 or 5 because symptoms are so varied; some patients aren't diagnosed until adulthood.
- It occurs in 3% to 5% of school-age children.
- It's three to four times more common in males than in females.
- It's also called *ADHD* and *ADD*.

PATHOPHYSIOLOGY

- Alleles of dopamine genes may alter dopamine transmission in the neural networks.
- During fetal development, bouts of hypoxia and hypotension may selectively damage neurons located in some of the critical regions of the anatomical networks.

CAUSES

- Exact cause unknown
- Believed to have genetic and neurobiologic causes or possibly result from altered neurotransmitter levels in the brain

Risk factors
- Family history of ADHD
- History of learning disability

- Mood or conduct disorder

ASSESSMENT FINDINGS

- Impulsive behavior
- Inattentiveness
- Disorganization in school
- Tendency to jump quickly from one partly completed project, thought, or task to another
- Difficulty meeting deadlines and keeping track of school or work tools and materials
- Symptoms of inattention
  - Makes careless mistakes
  - Struggles to sustain attention
  - Fails to finish activities
  - Has difficulty with organization
  - Avoids tasks that require sustained mental effort
  - Is distracted or forgetful
- Symptoms of hyperactivity
  - Fidgets
  - Can't sit still for a sustained period
  - Has difficulty playing quietly
  - Talks excessively
- Symptoms of impulsivity
  - Interrupts
  - Can't wait patiently

Diagnostic and Statistical Manual of Mental Disorders, Fourth Edition, Text Revision *criteria*
- Six or more symptoms from the inattention or hyperactivity-impulsivity categories
- Symptoms present for at least 6 months
- Some symptoms evident before age 7
- Some impairment from symptoms present in two or more settings

- Clear evidence of clinically significant impairment in social, academic, or occupational functioning
- Symptoms not accounted for by another mental disorder

TEST RESULTS

- Complete psychological, physical, and neurologic evaluations rule out other problems; specific tests include continuous performance test, behavior rating scales, and learning disability.

TREATMENT

- Education regarding the nature and effect of the disorder
- Behavior modification
- Control of external distractions
- Supportive psychotherapy
- Complementary therapy, such as chiropractic treatment, biofeedback, and dietary intervention
- Monitored activity (for safety purposes)
- Stimulants for core symptoms (first-line treatment)
- Tricyclic antidepressants considered after the failure of two or three stimulants (second-line treatment)
- Mood stabilizers for the treatment of coexisting conditions such as bipolar disorder
- Referral for family therapy

KEY PATIENT OUTCOMES

The patient will:
- demonstrate effective social interaction skills in one-on-one and group settings
- demonstrate effective injury prevention with decreased impulsivity
- demonstrate a decrease in disruptive behavior
- report improvement in family and social interactions
- demonstrate increasing independence and improved self-esteem
- demonstrate effective coping behavior.

NURSING INTERVENTIONS

- Set realistic expectations and limits.
- Maintain a calm and consistent manner.
- Keep all instructions short and simple; make one-step requests.
- Provide emotional support to the patient and his family.
- Decrease stimulation in the environment.
- Provide diversional activities suited to a short attention span.
- Monitor the patient's activity level, nutritional status, adverse drug reactions, response to treatment, and activity (for safety purposes).

PATIENT TEACHING

Be sure to cover with the parents:
- behavior therapy
- reinforcement of good behavior
- realistic expectations
- medication regimen and possible adverse reactions
- the importance of proper nutrition
- how to contact the Attention Deficit Disorder Association
- location and contact information for local support groups and services.

Autistic disorder

DESCRIPTION

- *Autistic disorder* is one type of pervasive developmental disorder that affects social interactions and communication.
- It has a varying degree of impairment.
- It's usually apparent before age 3.
- Prognosis varies depending on the degree of severity and access to treatment.
- It affects approximately 1 in 1,000 children.
- It's four to five times more common in males than in females, usually the firstborn male.

- It's sometimes called *Kanner's autism.*

PATHOPHYSIOLOGY

- Central nervous system (CNS) defects may arise from prenatal complications.

CAUSES

- Exact cause unknown
- Defects in CNS from prenatal complications such as rubella
- Hypotheses: include genetic or chromosomal abnormalities, obstetric complications, and exposure to toxic agents
- Theorized association with vaccinations implicated but no connection between vaccines and autism proved by research

ASSESSMENT FINDINGS

- Becoming rigid or flaccid when held
- Crying when touched
- Showing little or no interest in human contact; poor eye contact
- Delayed smiling response
- Severe language impairment
- Lack of socialization and imaginative play
- Echolalia
- Pronoun reversal (using "you" instead of "I")
- Bizarre or self-destructive behavior
- Extreme compulsion; rituals
- Abnormal reaction to sensory stimuli
- Cognitive impairment
- Eating, drinking, and sleeping problems
- Mood disorders
- Possible seizures

Diagnostic and Statistical Manual of Mental Disorders, Fourth Edition, Text Revision *criteria*

At least six of these 12 characteristics present, including at least two items from the first section, one from the second, and one from the third

- Qualitative impairment in social interaction
    - Impaired nonverbal behavior
    - Absence of peer relationships
    - Failure to seek or share enjoyment, interests, or achievements
    - Lack of social or emotional reciprocity
- Qualitative impairment in communication
    - Delay or lack of language development
    - Inability to initiate or sustain conversation
    - Idiosyncratic or repetitive language
    - Lack of appropriate imaginative play
- Restricted repetitive and stereotyped patterns of behavior, interests, and activities
    - Abnormal preoccupation with a restricted pattern of interest
    - Inflexible routines or rituals
    - Repetitive motor mannerisms
    - Preoccupation with parts of objects
- Diagnostic criteria also including delays or abnormal functioning in at least one of these areas before age 3
    - Social interaction
    - Language skills
    - Symbolic or imaginative play
- Not better accounted for by Rett syndrome or childhood disintegrative condition

TREATMENT

- Structured treatment plan
- Behavioral, educational, and psychological techniques
- Pleasurable sensory and motor stimulation
- Nutritional therapy (food intolerance, allergies, or vitamin deficiencies may contribute to behavioral issues)
- Monitored activities (for safety purposes)

- Speech therapy, sensory integration therapy, exercise, and physical therapy
- Physical restraint at times if the child is a danger to himself or others

KEY PATIENT OUTCOMES

The patient or his family will:
- identify and contact available resources as needed
- openly share feelings about the present situation
- demonstrate age-appropriate skills and behaviors as much as possible
- practice safety measures and take safety precautions in the home
- interact with family or friends.

NURSING INTERVENTIONS

- Institute safety measures when appropriate.
- Provide positive reinforcement.
- Encourage development of self-esteem.
- Encourage self-care.
- Prepare the patient for change by telling him about it.
- Help family members develop strong one-on-one relationships with the patient.
- Monitor the patient's response to treatment, adverse drug reactions, behavior patterns, nutritional status, social interaction, communication skills, and activity.
- Maintain the child's normal routine as strictly as possible.
- Encourage the parents to remain with the child as much as possible.

PATIENT TEACHING

Be sure to cover with the parents:
- physical care for the child's needs
- the importance of proper nutrition and exercise
- how to identify signs of excessive stress and useful coping skills
- the importance of bringing the child's favorite objects from home when going to a new environment

- how to locate the National Society for Children and Adults with Autism
- location and contact information for local support groups and services.

Cerebral palsy

DESCRIPTION

- *Cerebral palsy* is the most common crippling neuromuscular disease in children.
- It comprises several neuromuscular disorders.
- It results from prenatal, perinatal, or postnatal central nervous system (CNS) damage.
- It has three types, sometimes occurring in mixed forms.
  – *Spastic* affects about 70% of children with cerebral palsy.
  – *Athetoid* affects about 20%.
  – *Ataxic* affects about 10%.
- It causes minimal or severely disabling motor impairment.
- It has several associated defects, including seizures, speech disorders, mental retardation, and vision or hearing impairment. The patient may or may not experience these.
- The condition is nonprogressive and noncurable, but those who receive therapy have better outcomes.
- It's most common in premature neonates and in those who are small for their gestational age.
- It's slightly more common in boys than in girls.
- It's more common in whites.

PATHOPHYSIOLOGY

- A lesion or abnormality occurs in the early stages of brain development.
- Structural and functional defects occur, impairing motor or cognitive function.
- Defects may not be distinguishable until months after birth.

Types of cerebral palsy

Different types of cerebral palsy can be distinguished by specific assessment findings.

Spastic cerebral palsy
· Underdevelopment of affected limbs
· Characteristic scissors gait
· Crossing one foot in front of the other
· Hyperactive deep tendon reflexes
· Increased stretch reflexes
· Rapid alternating muscle contraction and relaxation
· Muscle weakness
· Impaired fine and gross motor skills
· Contractures of the involved limbs
· Muscle spasticity

Athetoid cerebral palsy
· Involuntary movements
· Grimacing
· Wormlike writhing
· Dystonia
· Sharp jerks impairing voluntary movement
· Involuntary facial movements (speech difficult)
· Drooling
· Exaggerated posturing

Ataxic cerebral palsy
· Lack of leg movement during infancy
· Wide, unsteady gait
· Disturbed balance
· Incoordination (especially of the arms)
· Hypoactive reflexes
· Nystagmus
· Muscle weakness
· Tremors

CAUSES
• Conditions that result in cerebral anoxia, hemorrhage, or other CNS damage

Prenatal causes
• Abnormal placental attachment
• ABO blood type incompatibility
• Anoxia
• Irradiation
• Isoimmunization
• Malnutrition
• Maternal diabetes
• Maternal infection (especially rubella in the first trimester)
• Rh factor incompatibility
• Gestational hypertension

Perinatal causes
• Asphyxia from the umbilical cord wrapping around the neck
• Depressed maternal vital signs from general or spinal anesthesia
• Multiple births (neonates born last in a multiple birth have an especially high rate of cerebral palsy)
• Premature birth
• Prolonged or unusually rapid labor
• Trauma during delivery

Postnatal causes
• Any condition resulting in cerebral thrombus or embolus
• Head trauma
• Infections, such as meningitis and encephalitis
• Hyperbilirubinemia
• Hypoglycemia
• Poisoning

ASSESSMENT FINDINGS
• Maternal or patient history revealing possible cause
• Hypotonia when the patient is younger than age 6 months, then tone gradually increases
• Retarded patient growth and delayed developmental milestones (see *Types of cerebral palsy*)
• Difficulty chewing and swallowing

TEST RESULTS
• Computed tomography scan and magnetic resonance imaging of the brain may show structural abnormalities such as cerebral atrophy.

- EEG may show the source of seizure activity.

TREATMENT

- Braces or splints
- Special appliances, such as adapted eating utensils and a low toilet seat with arms
- Range-of-motion (ROM) exercises
- Prescribed exercises to maintain muscle tone
- Anticonvulsants
- Muscle relaxants such as botulinum toxin (Botox) injections
- Antianxiety agents
- Referrals to specialists as needed, such as orthopedist, neurosurgeon, ophthalmologist, physical therapist, or counselor

KEY PATIENT OUTCOMES

The patient will:
- consume recommended daily caloric requirements
- express positive feelings about self
- maintain joint mobility and ROM
- develop adequate coping mechanisms (patient and family)
- develop effective communication skills.

NURSING INTERVENTIONS

- Speak slowly and distinctly.
- Give all care in an unhurried manner.
- Allow participation in care decisions.
- Provide a diet with adequate calories. Stroking the throat may aid swallowing.
- Provide frequent mouth and dental care.
- Provide skin care.
- Perform prescribed exercises.
- Provide care for associated hearing and vision disturbances, as necessary.
- Postoperatively, give analgesics as ordered.

- Provide a safe physical environment.
- Monitor the patient's pain relief, seizure activity, speech, visual and auditory acuity, respiratory status, swallowing function, reflexes, nutritional status, skin integrity, psychosocial status, motor development, and muscle strength.

PATIENT TEACHING

Be sure to cover with the patient and his family:
- the prescribed medication regimen
- adverse drug reactions
- the importance of daily skin inspection and massage
- the need to give the child small amounts of soft foods
- the need to chew food thoroughly
- drinking through a straw
- proper nutrition
- opportunities for learning, such as summer camps or Special Olympics
- correct use of assistive devices
- how to locate the United Cerebral Palsy Association
- location and contact information for local support groups and services.

Croup

DESCRIPTION

- *Croup* is a viral infection that causes severe inflammation and obstruction of the upper airway.
- It's a childhood disease manifested by acute laryngotracheobronchitis (most commonly), laryngitis, acute spasmodic laryngitis, and febrile rhinitis.
- Its incubation period is about 2 to 6 days.
- Recovery from croup is usually complete within 7 days.
- It occurs mainly in children ages 6 months to 3 years.

How croup affects the upper airways

In croup, inflammatory swelling and spasms constrict the larynx, thereby reducing airflow. This cross-sectional drawing (from chin to chest) shows the upper airway changes caused by croup. Inflammatory changes almost completely obstruct the larynx and significantly narrow the trachea.

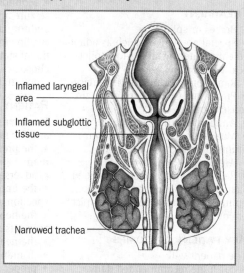

Inflamed laryngeal area

Inflamed subglottic tissue

Narrowed trachea

- It affects boys more commonly than girls.
- It usually occurs in late autumn and early winter.

PATHOPHYSIOLOGY
- Viral or bacterial invasion of the laryngeal mucosa leads to inflammation, hyperemia, edema, epithelial necrosis, and shedding.
- This leads to irritation and cough, reactive paralysis, and continuous stridor, or collapsible supraglottic or inspiratory stridor and respiratory distress.
- A thin, fibrinous membrane covers the mucosa of the epiglottis, larynx, and trachea. (See *How croup affects the upper airways*.)

CAUSES
- Adenoviruses
- Bacteria (*Staphylococcus aureus* and *Haemophilus influenzae*)
- Influenza viruses
- Measles viruses
- Parainfluenza viruses (most common)
- Respiratory syncytial virus (RSV)

ASSESSMENT FINDINGS
- Rhinorrhea
- Use of accessory muscles
- Nasal flaring
- Barklike cough
- Hoarse, muffled vocal sounds
- Inspiratory stridor; expiratory stridor, if severe
- Diminished breath sounds
- Symptoms worse at night
- Fever
- Dyspnea
- Rhonchi

Laryngotracheobronchitis
- Edema of the bronchi and bronchioles
- Decreased breath sounds
- Stridor
- Cyanosis

Steeple sign

The "steeple sign" is a long, narrowed area below the vocal cords that extends below the normal narrowing of the vocal cord.

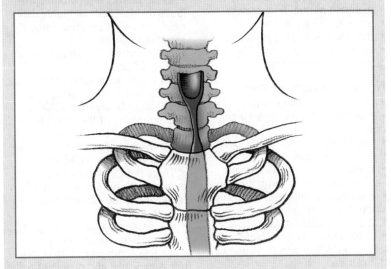

Laryngitis
- Suprasternal and intercostal retractions
- Inspiratory stridor
- Dyspnea, tachypnea
- Diminished breath sounds
- Severe dyspnea and exhaustion in later stages

Acute spasmodic laryngitis
- Labored breathing with retractions
- Clammy skin
- Rapid pulse rate

TEST RESULTS
- Throat cultures show bacteria and sensitivity to antibiotics.
- Neck X-ray may reveal upper airway narrowing and edema in subglottic folds and helps to differentiate croup from bacterial epiglottiditis.
- Neck X-ray may reveal a steeple sign. (See *Steeple sign*.)
- Computed tomography scan helps differentiate between croup, epiglottiditis, and noninfection.
- Laryngoscopy may reveal inflammation and obstruction in epiglottal and laryngeal areas.

TREATMENT
- Based on the degree of respiratory distress and cause of the croup
- Home or hospitalized care
- Humidification during sleep
- Intubation, if other means of preventing respiratory failure are unsuccessful
- Diet as tolerated, encourage fluids
- Parenteral fluids, if required
- Rest periods
- Oxygen therapy as needed
- Antipyretics
- Antibiotics (if bacterial cause)
- Aerosolized racemic epinephrine for moderately severe croup
- Corticosteroids for acute laryngotracheobronchitis (controversial)

- Tracheostomy (rare)

KEY PATIENT OUTCOMES

The patient or his family will:
- maintain adequate ventilation
- maintain normal temperature
- maintain a patent airway
- use effective coping strategies
- verbalize an understanding of the disorder and its treatment.

NURSING INTERVENTIONS

- Give the prescribed drugs.
- Provide quiet diversional activities.
- Engage the parents in the care of the infant or child.
- Position an infant in an infant seat, or prop him up with a pillow.
- Position the child in Fowler's position (if old enough).
- Provide humidification.
- Avoid mild-based fluids if the patient has thick mucus or swallowing difficulties.
- Provide frequent mouth care.
- Isolate the patient with RSV and parainfluenza infections.
- Use sponge baths and hypothermia blanket, as ordered, for temperatures above 102° F (38.9° C).
- Monitor the patient's vital signs, intake and output, and respiratory status. Also monitor for signs and symptoms of dehydration.

PATIENT TEACHING

Be sure to cover with the parents:
- the disorder, diagnosis, and treatment
- medications and possible adverse reactions
- when to notify the physician
- humidification
- hydration
- the signs and symptoms of secondary bacterial infection
- the signs and symptoms of pneumonia.

Cystic fibrosis

DESCRIPTION

- *Cystic fibrosis* is a chronic, progressive, inherited, incurable disease that affects exocrine (mucus-secreting) glands.
- It's transmitted as an autosomal recessive trait.
- It's a genetic mutation involving chloride transport across epithelial membranes (more than 1,300 specific mutations of the gene identified).
- It's the most common fatal genetic disease of White children.
- There is a 25% chance of transmission with each pregnancy when both parents are carriers of the recessive gene.
- It's most common in people of northern European ancestry.
- It's less common in Blacks, Native Americans, and people of Asian ancestry.
- It's equally common in both genders.
- It's characterized by major aberrations in sweat gland, respiratory, and GI functions.
- It accounts for almost all cases of pancreatic enzyme deficiency in children.
- Clinical effects appear soon after birth or may take years to develop.
- It can lead to death from pneumonia, emphysema, or atelectasis.

PATHOPHYSIOLOGY

- It stems from a defect in cystic fibrosis transmembrane conductance regulator (CFTR) gene.
- This results in abnormalities in chloride transport on mucosal surfaces, decreased secretion of chloride, and increased reabsorption of sodium and water.
- The viscosity of bronchial, pancreatic, and other mucous gland secretions increases, attracting bacte-

ria that result in infections and inflammation, and also obstructing glandular ducts.

• Accumulation of thick, tenacious secretions in the bronchioles and alveoli causes respiratory changes, eventually leading to severe atelectasis and emphysema.

• This disorder also causes characteristic GI effects in the intestines, pancreas, and liver.

• Obstruction of the pancreatic ducts results in a deficiency of trypsin, amylase, and lipase; it prevents the conversion and absorption of fat and protein in the intestinal tract and interferes with the digestion of food and the absorption of fat-soluble vitamins.

• In the pancreas, fibrotic tissue, multiple cysts, thick mucus, and fat replaces the acini, producing signs of pancreatic insufficiency, including diabetes.

CAUSES

• Autosomal recessive mutation of CFTR gene

• Causes of symptoms: increased viscosity of bronchial, pancreatic, and other mucous gland secretions, and consequent destruction of glandular ducts

ASSESSMENT FINDINGS

• Neonatal jaundice
• Salty-tasting skin (parents report)
• Recurring bronchitis, pneumonia, and sinusitis
• Nasal polyps
• Wheezing
• Coughing (may cause vomiting)
• Shortness of breath
• Abdominal distention, vomiting, constipation
• Frequent, bulky, foul-smelling, and pale stool with a high fat content
• Poor weight gain
• Poor growth
• Failure to thrive

• Ravenous appetite
• Hematemesis
• Dry, nonproductive, paroxysmal cough
• Dyspnea
• Tachypnea
• Bibasilar crackles and hyperresonance
• Barrel chest
• Distended abdomen
• Thin extremities
• Cyanosis; clubbing of the fingers and toes
• Sallow skin with poor turgor
• Delayed sexual development
• Hepatomegaly
• Rectal prolapse

TEST RESULTS

• Sweat test reveals increased sodium and chloride values (should be performed twice for confirmation).

• Genotyping reveals at least two CFTR mutations.

• Stool specimen analysis shows absence of trypsin.

• Deoxyribonucleic acid testing shows the presence of the delta F 508 mutation.

• Liver enzyme tests may reveal hepatic insufficiency.

• Sputum culture may show such organisms as *Pseudomonas aeruginosa* and *Staphylococcus aureus.*

• Serum albumin level is decreased.

• Serum electrolytes may show hypochloremia and hyponatremia.

• Arterial blood gas analysis shows hypoxemia.

• Chest X-ray may reveal hyperinflation and early signs of lung obstruction.

• Sinus X-ray reveals opacification of the sinuses.

• High-resolution chest computed tomography scan shows bronchial wall thickening, cystic lesions, and bronchiectasis.

• Pulmonary function tests show decreased vital capacity, elevated residual volume, and decreased forced expiratory volume in 1 second.

TREATMENT

• Based on organ systems involved
• Chest physiotherapy, nebulization, and breathing exercises several times per day
• Postural drainage
• Gene therapy (experimental)
• Annual influenza vaccination
• Salt supplements
• High-fat, high-protein, high-calorie diet
• Activity as tolerated
• Antibiotics
• Oxygen therapy as needed
• Oral pancreatic enzymes
• Bronchodilators
• Mucolytic agents
• Prednisone
• Vitamin A, D, E, and K supplements
• Lung transplantation

KEY PATIENT OUTCOMES

The patient or his family will:
• maintain a patent airway and adequate ventilation
• consume adequate calories daily
• use a support system to assist with coping
• express an understanding of the illness and treatment.

NURSING INTERVENTIONS

• Give the prescribed drugs.
• Administer pancreatic enzymes with meals and snacks.
• Perform chest physiotherapy and postural drainage.
• Administer oxygen therapy as needed.
• Provide a well-balanced, high-calorie, high-protein diet; include adequate fats.
• Provide vitamin A, D, E, and K supplements, if indicated.
• Ensure adequate oral fluid intake.
• Provide exercise and activity periods.

• Encourage breathing exercises.
• Enlist the help of the physical therapy department and play therapists, if available.
• Provide emotional support.
• Include family members in all phases of the patient's care.
• Monitor the patient's vital signs, intake and output, daily weight, hydration, pulse oximetry, and respiratory status.

PATIENT TEACHING

Be sure to cover with patient and his family:
• the disorder and its diagnosis and treatment
• medications and potential adverse reactions
• when to notify the physician
• aerosol therapy
• chest physiotherapy
• signs and symptoms of infection
• potential complications
• how to contact the Cystic Fibrosis Foundation
• location and contact information for local support groups and services.

Hemophilia

DESCRIPTION

• *Hemophilia* is a hereditary blood disorder characterized by greatly prolonged coagulation time, which can cause abnormal bleeding.
• It results from deficiency of specific clotting factors.
• Hemophilia A (classic hemophilia) affects more than 80% of individuals with hemophilia and results from factor VIII deficiency.
• Hemophilia B (Christmas disease) affects 15% of individuals with hemophilia and results from factor IX deficiency.
• It's the most common X-linked recessive genetic disease.

- It occurs in about 1 in 10,000 live male births in the United States.
- It's incurable.

PATHOPHYSIOLOGY

- A low level or absence of the blood protein necessary for clotting causes disruption of the normal intrinsic coagulation cascade.
- This produces abnormal bleeding, which may be mild, moderate, or severe, depending on the degree of protein factor deficiency.
- After a platelet plug forms at a bleeding site, the lack of clotting factors impairs formation of a stable fibrin clot.
- Hemorrhage isn't always immediate; delayed bleeding is common.

CAUSES

- Acquired immunologic process
- Hemophilia A and B inherited as X-linked recessive traits
- Spontaneous mutation

ASSESSMENT FINDINGS

- Familial history of bleeding disorders
- Prolonged bleeding with circumcision or from umbilical cord
- Concomitant illness
- Pain and swelling in a weight-bearing joint, such as the hip, knee, or ankle
- With mild hemophilia or after minor trauma, lack of spontaneous bleeding
- Moderate hemophilia producing only occasional spontaneous bleeding episodes
- Severe hemophilia causing spontaneous bleeding
- Prolonged bleeding after surgery or trauma or joint pain in spontaneous bleeding into muscles or joints
- Signs of internal bleeding, such as abdominal, chest, or flank pain; episodes of hematuria or hematemesis; and tarry stools

- Activity or movement limitations and the need for assistive devices, such as splints, canes, or crutches
- Hematomas on extremities, torso, or both
- Joint swelling in episodes of bleeding into joints (hemarthrosis)
- Limited and painful joint range of motion (ROM) in episodes of bleeding into joints

TEST RESULTS

Hemophilia A

- Factor VIII assay is 0% to 25% of normal.
- Partial thromboplastin time is prolonged.
- Platelet count and function, bleeding time, and prothrombin time are normal.

Hemophilia B

- Factor IX assay is deficient.
- Baseline coagulation results are similar to those of hemophilia A, with normal factor VIII.

Hemophilia A or B

- Degree of factor deficiency defines severity.
  - In mild hemophilia, factor levels are 5% to 25% of normal.
  - In moderate hemophilia, factor levels are 1% to 5% of normal.
  - In severe hemophilia, factor levels are less than 1% of normal.

TREATMENT

- Measures to prevent episodes of bleeding, such as close supervision and environmental control
- Quick treatment to control bleeding episodes by increasing plasma levels of deficient clotting factors
- Diet consisting of foods high in vitamin K (such as dark green, leafy vegetables and soybeans)
- Activity guided by degree of factor deficiency
- Aminocaproic acid before dental work

Hemophilia A
- Cryoprecipitated antihemophilic factor (AHF), lyophilized AHF, or both
- Recombinant factor VIII
- Desmopressin

Hemophilia B
- Factor IX concentrate

KEY PATIENT OUTCOMES

The patient will:
- maintain hemodynamic stability
- have peripheral pulses that remain palpable and strong
- express feelings of increased comfort and decreased pain
- maintain ROM and joint mobility
- demonstrate adequate coping skills
- verbalize an understanding of the disease process and treatment regimen.

NURSING INTERVENTIONS

- Follow standard precautions.
- Provide emotional support and reassurance when indicated.

During bleeding episodes
- Apply pressure to the bleeding sites.
- Give the deficient clotting factor or plasma, as ordered, until bleeding stops.
- Apply cold compresses or ice bags, and elevate the injured part.
- To prevent recurrence of the bleeding, restrict activity for 48 hours after bleeding is under control.
- Control the pain with prescribed analgesics.
- Avoid giving I.M. injections.
- Avoid giving aspirin, aspirin-containing drugs, and over-the-counter anti-inflammatory agents.

During bleeding into a joint
- Immediately elevate the joint.

- To restore joint mobility, encourage active ROM exercises at least 48 hours after the bleeding is controlled; avoid passive ROM.
- Restrict weight bearing until the bleeding stops and the swelling subsides.
- Give the prescribed analgesics for pain.
- Apply ice packs and elastic bandages to alleviate pain.
- Monitor the patient's coagulation studies, adverse reactions to blood products, signs and symptoms of decreased tissue perfusion, vital signs, and bleeding from the skin, mucous membranes, and wounds.

PATIENT TEACHING

Be sure to cover with the patient and his family:
- the benefits of regular isometric exercises
- the use of appropriate protective measures while avoiding unnecessary restrictions that impair normal development
- the need to avoid contact sports
- first aid measures for an injury
- the need to notify the physician immediately with any injury
- signs and symptoms of internal bleeding
- the importance of avoiding aspirin, combination medications that contain aspirin, and over-the-counter anti-inflammatory agents (use acetaminophen instead)
- the importance of good dental care and the need to check with the physician before dental extractions or surgery
- the need to wear medical identification jewelry at all times
- how to administer blood factor components at home, if appropriate
- adverse reactions that can result from replacement factor procedures
- signs, symptoms, and treatment of anaphylaxis

- referral for new patients to a hemophilia treatment center for evaluation
- how to contact the National Hemophilia Foundation
- location and contact information for local support groups and services.

Otitis media

DESCRIPTION

- *Otitis media* is a bacterial infection that causes inflammation of the middle ear associated with fluid accumulation.
- It peaks between ages 6 and 24 months.
- It subsides after age 3.
- It occurs most commonly during the winter months.
- It can be suppurative or secretory.

PATHOPHYSIOLOGY

- Suppurative otitis media occurs when nasopharyngeal flora reflux through the eustachian tube and colonize in the middle ear. (See *Site of otitis media*, page 564.)
- Chronic suppurative otitis media results from inadequate treatment of suppurative otitis media, infections by resistant strains of bacteria, or, rarely, tuberculosis.
- Secretory otitis media, also known as *otitis media with effusion*, results from obstruction of the eustachian tube.
  - Buildup of negative pressure in the middle ear permits sterile serous fluid from blood vessels to pass through the membrane of the middle ear.
  - Effusion may be secondary to eustachian tube dysfunction from viral infection or allergy.
  - Effusion may follow barotraumas (pressure injury caused by inability to equalize pressures between the environment and the middle ear).
- It occurs during rapid aircraft descent in a person with an upper respiratory tract infection.
- Chronic secretory otitis media follows persistent eustachian tube dysfunction, possibly resulting from mechanical obstruction (adenoidal tissue overgrowth, tumors), edema (allergic rhinitis, chronic sinus infection), or inadequate treatment of acute suppurative otitis media.

CAUSES

- Bacteria
  - Gram-negative bacteria
  - *Haemophilus influenzae*
  - *Moraxella catarrhalis*
  - Staphylococci
  - *Streptococcus pneumoniae*
- Disruption of eustachian tube patency

Risk factors (suppurative)

- Respiratory tract infection
- Allergic reaction
- Nasotracheal intubation
- Positional changes
- Predisposing factors of suppurative otitis media
  - Wider, shorter, more horizontal eustachian tubes and increased lymphoid tissue in children
  - Anatomic anomalies

ASSESSMENT FINDINGS

Acute suppurative

- Severe, deep, throbbing pain (from pressure behind the tympanic membrane)
- Signs of upper respiratory tract infection (sneezing and coughing)
- Mild to very high fever
- Hearing loss (usually mild and conductive)
- Tinnitus
- Dizziness
- Nausea
- Vomiting

Site of otitis media

The common site of otitis media is shown here.

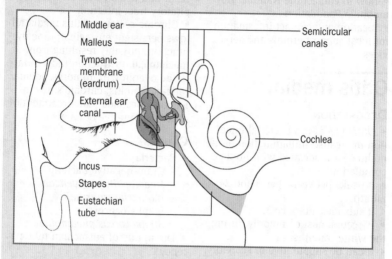

- Bulging of the tympanic membrane with erythema
- Purulent drainage in the ear canal, if the tympanic membrane ruptures
- Ruptured tympanic membrane accompanied by sudden stopping of pain
- Some patients asymptomatic

Acute secretory
- Possibly no symptoms in the first few months of life; irritability possibly the only indication of earache
- Severe conductive hearing loss; varying from 15 to 35 dB, depending on the thickness and amount of fluid in the middle ear cavity
- Sensation of fullness in the ear and popping, crackling, or clicking sounds on swallowing or with jaw movement
- Echo when speaking and vague feeling of top-heaviness due to the accumulation of fluid

- Ruptured tympanic membrane accompanied by sudden stopping of pain

Chronic
- Thickening and scarring of the tympanic membrane
- Decreased or absent tympanic membrane mobility
- Cholesteatoma (a cystlike mass in the middle ear)
- Painless purulent discharge
- Hearing loss
- History of ruptured tympanic membrane

Test results
Acute suppurative
- Otoscopy shows obscured or distorted bony landmarks of the tympanic membrane.
- Pneumatoscopy reveals decreased tympanic membrane mobility.
- Culture of ear drainage identifies the causative organism.

Acute secretory

• Otoscopy shows how bony landmarks appear more prominent because of tympanic membrane retraction.

• Clear or amber fluid appears behind the tympanic membrane.

• If hemorrhage has occurred, the membrane is blue-black.

Chronic

• Otoscopy shows thickening, scarring (sometimes), and decreasing mobility of the tympanic membrane.

• Pneumatoscopy reveals decreased or absent tympanic membrane movement.

TREATMENT

Acute suppurative

• Antibiotic therapy—ampicillin or amoxicillin (Amoxil)

• Myringotomy to treat severe, painful bulging of the tympanic membrane

• Single dose of ceftriaxone (Rocephin) effective against major pathogens (expensive and reserved for extremely sick infants)

• In recurring infection: antibiotics used with discretion; prevents the development of resistant strains of bacteria

Acute secretory

• Inflation of the eustachian tube using Valsalva's maneuver several times per day

• Nasopharyngeal decongestant therapy

• Possible myringotomy and aspiration of middle ear fluid followed by insertion of a polyethylene tube into the tympanic membrane for immediate and prolonged equalization of pressure

Chronic

• Broad-spectrum antibiotics, such as amoxicillin/clavulanate potassium (Augmentin) or cefuroxime (Ceftin)

• Elimination of eustachian tube obstruction

• Treatment of otitis externa

• Myringoplasty and tympanoplasty, which reconstructs middle ear structures when thickening and scarring is present

• Possibly, mastoidectomy

• Excision of cholesteatoma

KEY PATIENT OUTCOMES

The patient will:

• express feelings of increased comfort

• not exhibit signs or symptoms of infection

• verbalize an understanding of the disorder and treatment regimen

• regain hearing or develop compensatory mechanisms

• not experience injury or harm.

NURSING INTERVENTIONS

After tympanoplasty

• Reinforce dressings.

• Observe for excessive bleeding from the ear canal.

• Administer analgesics as needed.

With hearing loss

• Offer reassurance, when appropriate, that hearing loss caused by serious otitis media is temporary.

• Provide clear, concise explanations.

• Face the patient when speaking, and enunciate clearly and slowly.

• Allow time for the patient to grasp what was said.

• Provide a pencil and paper.

• Alert the staff to the patient's communication disorder.

After myringotomy

• Wash your hands before and after ear care.

• Place sterile cotton loosely in the patient's external ear, which absorbs drainage and prevents in-

fection. Change the cotton when damp. Avoid placing cotton or plugs deep in the ear canal.
• Give the prescribed analgesics.
• Give antiemetics after tympanoplasty, and reinforce dressings.
• Monitor the patient's pain level, response to treatment, and auditory acuity; monitor for excessive bleeding or discharge.

PATIENT TEACHING

Be sure to cover with the parents:
• proper instillation of ointment, drops, and ear wash, as ordered
• drug administration, dosage, and possible adverse effects
• the importance of taking antibiotics as prescribed
• adequate fluid intake
• correct instillation of nasopharyngeal decongestants
• use of fitted earplugs for swimming and bathing after myringotomy and tympanostomy tube insertion
• notification of the physician if the tube falls out and if patient experiences ear pain, fever, or pus-filled discharge
• recurrence prevention (Instruct the parents not to feed the patient when he's lying in a supine position and not to put him in his crib or bed with a bottle—doing so could cause reflux of nasopharyngeal flora.)

Respiratory syncytial virus infection

DESCRIPTION

• *Respiratory syncytial virus infection* is the leading cause of lower respiratory tract infection in infants and young children.
• It's the suspected cause of fatal respiratory diseases in infants.

• It almost exclusively affects infants (ages 1 to 6 months, peaking between ages 2 and 3 months) and young children, especially those in day-care settings.
• It may cause serious illness in patients with underlying cardiopulmonary disease.
• Its common characteristics include rhinorrhea, low-grade fever, tachypnea, shortness of breath, cyanosis, apneic episodes, and mild systemic symptoms accompanied by coughing and wheezing.
• It's also known as *RSV.*

PATHOPHYSIOLOGY

• Virus attaches to cells, eventually resulting in necrosis of the bronchiolar epithelium; in severe infection, peribronchiolar infiltrate of lymphocytes and mononuclear cells occurs.
• Intra-alveolar thickening and resultant fluid fill the alveolar spaces.
• Airway passages narrow on expiration, preventing air from leaving the lungs and causing progressive overinflation.

CAUSES

• Probably spread to infants and young children by school-age children, adolescents, and young adults with mild reinfections
• Reinfections common, typically producing milder symptoms than the primary infection
• Respiratory syncytial virus, a subgroup of myxoviruses resembling paramyxovirus
• Transmitted from person to person by respiratory secretions

ASSESSMENT FINDINGS

• Nasal congestion
• Nasal and pharyngeal inflammation
• Coughing
• Wheezing, rhonchi, and crackles
• Malaise
• Sore throat

- Earache
- Dyspnea
- Fever
- Otitis media
- Severe respiratory distress (nasal flaring, retraction, cyanosis, and tachypnea)

TEST RESULTS

- Cultures of nasal and pharyngeal secretions show RSV.
- Serum RSV antibody titers are elevated.
- Arterial blood gas values show hypoxemia and respiratory acidosis.
- In dehydration, blood urea nitrogen levels are elevated.

TREATMENT

- Respiratory support
- Adequate nutrition
- Avoidance of overhydration
- Rest periods when fatigued

KEY PATIENT OUTCOMES

The patient will:
- maintain a respiratory rate that supports adequate ventilation
- express or indicate feelings of increased comfort while maintaining adequate air exchange
- maintain adequate fluid volume.

NURSING INTERVENTIONS

- Institute contact isolation.
- Monitor respiratory status.
- Perform percussion, drainage, and suctions when necessary.
- Administer prescribed oxygen.
- Use a croup tent as needed.
- Place the patient in semi-Fowler's position (if he's able).
- Monitor fluid and electrolyte status.
- Promote rest periods and activity as tolerated.
- Offer diversional activities.

PATIENT TEACHING

Be sure to cover with the parents:

- the disorder, diagnosis, and treatment
- how the infection spreads
- drugs and possible adverse effects
- follow-up care.

Tracheoesophageal fistula and esophageal atresia

DESCRIPTION

- *Tracheoesophageal fistula* is a developmental anomaly characterized by an abnormal connection between the trachea and the esophagus; it usually accompanies esophageal atresia, in which the esophagus is closed off at some point.
- *Esophageal atresia* occurs in 1 of 1,500 to 3,000 live births; approximately one-third of these neonates are born prematurely.
- They both have numerous anatomic variations, most commonly esophageal atresia with fistula to the distal segment. (See *Types of tracheoesophageal anomalies,* page 568.)
- They're two of the most serious surgical emergencies in neonates and require immediate diagnosis and correction.

PATHOPHYSIOLOGY

- Tracheoesophageal fistula and esophageal atresia result from failure of the embryonic esophagus and trachea to develop and separate correctly.
- Respiratory system development begins at about day 26 of gestation; abnormal development of the septum (during this time) may lead to tracheoesophageal fistula.
- The most common abnormality is type C tracheoesophageal fistula with esophageal atresia, in which the upper section of the esophagus terminates in a blind pouch and the

Types of tracheoesophageal anomalies

Congenital malformations of the esophagus occur in 1 of 1,500 to 3,000 live births. The American Academy of Pediatrics classifies the anatomic variations of tracheoesophageal anomalies according to type.

Type A
Esophageal atresia without fistula (7.7%)

Type B
Esophageal atresia with tracheoesophageal fistula to the proximal segment (0.8%)

Type C
Esophageal atresia with fistula to the distal segment (86.5%)

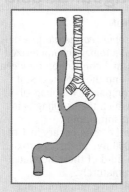 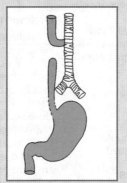 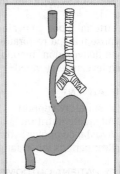

Type D
Esophageal atresia with fistula to both segments (0.7%)

Type E
Esophageal fistula without atresia (4.2%)

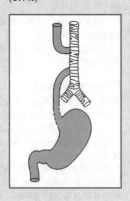 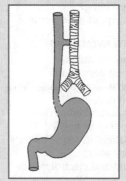

lower section ascends from the stomach and connects with the trachea by a short fistulous tract.
• In type A atresia, both esophageal segments are blind pouches and neither connects to the airway.

• In types B and D atresia, the upper portion of the esophagus opens into the trachea; infants with this anomaly may experience life-threatening aspiration of saliva or food.

• In type E (or H-type) tracheoe-sophageal fistula without atresia, the fistula may occur anywhere between the level of the cricoid cartilage and the midesophagus but is usually higher in the trachea than in the esophagus; such a fistula may be as small as a pinpoint.

CAUSES
• Embryonic developmental defect

ASSESSMENT FINDINGS
• Coughing and choking after eating
• Respiratory distress
• Drooling
• Tracheoesophageal fistula
  – Type B (proximal fistula) and Type D (fistula to both segments): immediate aspiration of saliva into the airway and bacterial pneumonitis
  – Type E (or H-type): repeated episodes of pneumonitis, pulmonary infection, and abdominal infection; choking followed by cyanosis
• Esophageal atresia
  – Type A: normal swallowing, excessive drooling, possible respiratory distress
  – Type C: seemingly normal swallowing followed shortly afterward by coughing, struggling, cyanosis, and lack of breathing

TEST RESULTS
• Chest X-rays may show a dilated, air-filled upper esophageal pouch, pneumonia in the right upper lobe, or bilateral pneumonitis; both pneumonia and pneumonitis suggest aspiration.
• Abdominal X-rays show gas in the bowel in a distal fistula (type C) but none in a proximal fistula (type B) or in atresia without fistula (type A).
• Cinefluorography may define the tip of the upper pouch and differentiate between overflow aspiration from a blind end (atresia) and aspiration from passage of liquids through a tracheoesophageal fistula.
• A size 6 or 8 French catheter passed through the nose meets an obstruction (esophageal atresia) about 4″ to 5″ (10 to 12.5 cm) distal to the nostrils; aspirate of gastric contents is less acidic than normal.

TREATMENT
• I.V. fluids
• Supine position with the head low to facilitate drainage or with the head elevated to prevent aspiration
• After surgery, placement of a suction catheter in the upper esophageal pouch to control secretions and prevent aspiration
• Antibiotics for superimposed infection
• Surgical correction: type and timing depend on the nature of the anomaly, the patient's general condition, and the presence of coexisting congenital defects
• In premature neonates who are poor surgical risks, correction of combined tracheoesophageal fistula and esophageal atresia occurring in two stages
  – Gastrostomy (for gastric decompression, prevention of reflux, and feeding) and closure of the fistula
  – 1 to 2 months later, anastomosis of the esophagus
• Correction of esophageal atresia alone requiring anastomosis of the proximal and distal esophageal segments in one or two stages; end-to-end anastomosis commonly producing postoperative stricture; end-to-side anastomosis less likely to do so
• If the esophageal ends are widely separated, possible colonic interposition (grafting a piece of the colon) or elongation of the proximal seg-

ment of the esophagus by bougien-
age

Key patient outcomes

The patient will:
• develop no respiratory complications
• remain hemodynamically stable
• express an understanding of the
disorder and its treatment (patient's
family).

Nursing interventions

• Monitor respiratory status, and
administer oxygen as needed.
• Perform pulmonary physiotherapy
and suctioning, as needed.
• Provide a humid environment.
• Administer antibiotics and parenteral fluids.
• Monitor intake and output.
• Maintain gastrostomy tube feedings.
• After surgery, monitor the chest
tubes and for signs of complications.
• Offer the parents support and
guidance in dealing with their infant's acute illness. Encourage them
to participate in care and to hold
and touch the infant as much as
possible to encourage bonding.
• Instruct the parents that X-rays
are required about 10 days after surgery, and again 1 and 3 months later, to evaluate the effectiveness of
surgical repair.

Patient teaching

Be sure to cover with the parents:
• the disorder, diagnosis, and treatment
• feeding procedures
• recognizing and reporting complications
• proper positioning.

III

Legal aspects of care

12 Standards of care 572

13 Ethical situations 591

12 Standards of care

To safeguard your practice, get to know the standards you're held to in the event of a legal issue.

Standard of care is a term used to specify what's reasonable under a certain set of circumstances. Standards are used to define certain aspects of a profession, such as the:

- focus of its pursuits
- beneficiaries of its service
- responsibilities of its practitioners.

In health care, the prevailing professional standard of care is defined as the level of care, skill, and treatment deemed acceptable and appropriate by similar health care providers. A standard is a yardstick against which effective care can be measured.

Sources of standards of care

The standards for patient care practice are derived from several sources:

- Agency for Healthcare Research and Quality (AHRQ) guidelines
- American Nurses Association (ANA) Standards of Clinical Nursing Practice
- Facility- and unit-specific policies and procedures
- Job descriptions
- The Joint Commission
- Patient Care Partnership
- State nurse practice acts and guidelines.

AGENCY FOR HEALTHCARE RESEARCH AND QUALITY GUIDELINES

Guidelines from the Agency for Healthcare Research and Quality (AHRQ)—formerly the Agency for Health Care Policy and Research—are a primary source of patient care standards for all health care practitioners.

The AHRQ supports research and provides evidence-based information related to health care. (See *Spotlight on the AHRQ.*) An Evidence-based Practice Centers program guides institutions in the United States and Canada to review scientific literature and produce reports that inform and help develop guidelines for nursing practice as well as identify areas of needed research. (See *Evidence-based Practice Centers.*)

The National Guideline Clearinghouse (NGC) is an initiative of the AHRQ that provides a public database of evidence-based practice guidelines to health care professionals or related professions such as health plan providers. The NGC's Web site (*www.guideline.gov*) supplies tools to obtain objective, specific information on available guidelines in an effort to promote their implementation and use.

AMERICAN NURSES ASSOCIATION STANDARDS OF CLINICAL NURSING PRACTICE

For professional nursing, the *Standards of Clinical Nursing Practice* outlines the expectancy of the comprehensive professional role within which all nurses must practice. Nursing practice standards ensure that the quality of nursing care, documentation, consistency, accountability, and professional credibility are upheld.

The ANA first published the *Standards of Nursing Practice* in 1973. Since then, specialty nursing organizations have developed their own standards of practice in various areas of nursing, such as emergency, perioperative, oncologic, and critical care nursing. Some of these standards were developed and published in collaboration with the ANA.

In 1991, the *Standards of Nursing Practice* was revised with participation from state nurses' associations and specialty nursing organizations. The revised publication is a comprehensive outline of expectations for all nurses. *Standards of Clinical Nursing Practice* is composed of authoritative statements describing a level of care or performance common to the nursing profession. It sets a standard by which the quality of nursing practice can be judged. (See *ANA standards of nursing practice,* pages 574.)

FACILITY- AND UNIT-SPECIFIC POLICIES AND PROCEDURES

The policies and procedures in your facility are also used to establish standards of care.

Policies and procedures are commonly used in litigation claims. Too often, practitioners are informed of policies and procedures but don't take time to examine and understand them. Deviating from facility policies and procedures suggests failure to meet the facility's standards of care.

Spotlight on the AHRQ

The Agency for Healthcare Research and Quality (AHRQ) is a federal agency that sponsors and conducts research on major areas of health care, including:
· quality improvement and patient safety
· outcomes and effectiveness of care
· clinical practice and technology assessment
· health care organization and delivery systems
· health care costs and sources of payment.

Evidence-based Practice Centers

These institutions currently participate in the Evidence-based Practice Centers (EPC) program and are funded by the Agency for Healthcare Research and Quality.
· Blue Cross and Blue Shield Association, Chicago
· Duke University, Durham, NC
· ECRI, Plymouth Meeting, PA
· John Hopkins University, Baltimore
· McMaster University, Ontario, Canada
· Oregon Health & Science University, Portland
· RTI International—University of North Carolina at Chapel Hill, NC
· Southern California Evidence-based Practice Center—RAND, Santa Monica, CA
· Stanford University, Stanford, CA
· Tufts–New England Medical Center, Boston, MA
· University of Alberta, Alberta, Canada
· University of California, San Francisco, CA
· University of Minnesota, Minneapolis
· University of Ottawa, Canada

ANA standards of nursing practice

The American Nurses Association (ANA) developed these standards (last revised in 2003) to provide registered nurses with guidelines for determining quality nursing care. The courts, hospitals, nurses, and patients may refer to these standards. The standards of nursing practice are divided into the "standards of practice," which identify the care that's provided to recipients of nursing services, and the "standards of professional performance," which explain the level of behavior expected in professional role activities. This doesn't present the standards that are specific to only advanced practice nurses.

Standards of Practice

Standard 1: Assessment
The nurse collects patient health data.

Standard 2: Diagnosis
The nurse analyzes the assessment data in determining the diagnosis.

Standard 3: Outcomes identification
The nurse identifies expected outcomes individualized to the patient.

Standard 4: Planning
The nurse develops a care plan that prescribes interventions to attain expected outcomes.

Standard 5: Implementation
The nurse implements the plan.

Standard 5a: Coordination of care
The nurse coordinates care delivery.

Standard 5b: Health teaching and health promotion
The nurse promotes health and a safe environment.

Standard 6: Evaluation
The nurse evaluates the patient's progress toward attainment of outcomes.

Standards of professional performance

Standard 7: Quality of practice
The nurse systematically enhances the quality and effectiveness of nursing practice.

Standard 8: Education
The nurse acquires current knowledge and competency in nursing practices.

Standard 9: Professional practice evaluation
The nurse evaluates her own nursing practice in relation to professional practice standards and relevant statutes and regulations.

Standard 10: Collegiality
The nurse interacts with and contributes to the professional development of peers and colleagues.

Standard 11: Collaboration
The nurse collaborates with the patient, family, and others in providing patient care.

Standard 12: Ethics
The nurse integrates ethics in all areas of practice.

Standard 13: Research
The nurse uses research findings in practice.

Standard 14: Resource utilization
The nurse considers factors related to safety, effectiveness, cost, and impact in planning and delivering patient care.

Standard 15: Leadership
The nurse shows leadership in the practice setting and in the profession.

Adapted and summarized with permission from American Nurses Association, *Nursing: Scope and Standard of Practice*, @0024 Nursebooks.org, Silver Spring, MD

Job descriptions

Job descriptions are also used to set standards of care.

How does your employer define the health care team's roles and relationships? Depending on the practice setting—such as a hospital, home, or extended care facility— your role may vary.

To protect patients and staff members, firm practice guidelines for all personnel are needed to make sure that job descriptions are accurate. If health care employees provide care duties outside of their formal job descriptions and a patient incurs harm as a result of this care, the facility's legal counsel or an insurance company could win a judgment against those employees to recover some of the losses incurred.

The Joint Commission

The Joint Commission is a private, nongovernmental agency that's responsible for evaluating and accrediting more than 17,000 health care organizations in the United States, such as hospitals, nursing homes, health care networks, home health care providers, and long-term care facilities. It has also developed nursing standards to be used in hospital audit systems. In some states, The Joint Commission's standards have been incorporated into law, resulting in broadly applicable standards of patient care. (See *The Joint Commission's standards,* pages 576 to 578.) In addition, state nursing associations and specialty nursing organizations actively work with hospital nursing administrators for adoption of standards.

The Joint Commission continually creates and publishes new standards and goals to improve patient safety. Hospitals and other health care organizations must comply with these standards to receive the Joint Commission's accreditation. The "National Patient Safety Goals" were established to create an environment of safety and focus on the prevention of health care errors. (See *The Joint Commission's National Patient Safety Goals,* pages 579 and 580.)

Patient Care Partnership

The Patient Care Partnership (formerly the Patient's Bill of Rights) is another recognized basis for standards of care. The American Hospital Association first sanctioned a Patient's Bill of Rights in 1973 to establish standards of treatment that each patient can expect. The Patient Care Partnership, its current title, communicates patients' rights in an easy-to-understand format and in several languages. (See *Patient Care Partnership,* page 581.)

State nurse practice acts and guidelines

Nurse practice acts and guidelines set by each state are also used to establish standards of care for nurses.

State nurse practice acts are laws that define which treatments, actions, and functions can be performed or delegated in each state. (See *Nurse practice acts,* page 582.)

The range of a nurse's legal responsibilities may vary from state to state. It's each nurse's professional responsibility to understand her scope of practice. If a nurse is licensed in more than one state, she needs to make sure that she's familiar with the specific guidelines of the state in which she's practicing. (See *State boards of nursing,* pages 583 to 586.)

(Text continues on page 580.)

The Joint Commission's standards

These standards are based on the *Comprehensive Accreditation Manual for Hospitals* published by The Joint Commission. They are used by The Joint Commission to evaluate and monitor the clinical and organizational performance of health care facilities.

Standards for patient assessment
• Patients should receive nursing care based on a documented assessment of their needs.

Structure supporting the assessment of patients
• The activities that comprise the patient assessment function should be defined in writing.
• A registered nurse (RN) should assess the patient's need for nursing care in all settings in which nursing care is to be provided.

Standards for planning and providing care
• The care, treatment, and rehabilitation planning process should ensure that care is appropriate to the patient's specific needs and the severity level of his disease, condition, impairment, or disability.
• Qualified individuals must plan and provide care, treatment, and rehabilitation in a collaborative and disciplined manner, as appropriate to the patient.

Care decisions
• The information generated through the analysis of assessment data should be used to identify and prioritize the patient's needs for care.
• Care decisions should be based on the identified patient needs and on care priorities.

Patient's rights
• The organization should have a functioning process to address ethical issues.
• The process should be based on a framework that recognizes the interdependence of patient care and organizational ethical issues.

• The process should include mechanisms that address the patient's involvement in all aspects of care.

Standards for human resources planning
• The organization's leaders should define for their respective areas the qualifications and job expectations of the staff and develop a system to evaluate how well the expectations are met.
• The organization should provide an adequate number of staff members whose qualifications are commensurate with defined job responsibilities and applicable licensure, law, and regulation and certification.
• Processes should be designed to ensure that the competence of all staff members is assessed, maintained, demonstrated, and improved on an ongoing basis.
• The organization should assess each individual's ability to achieve job expectations as stated in his or her job description.

Initial assessment
• An initial assessment of each patient's physical, psychological, and social status should be performed to determine the need for care, the type of care to be provided, and the need for further assessment.
• The need for an assessment of the patient's nutritional status should be determined.
• The need for a discharge planning assessment of the patient should be determined.
• The initial assessment of each patient admitted should be conducted within a certain time frame preceding or following admission, as specified by policy.
• The patient's history and physical examination, nursing care assessment, and other screening assessments should be completed within the first 24 hours of admission as an inpatient.

The Joint Commission's standards *(continued)*

Reassessment
· Each patient should be reassessed periodically.
· The patient should be reassessed when a significant change occurs in his condition.

Standards for organizational planning
· The leadership should provide for organizational planning.
· Planning should include setting a mission, a vision, and values for the organization and providing strategic, operational, programmatic, and other plans and policies to achieve the mission and vision.
· When the larger organization is composed of many subunits, there should be a mechanism for leaders of individual units to participate in policy decisions affecting their organization.

Patient care services
· The plan for the provision of patient care should respond to identified patient needs and be consistent with the organization's mission.
· The organization's leaders and, as appropriate, community leaders and heads of other organizations should collaborate to design services.
· The design of patient care services to be provided throughout the organization should be appropriate to the scope and level of care required by the patients served.
· The leaders should collaborate with representatives from the appropriate disciplines and services to develop an annual operating budget and, at least as required by applicable law and regulation, a long-term capital expenditure plan, including a strategy to monitor the plan's implementation.
· The budget review process should include consideration of the appropriateness of the organization's plan for providing care to meet patient needs.
· The leaders and other representatives of the organization should participate, as appropriate, in the organization's decision-making structure and processes.
· The organization's leaders should develop programs to promote the recruitment, retention, development, and continuing education of all staff members. These programs should include mechanisms for promoting the job-related educational and advancement goals of staff members.

Directing departments
· Each department of the organization should have effective leadership. Department directors are responsible, either personally or through delegation, for:
– developing and implementing policies and procedures that guide and support the provision of services
– recommending a sufficient number of qualified and competent persons to provide care, including treatment
– continuously assessing and improving the performance of care and services provided
– maintaining quality control programs as appropriate
– orienting and providing inservice training and continuing education of all persons in the department.

Integrating services
· Patient care services must be appropriately integrated throughout the organization. The leaders should individually and jointly develop and participate in systematic and effective mechanisms for:
– fostering communication among individuals and components of the organization and coordinating internal activities
– communicating with the leaders of any health care delivery organization that's corporately or functionally related to the organization seeking accreditation.

Improving performance
· The organization's leaders should set expectations, develop plans, and manage processes to assess, im-

(continued)

The Joint Commission's standards *(continued)*

prove, and maintain the quality of the organization's governance, management, clinical, and support activities.

Standards for information management planning

• Information management processes should be planned and designed to meet the health care organization's internal and external information needs.
• The information management processes within and among departments, the medical staff, the administration, and the governing body, and with outside services and agencies, should be appropriate for the organization's size and complexity.
• Based on the organization's information needs, appropriate staff members should participate in assessing, selecting, and integrating health care information technology and, as appropriate, use efficient interactive information management systems for clinical and organizational information.
• The information management function must provide for information confidentiality, security, and integrity.
• The organization should determine how data and information could be retrieved easily and on a timely basis without compromising security and confidentiality.

Patient information

• The information management function should provide for the definition, capture, analysis, transformation, transmission, and reporting of individual patient information related to the process and outcome of the patient's care.
• The medical record must contain sufficient information to identify the patient, support the diagnosis, justify the treatment, document the course and results accurately, and facilitate continuity of care among health care providers. Each medical record should contain at least the following:
– the diagnosis or diagnostic impression

– diagnostic and therapeutic orders, if any
– all diagnostic and therapeutic procedures and tests performed and the results
– goals of treatment plan
– progress notes made by authorized individuals
– all necessary reassessments
– the response to the care provided.
• At discharge, a summary should contain the reason for hospitalization, any significant findings, the procedures performed and treatment rendered, the patient's condition on discharge, and discharge instructions given to the patient and family.

Standards for nursing

• A nurse-executive who's an RN, qualified by advanced education and management experience, should direct nursing services.

The nurse-executive

• If the organization's structure is decentralized, an identified nurse leader at the executive level should provide authority and accountability for, and coordination of, the nurse-executive functions.
• The nurse-executive has the authority and responsibility for establishing standards of nursing practice.
• The nurse-executive and other nursing leaders should participate with leaders from the governing body, management, medical staff, and clinical areas in planning, promoting, and conducting organization-wide performance improvement activities.

Policies and procedures

• Nursing policies and procedures, nursing standards of patient care, and standards of nursing practice must be created in a set sequence.
• Policies, procedures, and standards should be developed in writing by the nurse-executive, RNs, and designated nursing staff members. Documents should be approved by the nurse-executive or a designee.

Adapted with permission from The Joint Commission. *EC Standards*. Oakbrook Terrace, Ill.: The Joint Commission.

The Joint Commission's National Patient Safety Goals

The 2007 National Patient Safety Goals, published by The Joint Commission, were established to help accredited organizations address specific areas of concern in regard to patient safety. These goals cover the hospital setting only.

· Improve the accuracy of patient identification by:
  – using at least two patient identifiers (not the patient's room number or location) whenever taking blood samples or other specimens for testing, or administering medications or blood products
  – labeling the sample or specimen containers in the presence of the patient

· Improve the effectiveness of communication among caregivers by:
  – utilizing a "read-back" system to verify verbal or telephone orders or reports of critical test results after writing the information down; confirmation of the information is supplied by the person giving the order or results
  – standardizing abbreviations, acronyms, symbols, and dose designations used throughout the facility
  – establishing a do-not-use list and applying it to all medication-related orders and documents
  – assessing and improving the timeliness of reporting critical test results values to appropriate licensed caregivers
  – establishing a "handoff" system to communicate patient information to appropriate personnel, allowing time for questions and verification of information, and limiting interruptions during this process

· Improve the safety of medication use by:
  – standardizing and limiting the number of drug concentrations available to the facility
  – preventing medication interchange by establishing a list of look-alike

and sound-alike medications used by the facility
  – labeling all medications, containers or solutions on and off the sterile field with the medication name, strength, amount, and expiration date or time; having two qualified people verify the labels verbally and visually when the person administering the medication did not prepare the medication
  – discarding non-labeled medications, containers, or solutions
  – keeping the original containers for medications or solutions to use as reference until the procedure is complete
  – discarding all medications and solutions when the procedure is complete.

· Reduce the risk of health care–associated infections by:
  – complying with current Centers for Disease Control and Prevention hand hygiene guidelines
  – reporting all identified deaths or major permanent losses of function caused by health care–associated infection as a sentinel event.

· Accurately and completely reconcile medications across the continuum of care by:
  – establishing a process for comparing a patient's current medications on admission to those ordered while in a facility
  – providing a list of patient's medications to the patient upon discharge, or to a transferring facility, practitioner or level of care within or outside the facility.

· Reduce the risk of patient harm resulting from falls by:
  – establishing and implementing a fall reduction program that includes staff education, patient and family education, interventions to reduce patient risk, and evaluation of the program.

· Encourage patients' active involvement in their own care as a patient

(continued)

■

The Joint Commission's National Patient Safety Goals
(continued)

safety strategy by:
– educating and encouraging patients and families to report concerns regarding care, treatments, services, and patient safety issues.
• The organization identifies safety risks inherent in its patient population by:
– assessing the psychiatric patient's risk of suicide, identifying appropriate safety needs, and supplying crisis information to the patient and family.

Universal protocol
The universal protocol was developed with the intention of preventing wrong site, wrong procedure, wrong person surgery. It contains these principles.
• Involvement and communication among all members of the surgical team
• Involvement of the patient to the highest possible extent
• Consistent use of a standardized system using a universal protocol
• Flexibility of protocol possible when needed for specific patient situations
• Required site marking with cases involving right or left, multiple digits, or levels (such as the spine)
• The universal protocol should adapt for all invasive procedures, including

those performed outside of the operating room
The universal protocol contains these steps.

Preoperative verification process
• Gather and verify information involved with performing a procedure, maintain communication of information through all settings and interventions occurring during the preoperative period, and have a "time out" immediately before initiating the procedure.

Marking the operative site
• When a procedure involves a specific site, digit, or level, the intended site must be marked in such a way as to be visible after the patient has been prepared for the procedure; the method of marking should be consistent throughout the facility.

"Time out" immediately before the procedure
• A designated team member initiates a communication session among all members of the surgical team to correctly identify the patient, procedure site, procedure, patient position, implants or special equipment for procedure as well as resolve any questions or concerns prior to staring the procedure.

Litigation

Litigation is a lawsuit that's contested in court to enforce a right or pursue a resolution.

Negligence, which is now recognized as a form of malpractice, is defined as failure to meet a standard of care—in other words, failure to do what another reasonably prudent health care provider would do in similar circumstances. Examples of legal liability specifically related to

patient care usually involve claims of negligence, such as:
• failure to prevent
• failure to treat
• failure to heal.

Malpractice is a health care professional's wrongful conduct, improper discharge of professional duties, or failure to meet standards of care that result in harm to another person. Practitioners are being sued individually for malpractice with increasing frequency. Most malpractice litigation comes as a result of

Patient Care Partnership

The American Hospital Association established and created a Patient Care Partnership, a brochure informing patients of their rights and responsibilities on admission to a medical facility. In addition to English, the brochure is available in Spanish, Russian, Vietnamese, Tagolog, Arabic, and Chinese. Upon admission to a medical facility, a patient has the right to:

• high-quality patient care
• know the identity of doctors, nurses, students, and others involved in care
• a clean, safe environment
• know about unexpected events that occur and how they affect care
• involvement in care
• know about his medical condition and appropriate treatment choices in order to make an informed decision regarding a treatment plan

• be provided information about health history and insurance coverage to help decision making regarding care
• understand who has the authority to make decisions on his behalf as well as assistance from counselors, chaplains, and others in making difficult decisions
• privacy protection
• confidentiality regarding health care information
• preparation for him and his family when he leaves the hospital
• information or training regarding appropriate care outside the hospital
• help with his bill and with filing insurance claims
• information and assistance regarding health care coverage and billing for patients without insurance.

claims that a health care provider failed to:

• provide physical protection
• monitor or assess
• promptly respond
• properly administer a medication.

Practitioners in critical care, emergency, trauma, and obstetrics and those who practice as specialists are most vulnerable.

Four criteria must be verified to determine whether a medical malpractice claim is merited.

• A duty must be established with the patient. This means that the practitioner accepts accountability for the care and treatment of the patient.
• A breach of duty or standard of care by the practitioner must be determined to evaluate whether there has been an act of negligence or a breach of duty that resulted in harm to the patient.
• Proximate cause or causal connection must be established between the breach of duty or standard of care and the damages or injuries to the patient. The patient must prove that damages were caused directly by the practitioner's negligence and that the damages were foreseeable. In other words, were the damages a direct result of the negligence?
• Damages, or injuries, to the patient must be presented as evidence as a result of the alleged negligence. These damages can be physical (disfigurement or pain and suffering), mental (mental anguish), or financial (past, present, or future medical expenses).

If the patient-plaintiff can establish these four components, malpractice litigation is merited.

AVOIDING LITIGATION

The key to reducing your risk of involvement in malpractice litigation is prevention. However, even if you provide optimum care to every patient, there's no guarantee that your actions will never be called into question in a litigation case. If that

Nurse practice acts

A nurse should be aware of the nurse practice act for each state in which she practices.

State statutes

• Each state has statutes, or nurse practice acts, that define the levels of nursing (for example, advanced practice nurse [nurse practitioner, clinical nurse specialist, certified nurse midwife, certified nurse anesthetist], registered nurse, licensed practical nurse, and nursing assistant); they're the most important laws governing nurses and nursing practice.

– Most statutes set licensure requirements for each level of nursing.
– They may prescribe minimum educational qualifications for licensure.

• Regulatory boards created by the nurse practice acts govern nursing practice in the state.

• Nurse practice acts may provide for a board of nursing accreditation and approval of educational programs in the state.

Disciplinary actions

• The state board of nursing may take action against a nurse who violates the nurse practice act or the licensing board's regulations.

– A nurse can be disciplined for habitual substance abuse affecting the ability to practice, fraud or deceit in obtaining a nursing license, incompetence, criminal felony conviction, and unprofessional conduct.

– Other actions or conditions that would inhibit the nurse's safe and effective nursing practice also are grounds for discipline.

• A licensed nurse has a limited property right to her license.

– The state must follow specific procedures to determine whether a nurse's license should be revoked to protect public safety.

– The licensee must be notified of the complaint, must have an opportunity to respond to the complaint and present evidence, and must be allowed to have a hearing before an impartial panel and a process to appeal the panel's decision.

Possible sanctions

• The nurse's license may be revoked.

• The license may be suspended for a predetermined time.

• The license may be suspended for an undetermined time, and the nurse may reapply after completing a course of study or treatment.

• Conditions may be placed on the license to limit the nurse's practice.

• The nurse may voluntarily surrender the license or enter into a consensual agreement with the nursing board, agreeing to limitations on the license or supervision of practice for a time.

• The nurse may receive a disciplinary warning or reprimand.

happens, you must be aware of how you're protected.

Many practitioners practice under the perception that they're protected by their facility's or employer's insurance policy. In most legal claims, your interests and the interests of your employer are comparable. However, the insurance company that provides your employer's coverage may be more allegiant to the employer than to you. In addition, the employer's insurance may not cover you if your performance fell outside of your job description or if you didn't follow written policy and procedure.

Practicing without your own malpractice insurance is risky. Malpractice insurance doesn't keep you from getting sued, but it may lift most of the financial burden and fear of a lawsuit off your shoulders. (See *Choosing liability insurance,* pages 587 and 588.)

(Text continues on page 588.)

State boards of nursing

Alabama Board of Nursing
RSA Plaza, Suite 250
770 Washington Ave.
Montgomery, AL 36104
Phone: (334) 242-4060
Web site: www.abn.state.al.us/

Alaska Board of Nursing
Division of Occupational Licensing
  Department of Community & Econo-
  mic Development
Robert B. Atwood Building
550 W. 7th Ave., Suite 1500
Anchorage, AK 99501-3567
Phone: (907) 269-8161
Web site: www.dced.state.ak.us/occ/
pnur.htm

American Samoa Health Services
Regulatory Board
LBJ Tropical Medical Center
Pago Pago, AS 96799
Phone: (684) 633-1222

Arizona State Board of Nursing
4747 N. 7th St., Suite 200
Phoenix, AZ 85014
Phone: (602) 889-5150
Web site: www.azbn.gov

Arkansas State Board of Nursing
University Tower Building
1123 S. University, Suite 800
Little Rock, AR 72204-1619
Phone: (501) 686-2700
Web site: www.arsbn.org

California Board of Registered Nursing
1625 N. Market Blvd., Suite N217
Sacramento, CA 95834
Phone: (916) 322-3350
Web site: www.rn.ca.gov/

California Board of Vocational Nursing
  and Psychiatric Technicians
2535 Capitol Oaks Dr., Suite 205
Sacramento, CA 95833
Phone: (916) 263-7800
Web site: www.bvnpt.ca.gov/

Colorado Board of Nursing
1560 Broadway, Suite 1350
Denver, CO 80202
Phone: (303) 894-2430
Web site: www.dora.state.co.us/
  nursing/

Connecticut Board of Examiners for
  Nursing
Department of Public Health
410 Capitol Ave.
P.O. Box 340308
Hartford, CT 06134-0308
Phone: (860) 509-8000
Web site: www.state.ct.us/dph

Delaware Board of Nursing
Cannon Building, Suite 203
861 Silver Lake Blvd.
Dover, DE 19904
Phone: (302) 744-4515
Web site: www.professionallicensing.
  state.de.us/boards/nursing/index.
  shtml

District of Columbia Board of Nursing
Department of Health
717 14th St. N.W., Suite 600
Washington, DC 20005
Phone: (877) 672-2174
Web site: www.dchealth.dc.gov/

Florida Board of Nursing
4052 Bald Cypress Way
BIN C00
Tallahassee, FL 32399-3250
Phone: (850) 245-4125
Web site: www.doh.state.fl.us/mqa/

Georgia Board of Nursing
237 Coliseum Dr.
Macon, GA 31217-3858
Phone: (478) 207-1640
Web site: www.sos.state.ga.us/plb/rn

Guam Board of Nurse Examiners
P.O. Box 2816
Hagatna, GU 96932
Phone: (671) 735-7406

Hawaii Board of Nursing
King Kalakaua Building
335 Merchant St., 3rd Floor
Honolulu, HI 96813
Phone: (808) 586-3000
Web site: www.hawaii.gov/dcca/areas/
  pvl/boards/nursing

(continued)

State boards of nursing (continued)

Idaho Board of Nursing
280 N. 8th St., Suite 210
P.O. Box 83720
Boise, ID 83720-0061
Phone: (208) 334-3110
Web site: www2.state.id.is/ibn/
ibnhome.htm

Illinois Department of Professional
Regulation
James R. Thompson Center
100 W. Randolph, Suite 9-300
Chicago, IL 60601
Phone: (312) 814-2715
Web site: www.dpr.state.il.us/

Indiana State Board of Nursing
Professional Licensing Agency
402 W. Washington St., Room W072
Indianapolis, IN 46204
Phone: (317) 234-2043
Web site: www.in.gov/pla/

Iowa Board of Nursing
River Point Business Park
400 S.W. 8th St., Suite B
Des Moines, IA 50309-4685
Phone: (515) 281-3255
Web site: www.state.ia.us/
government/nursing/

Kansas State Board of Nursing
Landon State Office Building
900 S.W. Jackson, Suite 1051
Topeka, KS 66612-1230
Phone: (785) 296-4929
Web site: www.ksbn.org

Kentucky Board of Nursing
312 Whittington Pkwy., Suite 300
Louisville, KY 40222
Phone: (502) 429-3300
Web site: www.kbn.ky.gov

Louisiana State Board of Nursing
5207 Essen Lane, Suite 6
Baton Rouge, LA 70809
Phone: (225) 763-3570
Web site: www.lsbn.state.la.us/

Maine State Board of Nursing
158 State House Station
Augusta, ME 04333
Phone: (207) 287-1133
Web site: www.maine.gov/
boardofnursing

Maryland Board of Nursing
4140 Patterson Ave.
Baltimore, MD 21215
Phone: (410) 585-1900
Web site: www.mbon.org

Massachusetts Board of Registration
in Nursing
Commonwealth of Massachusetts
239 Causeway St., 2nd Floor
Boston, MA 02114
Phone: (617) 973-0800
Web site: www.mass.gov/dpl/boards/
RN/

Michigan DCH/Bureau of Health
Professions
Ottawa Towers N.
611 W. Ottawa, 1st Floor
Lansing, MI 48933
Phone: (517) 335-0918
Web site: www.michigan.gov/
healthlicense

Minnesota Board of Nursing
2829 University Ave. S.E.
Minneapolis, MN 55414
Phone: (612) 617-2270
Web site: ww.nursingboard.state.mn.
us/

Mississippi Board of Nursing
1935 Lakeland Dr., Suite B
Jackson, MS 39216-5014
Phone: (601) 987-4188
Web site: www.msbn.state.ms.us/

Missouri State Board of Nursing
3605 Missouri Blvd.
P.O. Box 656
Jefferson City, MO 65102-0656
Phone: (573) 751-0681
Web site: www.pr.mo.gov/nursing.asp

Montana State Board of Nursing
301 South Park
P.O. Box 200513
Helena, MT 59620-0513
Phone: (406) 841-2340
Web site: www.discoveringmontana.
com/dli/bsd/license/bsd_boards/
nur_board/board_page.asp

State boards of nursing *(continued)*

Nebraska Health and Human Services
  Department of Regulation and
  Licensure
Nursing and Nursing Support
301 Centennial Mall S.
Lincoln, NE 68509-4986
Phone: (402) 471-4376
Web site: *www.hhs.state.ne.us/crl/
nursing/nursingindex.htm*

Nevada State Board of Nursing
5011 Meadowwood Mall Way #201
Reno, NV 89502-6547
Phone: (702) 688-2620
Web site: *www.nursingboard.state.nv.
  us/*

New Hampshire Board of Nursing
21 S. Fruit St., Suite 16
Concord, NH 03301-2341
Phone: (603) 271-2323
Web site: *www.state.nh.us/nursing/*

New Jersey Board of Nursing
124 Halsey St., 6th Floor
P.O. Box 45010
Newark, NJ 07101
Phone: (973) 504-640
Web site: *www.state.nj.us/lps/ca/
  medical/nursing.htm*

New Mexico Board of Nursing
6301 Indian School Rd. N.E.,
Suite 710
Albuquerque, NM 87109
Phone: (505) 841-8340
Web site: *www.bon.state.nm.us/
  index/html*

New York State Board of Nursing
Education Building
89 Washington Ave.
2nd Floor West Wing
Albany, NY 12234
Phone: (518) 474-3817, ext. 120
Web site: *www.nysed.gov/prof/nurse.
  htm*

North Carolina Board of Nursing
3724 National Dr., Suite 201
Raleigh, NC 27602
Phone: (919) 782-3211
Web site: *www.ncbon.com*

North Dakota Board of Nursing
919 S. 7th St., Suite 504
Bismarck, ND 58504
Phone: (701) 328-9777
Web site: *www.ndbon.org*

Commonwealth Board of Nurse
  Examiners (Northern Mariana
  Islands)
P.O. Box 501458
Saipan, MP 96950
Phone: (670) 664-4812

Ohio Board of Nursing
77 South High St., Suite 400
Columbus, OH 43215-3413
Phone: (614) 466-3947
Web site: *www.nursing.ohio.gov*

Oklahoma Board of Nursing
2915 N. Classen Blvd., Suite 524
Oklahoma City, OK 73106
Phone: (405) 962-1800
Web site: *www.youroklahoma.com/
nursing*

Oregon State Board of Nursing
800 Oregon St. N.E., Suite 465
Portland, OR 97232
Phone: (971) 673-0685
Web site: *www.osbn.state.or.us*

Pennsylvania State Board of Nursing
P.O. Box 2649
Harrisburg, PA 17105-2649
Phone: (717) 783-7142
Web site: *www.dos.state.pa.us/bpoa/
cwp/view.asp?a=1004&q=432869*

Commonwealth of Puerto Rico
Board of Nurse Examiners
800 Roberto H. Todd Ave.
Room 202, Stop 18
Santurce, PR 00908
Phone: (787) 725-7506

Rhode Island Board of Nurse Registration and Nursing Education
105 Cannon Building
3 Capitol Hill
Providence, RI 02908
Phone: (401) 222-5700
Web site: *www.health.ri.gov/*

(continued)

State boards of nursing *(continued)*

South Carolina State Board of Nursing
P.O. Box 12367
Columbia, SC 29211
Phone: (803) 896-4550
Web site: *www.llr.state.sc.us/doh/ nursing*

South Dakota Board of Nursing
4305 S. Louise Ave., Suite 201
Sioux Falls, SD 57106-3124
Phone: (605) 362-2760
Web site: *www.state.sd.us/doh/ nursing/*

Tennessee State Board of Nursing
227 French Landing, Suite 300
Heritage Place Metrocenter
Nashville, TN 37243
Phone: (615) 532-5166
Web site: *www.tennessee.gov/health*

Texas Board of Nurse Examiners
333 Guadalupe St., Suite 3-460
Austin, TX 78701
Phone: (512) 305-7400
Web site: *www.bne.state.tx.us*

Utah State Board of Nursing
Heber M. Wells Building, 4th Floor
160 East 300 S.
Salt Lake City, UT 84111
Phone: (801) 530-6628
Web site: *www.dopl.utah.gov/ licensing/nurse.html*

Vermont State Board of Nursing
Heritage Building
81 River St.
Montpelier, VT 05609-1106
Phone: (802) 828-2396
Web site: *www.vtprofessionals.org/ opr1/nurses*

Virgin Islands Board of Nurse
  Licensure
P.O. Box 4247
St. Thomas, VI 00803
Phone: (340) 776-7397

Virginia Board of Nursing
6603 W. Broad St., 5th Floor
Richmond, VA 23230-1712
Phone: (804) 662-1712
Web site: *www.dhp.virginia.gov/ nursing/*

Washington State Nursing Care
  Quality Assurance Commission
Department of Health
HPQA #6
310 Israel Rd. S.E.
Tumwater, WA 98501-7864
Phone: (360) 236-4700
Web site: www.fortress.wa.gov/doh/ hpqa1/hps6/Nursing/default.htm

West Virginia State Board of Examin-
  ers for Licensed Practical Nurses
101 Dee Dr.
Charleston, WV 25311
Phone: (304) 558-3572
Web site: *www.lpnboard.state.wv.us*

West Virginia Board of Examiners for
  Registered Professional Nurses
101 Dee Dr.
Charleston, WV 25311
Phone: (304) 558-3596
Web site: *www.wvrnboard.com/*

Wisconsin Department of Regulation
  and Licensing
1400 E. Washington Ave., Room 173
Madison, WI 53708
Phone: (608) 266-0145
Web site: *www.drl.state.wi.us*

Wyoming State Board of Nursing
1810 Pioneer Ave.
Cheyenne, WY 82001
Phone: (307) 777-7601
Web site: www.nursing.state.wy.us

Choosing liability insurance

To find professional liability coverage that fits your needs, compare the coverage of a number of different policies. Make sure your policy provides coverage for in-court and out-of-court malpractice suits and expenses and for defense of a complaint or disciplinary action made to or by your board of nursing. Understanding insurance policy basics will enable you to shop more aggressively and intelligently for the coverage you need. You should work with an insurance agent who's experienced in this type of insurance. If you already have professional liability insurance, the information below may help you better evaluate your coverage.

Type of coverage

Ask your insurance agent whether the policy covers only claims made before the policy expires (claims-made coverage) or if it covers any negligent act committed during the policy period, regardless of when it's reported (occurrence coverage). Keep in mind that the latter type offers better coverage.

Coverage limits

All malpractice insurance policies cover professional liability. Some also cover representation before your board of nursing, general personal liability, medical payments, assault-related bodily injury, and property damage.

The amount of coverage varies, as does your premium. Remember that professional liability coverage is limited to acts and practice settings specified in the policy. Be sure your policy covers your nursing role, whether you're a student, a graduate nurse, or a working nurse with advanced education and specialized skills.

Options

Check whether the policy would provide coverage for these incidents:
· negligence on the part of nurses under your supervision
· misuse of equipment
· errors in reporting or recording care
· failure to provide patient education
· errors in administering medication
· mistakes made while providing care in an emergency, outside your employment setting.

Also ask whether the policy provides protection if your employer sues you.

Definition of terms

Definition of terms can vary from policy to policy. If your policy includes restrictive definitions, you won't be covered for actions outside those guidelines. Therefore, for the best protection, seek the broadest definitions possible and ask the insurance company for examples of actions the company hasn't covered.

Duration of coverage

Insurance is an annual contract that can be renewed or canceled each year. Most policies specify how they can be canceled—for example, in writing by either you or the insurance company. Some contracts require a 30-day notice for cancellation. If the company is canceling the policy, you'll probably be given at least 10 days' notice.

Exclusions

Ask the insurer about exclusions—areas not covered by the insurance policy. For example: "This policy doesn't apply to injury arising out of performance of the insured of a criminal act" or "This policy doesn't apply to nurse anesthetists."

Other insurance clauses

All professional liability insurance policies contain "other insurance" clauses that address payment obligations when a nurse is covered by more than one insurance policy, such as the employer's policy and the nurse's personal liability policy.
· The *pro rata* clause states that two or more policies in effect at the same time will pay any claims in accordance with a proportion established in the individual policies.

(continued)

Choosing liability insurance *(continued)*

• The *in excess* clause states that the primary policy will pay all fees and damages up to its limits, at which point the second policy will pay any additional fees or damages up to its limits.

• The *escape* clause relieves an insurance company of all liability for fees or damages if another insurance policy is in effect at the same time; the clause essentially states that the other company is responsible for all liability.

If you're covered by more than one policy, be alert for "other insurance" clauses and avoid purchasing a policy with an escape clause for liability.

Additional tips
Here's some additional information that will guide you in the purchase of professional liability insurance.
• The insurance application is a legal document. If you provide false information, it may void the policy.
• If you're involved in nursing administration, education, research, or ad-

vanced or nontraditional nursing practice, be especially careful in selecting a policy because many policies don't cover these activities.
• After selecting a policy that ensures adequate coverage, stay with the same policy and insurer, if possible, to avoid potential lapses in coverage that could occur when changing insurers.
• No insurance policy will cover you for acts outside of your scope of practice or licensure; nor will insurance cover you for intentional acts that you know will cause harm.
• Be prepared to uphold all obligations specified in the policy; failure to do so may void the policy and cause personal liability for any damages. Remember that an act of willful wrongdoing on your part renders the policy null and void and may lead to a breach-of-contract lawsuit.
• Check out the insurance company by calling your state division of insurance to inquire about the company's financial stability.

Documentation

Excellent documentation is the key to minimizing your liability; it is direct evidence of your evaluation and care of the patient. The medical record is your best protection and first line of defense. (See *Documentation tips* and *Uses of documentation,* page 590.)

A patient's satisfaction with care also reduces liability. Typically, a malpractice claim represents the connection between patient injury and patient anger. Good communication with the patient and his family is essential to maintaining a good connection. (See *Reducing the risk of a lawsuit,* page 590.)

Health care is a service industry, so you need to incorporate good

customer service into your daily practice, including:
• being respectful and courteous—people become angry when treated rudely.
• being attentive—give patients the time that they need.
• being sympathetic and empathetic—concern pays off in the long run.
• being considerate and honest—patients recognize honesty, which makes them feel better about the care they receive.
• recognizing your limits—ask for help or a second opinion if you have doubts.
• staying current—continuing education is a professional responsibility.

Documentation tips

If you're ever involved in a malpractice lawsuit, how you document, what you document, and what you didn't document will heavily influence the jury and the outcome of the trial. Following these tips can ensure that your records don't tip the scales of justice against you.

How to document
• Use the appropriate form, and document in ink.
• Record the patient's name and identification number on every page of his chart.
• Record the complete date and time of each entry.
• Document the care given in a timely manner.
• Include patient statements in quotations when significant.
• Be specific. Avoid general terms and vague expressions.
• Use standard abbreviations only.
• Use a medical term only if you're sure of its meaning.
• Document symptoms by using the patient's own words.
• Document objectively.

What to document
• Document all nursing actions you take in response to a patient's problem. For example: "8 p.m. medicated for incision pain." Be sure to include the medication name, dose, route, and site.
• Document the patient's response to medications and other treatment.
• Document safeguards you use to protect the patient. For example: "raised side rails" or "applied safety belt."
• If there is an abnormal incident to report, document the incident in two

places: in your progress notes and in an incident report. Don't mention the incident report in the patient's record, unless your facility or state requires it.
• Document each observation. Failure to document observations will produce gaps in the patient's records. These gaps will suggest that you neglected the patient.
• Document procedures after you perform them, never in advance.
• Write on every line. Don't insert notes between lines or leave empty spaces for someone else to insert a note.
• If you have empty spaces, place a line through them so that someone else can't insert information in the middle of your notes.
• Sign every entry.
• Chart an omission as a new entry. Never backdate or add to previously written entries. Within the body of the note, reference the time and date of omission.
• Correct errors according to your facility's policies and procedures.
• Draw a thin line through an error and mark "error" above it, with the date and your initials. Never erase or obliterate an erroneous entry.
• Document only the care you provide. Never document for someone else.
• Understand and follow the documentation standards of your facility and your state or province. These standards are usually defined in state or provincial nurse practice acts (the statutes governing nursing practice) and in state or provincial administrative codes (the rules and regulations governing nursing practice).

Uses of documentation

Complete, accurate, and timely documentation is crucial to the continuity of patient care. The medical record is also a legal and business record. A well-documented medical record:
• reflects the patient care given
• demonstrates the results of treatment
• helps to plan and coordinate the care contributed by each professional
• allows interdisciplinary exchange of information about the patient
• provides evidence of the nurse's legal responsibilities toward the patient
• demonstrates standards, rules, regulations, and laws of nursing practice
• supplies information for analysis of cost-to-benefit reduction
• reflects professional and ethical conduct and responsibility
• furnishes data for a variety of uses—continuing education, risk management, diagnosis-related group assignment and reimbursement, continuous quality improvement, case management monitoring, and research.

Reducing the risk of a lawsuit

Patients who are more likely to file lawsuits against nurses share certain personality traits and behaviors. Additionally, nurses who are more likely to be named as defendants also have certain characteristics in common.

Beware of these patients
Although not all persons displaying the behaviors listed here will file a lawsuit, a little extra caution in your dealings with them won't hurt. Providing professional and competent care to such patients will lessen their tendency to sue.

A patient who's likely to file a lawsuit may:
• persistently criticize all aspects of the nursing care provided
• purposefully not follow the care plan
• overreact to any perceived slight or negative comment, real or imagined
• unjustifiably depend on nurses for all aspects of care and refuse to accept any responsibility for his own care
• openly express hostility to nurses and other health care personnel
• project his anxiety or anger onto the nursing staff, attributing blame for all negative events to health care providers
• have previously filed lawsuits.

Nurses at risk
Nurses who are most likely to be named as defendants in a lawsuit display certain characteristic behaviors. If you recognize any of these attributes within yourself, changing your behavior will reduce your risk of liability.

A nurse who's likely to be a defendant in a lawsuit may:
• be insensitive to the patient's complaints or fail to take them seriously
• fail to identify and meet the patient's emotional and physical needs
• refuse to recognize the limits of her nursing skills and personal competency
• lack sufficient education for the tasks and responsibilities associated with a specific practice setting
• display an authoritative and inflexible attitude when providing care
• inappropriately delegate responsibilities to subordinates.

13 Ethical situations

The goal of nursing is to promote, restore, and maintain the health of people, who are regarded as holistic beings. Although the number of expectations for providing nursing care has grown, this goal remains.

In adapting to changing health care needs, nurses assume various roles in health care settings. (See *Practice roles*, page 592.) Each role has specific responsibilities, but some aspects of nursing are common to all positions. In addition to assuming various roles, the nurse must always uphold the ethical aspects of her profession.

Ethical decisions

Every day, nurses make ethical decisions in their practice. These may involve patient care, actions related to coworkers, or nurse-physician relations. There are no automatic guidelines for solving ethical conflicts. Legally, nurses are responsible for using their knowledge and skills to protect and promote the comfort and safety of patients. Ethically, nurses are responsible as patient advocates for safeguarding their patients' rights.

As the basis for professional codes of ethics, ethical theories attempt to provide a system of principles and rules for resolving ethical dilemmas. Ethical theories consist of fundamental beliefs about what's morally right or wrong, and propose reasoning for maintaining those beliefs. (See *Ethical theories*, pages 592 and 593.) Professional organiza-

tions, such as the International Council of Nurses, have looked at ethical theories and developed a code of ethics to guide nursing decisions (See *International Council of Nurses code of ethics*, page 594.) Ultimately, the nurse needs to combine these guidelines and theories with other objective and personal reflections to make ethical decisions in certain aspects of nursing care. (See *Basis of ethical decisions*, page 595.) Some hospital systems have set up mandatory education regarding ethical behavior in the workplace in order to provide guidance.

ETHICAL CONFLICTS IN PRACTICE

Rapid advances in medical research have outpaced society's ability to solve the ethical problems associated with new health care technology. For nurses, sociocultural factors, legal controversies, growing professional autonomy, and consumer involvement in health care complicate ethical decision making in clinical practice.

Ethical dilemmas resist easy resolution. The choice is typically between a desirable alternative and an undesirable alternative (such as withdrawing life care if it is not your personal belief). By learning as much as possible about the underlying ethical principles, you'll be better equipped to participate in the decision-making process. The more you practice ethical thinking, the more confident you'll become in your decision-making ability.

Practice roles

No matter what the practice setting, the nurse can assume various roles.

Caregiver

As a caregiver, the nurse assesses the patient, analyzes his needs, develops nursing diagnoses, and plans, delivers, and evaluates nursing interventions.

Advocate

As an advocate, the nurse helps the patient and his family members interpret information from other health care providers and make decisions about health-related needs.

Educator

As an educator, the nurse educates the patient and his family members by providing knowledge of health-promoting activities, disease-related conditions, and specific treatments. Education can take place in planned individual or group sessions or informally when caring for the patient.

Coordinator

As a coordinator, the nurse coordinates the patient's care plan with various health care providers. Many organizations recognize this nursing role, which requires good communication and management skills, by appointing nurses as case managers for patients.

Discharge planner

As a discharge planner, the nurse assesses the patient's needs at discharge, including the patient's support systems and living situation. The nurse also links the patient with available community resources.

Change agent

As a change agent, the nurse works with the patient and staff members to address organizational and community concerns. This role demands knowledge of change theory, which provides a framework for understanding the dynamics of change, human responses to change, and strategies for effecting change.

Ethical theories

Deontology

Deontologic theory emphasizes moral obligation or commitment, giving most weight to obeying moral laws such as "Always tell the truth" and "Never harm a patient." Using this theory, honoring ethical obligations ensures the greatest good.

Limitations
• Complications can arise when duties conflict with one another and a decision as to which duty takes precedence must be made such as keeping a patient's promise not to tell his family about his diagnosis.
• Decisions may be difficult and consequences painful.

Egoism

Egoism considers self-interest and self-preservation as the only proper goals of all human actions, insisting that the only right decision is the one that maximizes the autonomy of the decision-maker.

Limitations
• Egoism ignores moral principles or rules outside the individual's point of view.
• Inconsistencies arise from one decision to the next, even in similar situations.
• Social chaos can result when individuals act solely in their own interests.
• Because it ignores the rights of others, egoism is unacceptable for most ethical decisions in health care.

Ethical theories *(continued)*

Obligationism

Obligationism attempts to resolve ethical dilemmas by balancing distributive justice (dividing equally among all) with beneficence (doing good and not harm). This theory holds that benefits and burdens should be distributed equally, according to merits and needs.

Limitations
· The two basic principles of obligationism—justice and beneficence—may conflict in certain situations.
· The theory can be useful in determining public policy, but it's impractical for decisions that affect one person.

Social contract theory

Social contract theory is based on the concept of original position. The least advantaged people (such as children and the disabled) are considered the norm. Whether an act is right or wrong is determined from the norm's point of view.

Limitations
· Without specific guidelines, the theory is useless in day-to-day health care decisions.
· Social inequalities are persistent.

Teleology

Teleologic theory determines what's right or wrong based on an action's consequences. Ethical decisions are usually made through a process called *risk-benefits analysis,* in which the action chosen is that which will result in maximized good.

Limitations
· Determining the maximized good is highly subjective and can result in inconsistent decisions.
· Assuming that good and harm can be quantified and evaluated is a less than ideal approach to resolving health care issues.

Theological ethics

Ethical theories and moral-legal principles can be based in religious traditions—for example, Good Samaritan acts are based on the biblical concept of altruism and selflessness.

Limitations
· It may be difficult for someone who doesn't share a particular religious faith to understand its beliefs or to apply its teachings to health care situations.

Virtue ethics

Virtue ethics encourage and focus on traits of character, such as trustworthiness, loyalty, helpfulness, friendliness, kindness, bravery, generosity, cleanliness, reverence, and the like.

Limitations
· Virtue ethics tend to neglect conduct and outcome, and don't provide a formula for resolving conflict cases.

Getting help

When ethical problems arise, discuss them candidly with other members of the health care team, especially the patient's physician. Also consider calling on social workers, psychologists, clergy, and ethics committee members.

By learning as much as possible, you can facilitate the decision-making process for the patient, his family, his physician, and yourself.

(See *The ethics committee,* page 596.)

Right to die

The most difficult ethical decisions in health care involve whether to initiate or withhold life-sustaining treatment for patients who are irreversibly comatose or vegetative, or suffering with end-stage terminal ill-

International Council of Nurses code of ethics

The International Council of Nurses (ICN), an organization based in Geneva, Switzerland, that seeks to improve the standards and status of nursing worldwide, has published a code of ethics. The American Nurses Association (ANA) and the Canadian Nurses Association (CNA) have also developed codes of ethics. For more information on these codes, go to the ANA Web site *(http://nursingworld.org)* or the CNA Web site *(www.cna-nurses.ca/cna.)*

The ICN Code

The ICN Code of Ethics for Nurses has four pricipal elements that outline the standards of ethical conduct.

1. Nurses and people
• The nurse's primary professional responsibility is to people requiring nursing care.
• In providing care, the nurse promotes an environment in which the human rights, values, customs, and spiritual beliefs of the individual, family, and community are respected.
• The nurse ensures that the individual receives sufficient information on which to base consent for care and related treatment.
• The nurse holds in confidence personal information and uses judgment in sharing this information.
• The nurse shares with society the responsibility for initiating and supporting action to meet the health and social needs of the public, in particular those of vulnerable populations.
• The nurse also shares responsibility to sustain and protect the natural environment from depletion, pollution, degradation, and destruction.

2. Nurses and practice
• The nurse carries personal responsibility and accountability for nursing practice, and for maintaining competence by continual learning.
• The nurse maintains a standard of personal health such that the ability to provide care isn't compromised.
• The nurse uses judgment regarding individual competence when accepting and delegating responsibility.
• The nurse at all times maintains standards of personal conduct which reflect well on the profession and enhance public confidence.
• The nurse, in providing care, ensures that the use of techology and scientific advances are compatible with the safety, dignity, and rights of people.

3. Nurses and the profession
• The nurse assumes the major role in determining and implementing acceptable standards of clinical nursing practice, management, research, and education.
• The nurse is active in developing a core of research-based professional knowledge.
• The nurse, acting through the professional organization, participates in creating and maintaining safe, equitable social and economic working conditions in nursing.

4. Nurses and coworkers
• The nurse sustains a cooperative relationship with coworkers in nursing and other fields.
• The nurse takes appropriate action to safeguard individuals, families, and communities when their health is endangered by a coworker or any other person.

ness. Treatment decisions for these patients can be morally troubling. The patient, his family, and the health care team may be asked to choose between a potentially painful extension of life and probable death if treatment is not provided. Surrogate decision makers—people who are designated to act when a patient is no longer capable of deciding his own fate—also face tremendous moral and emotional pressures.

Sometimes, the patient's expressed wishes to withhold life-sustaining treatment are ignored or overridden by physicians and family members. As a nurse, you may feel caught in the middle, frustrated and demoralized by the demands of caring for an unresponsive patient who had expressly wished to withhold life-sustaining treatment.

DEFINING DEATH

Part of the problem stems from a lack of consensus about what constitutes death. Some people define *death* as the loss of all vital functions, whereas others define it by neurologic criteria such as *brain death*—the irreversible cessation of brain functioning accompanied by ongoing biological functioning in all other parts of the body that's only maintained by life-support measures.

Some people maintain a strong ethical belief in the absolute sanctity of life. Others argue that it's wrong and wasteful to continue life support when a patient's life is devoid of dignity. To function effectively when caring for critically ill patients, you'll need to be aware of your personal feelings about death and quality-of-life issues.

Ordinary vs. extraordinary treatment

Ordinary means of medical treatment are medications, procedures, and surgeries that offer the patient some hope of benefit without incurring excessive pain or expense. In contrast, extraordinary means, sometimes called *heroic measures*, maintain or prolong a patient's life and may cause suffering for the patient and his family. Because of con-

---

■
Basis of ethical decisions

Ethical decision making most commonly involves reflection on:
• options or courses of action available
• options that seem unavailable
• consequences, both good and bad, of all possible options
• rules, obligations, and values that should direct choices
• who should make the choices
• desired goal or outcome.

Equally important is the process of self-reflection. This involves uncovering, sharing, and discussing:
• personal and professional values relevant to the situation
• cultural considerations
• prejudices or biases that affect objectivity
• previous experiences with similar situations and decisions
• limitations that affect skills or understanding
• motives and intentions, particularly those of self-interest and convenience.

---

tinuing advances in medicine and technology, the distinction between "ordinary" and "extraordinary" treatments is becoming less defined.

In 1983, the President's Commission for the Study of Ethical Problems in Medicine and Behavioral Research defined ordinary and extraordinary treatments this way: "The Commission believes that extraordinary treatment is that which, in the patient's view, entails significantly greater burdens than benefits and is therefore undesirable and not obligatory, while ordinary treatment is that which, in the patient's view, produces greater benefits than burdens."

The commission further stated that health care professionals aren't

The ethics committee

The ethics committee addresses ethical issues regarding the clinical aspects of patient care. It provides a forum for the patient, his family, and health care providers to resolve difficult conflicts.

The functions of an ethics committee include:

• policy development (such as developing policies to guide deliberations over individual cases)

• education (such as inviting guest speakers to visit your health care facility and discuss ethical concerns)

• case consultation (such as debating the prognosis of a patient who's in a persistent vegetative state)

• addressing a single issue (such as reviewing all cases that involve a no-code, or do-not-resuscitate [DNR] order)

• addressing problems of a specific population group (for example, the American Academy of Pediatrics recommending that hospitals have a standing committee called the "infant bioethical review committee")

• addressing issues of organization ethics (such as business practice, marketing, admission, and reimbursement).

Pros and cons

Properly run, an ethics committee provides a safe outlet for venting opposing views on emotionally charged ethical conflicts. The committee process can help to lessen the bias that interferes with rational decision making. It allows for members of disparate disciplines, including physicians, nurses, clergy, social workers, hospital administrators, and ethicists, to express their views on treatment decisions.

Critics of the ethics committee think that committee decision making is too bureaucratic and slow to be useful in clinical crises. They also point out that one dominating committee member may intimidate others with opposing views. Furthermore, they contend that physicians may view the committee as a threat to their autonomy in patient-

care decisions. For these reasons, many ethics committees use a "rapid response team" of committee members who are on call to respond quickly in emergent ethical dilemmas. The rapid-response team usually consists of three or four committee members, including a physician, who have had special training in negotiation and mediation. The entire committee will retrospectively review each case.

Selection of committee members

Committee members should be selected for their ability to work cooperatively in a group. The American Hospital Association recommends the following ratio of committee members: one-third physicians, one-third nurses, and one-third others, including laypersons, clergy, and other health professionals. Joint Commission regulations require that nursing staff members participate in the hospital ethics committee.

The nurse's role on a hospital ethics committee

Because of the nurse's close contact with the patient, his family, and other members of the health care team, she's frequently in a position to identify ethical dilemmas such as when a family is considering a DNR order for a relative. In many cases, the nurse is the first to recognize conflicts among family members or between the physician and the patient or his family.

Before ethics committees were widely used, nurses had no official outlet for voicing their opinions in ethical debates. In many situations, physicians made ethical decisions about patient care behind closed doors. Nursing supervisors would frequently call meetings to alert nursing staff on treatment decisions and to discourage protest. Now, ethics committees provide nurses with a means to express their views, hear the opinions of others, and better understand the rationales behind ethical decisions.

obligated to provide treatment that's considered useless or futile.

Discontinuing treatment

Despite the commission's recommendations, countless terminally ill patients continue to receive treatment that's unlikely to benefit them. Determining whether a particular treatment is futile is highly subjective. Such decisions are often based not only on incomplete information, but also value judgments about quality of life. One method being considered to help with these subjective decisions is a computerized mortality prediction system called the *Acute Physiology and Chronic Health Evaluation System.*

When deciding whether to terminate life-sustaining treatment, health care providers face incredible emotional pressure. Nurses do have one ethically sound option: helping patients determine their own fate by educating them about their right to refuse extraordinary treatment.

RIGHT TO REFUSE TREATMENT

The right to refuse treatment is grounded in the ethical principle of respect for the autonomy of the individual. This principle of autonomy has led to the concept of *informed consent*—the obligation of health care providers to inform the patient of the risks and benefits of a procedure and to obtain permission before the procedure is carried out. Terminally ill patients who receive life-sustaining treatment have a right to informed consent.

Because the nursing profession is oriented to saving and prolonging lives, you may find it difficult to agree with a patient's decision to withhold life-sustaining treatment. Limiting treatment doesn't mean abandoning the patient. Supportive measures aren't considered extraordinary treatment. A patient who has

chosen to forgo life-sustaining treatment still has the right to receive care that preserves his comfort, hygiene, and dignity. In particular, he has the right to adequate pain control.

Health care workers' rights

Although patients have the right to decide whether to accept or forgo heroic measures, they don't have the right to insist on treatments that provide no medical benefit. If you believe that you'll violate your own values by implementing a certain treatment, you have an obligation to arrange for the transfer of the patient's care to another provider. Likewise, if you believe that you will violate your values by withholding treatment, you should request a transfer. This right, also known as *the conscience clause* or *conscientious objection,* applies to assisting in abortions as well as to noninitiation or withdrawal of life-sustaining treatment or euthanasia.

DOCUMENTING A PATIENT'S WISHES

A patient who has a strong desire to request or reject aggressive treatment measures should document his wishes. He should also designate a surrogate decision maker to speak for him if he can no longer make his own health care decisions. Statements that indicate a patient's wishes in the event he loses his decision-making capability are known as *advance directives,* the patient's best means of ensuring that his wishes will be respected. The advance directive includes a living will, which goes into effect when the patient can no longer make health care decisions, and the durable health care power of attorney, which authorizes another person to make those decisions. If a patient has both, the person with

Helping the patient plan ahead

Of the many professionals who care for the critically ill, nurses have the best chance to act as true patient advocates. The patient may look to you as well as his physician for guidance. You can't make the ultimate medical decisions to initiate or limit treatment, but you can help the patient express his wishes about his health care and guide him in translating these desires into advance directives.

When you're discussing limiting treatment with a patient, consider these suggestions.
• Present options, such as do-not-resuscitate orders, in a realistic but positive context. Reassure the patient that he'll continue to receive supportive care and pain medication.
• Pay attention to the patient's questions and misunderstandings. Be especially alert to unexpressed fears.
• During your discussions with the patient, note his nonverbal cues and emotional responses.

Despite your best efforts to provide objective advice, the patient may not be able to reach a decision about initiating or terminating care. Remember that you must respect the patient's explicit refusal to participate in health care decisions.

Standards for judging decision-making ability

Commonly used standards for judging decision-making capability include:
• the ability to indicate a choice
• a clear understanding of the issues at hand
• the ability to reason based on the information given
• an appreciation of the true nature of the situation.

If a patient is incapable of making a decision, it becomes the duty of a surrogate decision-maker or the health care team to act in his best interest.

---

durable power should support the patient's wishes. Other family members or health care providers can't override the person with the durable health care power of attorney.

Although specific treatments (such as feedings through a tube) can be requested in an advance directive, most people execute a living will to ensure that no extraordinary means are used to sustain or prolong life. A durable health care power of attorney designates a surrogate decision-maker who will have full authority to carry out the patient's wishes regarding health care decisions. The authority of this surrogate decision maker is based on the principle of *substituted judgment*— allowing the surrogate to make the same decisions the patient would if he were able.

Advance directives, although useful, haven't ended the controversy over a patient's right to limit treatment. Critics contend that they represent the first step toward active euthanasia, or *mercy killing.* These people believe that advance directives, such as living wills, should be restricted to a narrow range of circumstances.

Although many states have enacted so-called "natural death acts" to encourage practitioners to abide by a living will by granting statutory enforcement, these laws vary from state to state. Several require a "reasonable effort by the physician" to transfer the patient to a physician who will abide by the living will. (See *Helping the patient plan ahead.*)

Organ transplantation

The benefits of organ transplantation are widely recognized by health care professionals and the general public. Nevertheless, organ transplantation poses serious ethical concerns. Transplant procedures affect families of the donor and the recipient, nurses, physicians, and even ambulance attendants at a deep emotional level. In such a highly charged atmosphere, conflicts of rights can easily develop:

• If the potential donor is a child, questions may arise as to the validity of informed consent.

• Controversy may occur over when to declare a potential donor's death.

• The wishes of a potential donor's family may conflict with the needs of a transplant patient.

• Because the number of available donor organs is limited, difficult choices must be made about which patients should receive transplants.

• Many transplants are prohibitively expensive; questions arise as to whether subsidizing the procedure is a just allocation of health care resources.

• In light of the limited number of available donor organs and the high cost of the procedure, questions arise as to the patient's right to multiple transplants.

Even if you don't make the ultimate medical decisions about an organ transplant, you may play a critical role in resolving ethical conflicts.

PROTECTING THE RIGHTS OF POTENTIAL DONORS

Some transplantation procedures pose few ethical problems. An autograft, in which tissue is transplanted from one part of the patient's body to another (such as a skin graft to treat a third-degree burn), is a good example. Certain types of transplants from one person to another (allograft), including blood transfusions and cornea or bone marrow transplants, are widely accepted and ethically untainted.

The most difficult ethical issues surround the procurement of essential organs, such as hearts, kidneys, livers, and lungs. In these instances, organ procurement remains ethical only if steps are taken to ensure that the donor's life and functional integrity aren't compromised and the recipient process follows a standard procedure.

Nonmaleficence

At first glance, removing an organ from a healthy person who has nothing to gain from the procedure seems to violate the ethical principle of *nonmaleficence*—the obligation to "do no harm." However, when providing care, there are many instances in which the principle of nonmaleficence can't be strictly applied. Some harm, in the form of an invasive or a potentially risky procedure, must be incurred in diagnosing and treating many diseases.

When a living person donates an organ, the key issue is informed consent. From both an ethical and a legal standpoint, informed consent requires the donor to be fully aware of all risks and benefits that can result from the transplant procedure. Because relatives, particularly identical twins or full siblings, typically provide the closest match for a transplanted organ, emotional pressure may be exerted on a potential donor. Guilt and emotional distress may disturb a potential donor's ability to render informed consent.

CADAVERIC DONORS

Harvesting organs from a deceased donor poses a different set of ethical problems. Perhaps the most fundamental issue involves the actual definition of *death*. Although some organs and tissues, such as bone, skin, corneas, and kidneys, can be transplanted after complete cardiac arrest, other organs, including the heart, lungs, liver, and pancreas, aren't viable unless they're taken from a patient with brain death, also known as a *beating heart cadaver*.

Most states recognize the definition of brain death set forth by the Uniform Determination of Death Act as the legal definition of death. In general terms, a patient is pronounced brain-dead when all functional activity in every area of the brain, including the brain stem, stops. Significantly, this definition isn't universally accepted by health care workers, ethicists, or laypersons. Some may find it difficult to accept pronouncement of death when other aspects of bodily function continue, even if by artificial support.

The issue of declaring brain death must be approached cautiously. The determination that a person is brain-dead should be made by neurologic consult and never by a physician who's involved in organ removal. The request for organ donation shouldn't be made until the potential donor's family understands the definition, diagnosis, and outcome of brain death.

Informed consent

The Uniform Anatomical Gift Act allows a person to donate specific organs or even his entire body for organ transplantation. A patient may have indicated his willingness to be an organ donor prior to his brain death, and this permission may be denoted on a driver's license or official signed donor document. This is called *first person consent* and it gives the hospital legal authority to proceed with organ procurement without consent from the family.

Approaching a potential donor's family

All states have enacted required request acts. These laws require hospitals to ask families of potential organ donors to permit donation. The required request laws are intended to increase organ availability. (See *National Organ Transplant Act.*)

Most required request laws are fair to the families of potential donors. Family members are under no obligation to grant permission to donate organs. Most required request acts grant exclusion if the request will cause the family severe emotional distress.

These laws may create serious ethical conflicts, however, for a nurse who opposes organ transplantation or who finds the idea of approaching a grieving family offensive or inappropriate. Should a nurse be forced to request organ donation regardless of her feelings? The solution is to assign the job of approaching the donor's family to an organ procurement team, whose members have been specially trained to deal with this emotional situation.

If you're making the request for an organ donation from a patient's family, approach family members tactfully and be sufficiently informed to answer their questions. You should be able to explain the potential benefits to others. Remember that the decision of the family must be respected.

National Organ Transplant Act

In response to widespread public interest in organ transplantation, Congress enacted the National Organ Transplant Act of 1984 (PL 98-507). This act:
- prohibits the sale of organs
- provides funding for grants to organ procurement agencies
- establishes a national organ-sharing system.

Task Force on Organ Transplantation
This act also convened the 25-member Task Force on Organ Transplantation, with members representing medicine, law, theology, ethics, allied health, the health insurance industry, and the general public.

Representatives from the Office of the Surgeon General, the National Institutes of Health, the Food and Drug Administration, and the Health Care Financing Administration were also appointed to the task force. This task force examined the medical, legal, ethical, economic, and social issues created by organ transplantation.

In its final report, the task force concluded that the best way to close the gap between the small number of organ donors and the large number of potential transplant recipients was to actively solicit donations from bereaved families. As a result, the task force recommended that all state legislatures introduce and enact legislation requiring health care professionals to present organ donation as an option to families ("required request").

Assertive approach
Required request policies are legally mandated in many states. This assertive approach to organ procurement has proved highly successful; as many as 80% of families given the option to become donor families ultimately do so. Significantly, studies show that organ donation can facilitate the grieving process and speed recovery for the bereaved family.

HIV and AIDS

Nurses have always honored their professional responsibility to care for all patients, regardless of personal attributes, lifestyle, or the nature of the illness. Today, human immunodeficiency virus (HIV) and acquired immunodeficiency syndrome (AIDS) challenge this long-standing professional ethic. No other contagious illness incites such emotionally charged ethical debate.

HIV and AIDS touch on two highly controversial social issues: sexuality and drug use. It isn't surprising that many nurses experience value conflicts when working to meet their professional obligations.

Prejudice, fear, and misunderstanding surround HIV and AIDS.

An HIV-positive test result may mean the loss of a job, medical insurance, financial security, and even housing. Family, friends, and even the public may shun the HIV or AIDS patient. As a result, maintaining confidentiality is a serious concern for people with HIV and AIDS.

Mandatory testing
Testing for HIV isn't the same as testing for other infectious diseases. The patient with a positive gonorrhea culture doesn't face the same likelihood of discrimination as the patient who is HIV-positive.

Some organizations, including the military and prisons, and many insurance companies insist on mandatory HIV testing. Several states attempted to institute mandatory testing to obtain a marriage license and then abandoned the policy because

Testing guidelines

Following these guidelines can help to ensure that human immunodeficiency virus (HIV) testing is carried out in an ethically responsible manner.

• The sole purpose of any screening program should be to prevent the spread of HIV.

• The confidentiality of the test results must be ensured. If it's necessary to disclose the results (when a blood donor tests positive), the affected person should be notified.

• The patient should receive adequate pretest and posttest counseling.

• The diagnostic laboratory must be reliable.

• Informed consent should be obtained before a patient is allowed to participate in a voluntary screening program.

of high costs and the low percentage of positive results. Most states now mandate written consent for testing and mandate pretest and posttest counseling.

Does mandatory testing violate the ethical principles of autonomy (the patient's right to control his own fate) and justice (his right to be treated fairly)? Does it violate his right to privacy? Many nurses believe that it doesn't. Health care workers, they argue, have a right to protect themselves and need a complete picture of the patient's health status to deliver quality care.

Public health officials contend that mandatory testing would improve our understanding of the spread of the disease and aid in prevention. Hospital administrators say that knowing a patient's HIV status could lower health care costs by pinpointing those who require extra precautions. The solution to this dilemma is to teach healthcare workers to treat all patients' secre-

tions as infectious and to maintain standard precautions with every patient contact.

Opponents of mandatory testing emphasize the risk of discrimination and the high cost of screening all patients. They also believe that testing drives away patients who need care because many people fear being tested.

Mandatory testing can also backfire. An exposed person can take 12 weeks or longer to develop HIV antibodies. During this time, he's contagious but seronegative. (See *Testing guidelines*.)

HIPAA

The Health Insurance Portability and Accountability Act (HIPAA) of 2003 protects the privacy, confidentiality, and security of medical information. Under HIPAA, only those who have a "need to know" are authorized to access patient information. Some state practice acts impose an ethical duty to guard the patient's privacy, and the federal government also imposes a fine on individuals who violate confidentiality. However, no one can fully guarantee that unauthorized individuals won't gain access to medical records, especially with more institutions converting to computerized records.

The patient's right to privacy may conflict with your duty to prevent the spread of HIV. You may request that the patient inform his partner of his HIV status, but legally you must respect the patient's right to confidentiality. The Centers for Disease Control and Prevention and state regulations require reporting cases of HIV/AIDS; however, they uphold patient privacy rights and these cases must be reported utilizing established guidelines.

Personal safety in the workplace

Health care workers are entitled to work in a safe environment. The ethical principle of justice or fairness supports the position that employers should provide security measures, whether in an institution or in the community. Without those safeguards, an ethical dilemma arises. Although nurses must provide care to patients (nonabandonment and fidelity), they also need to protect themselves.

Policies that address appropriate staffing levels, adequate training, and security escorts minimize the ethical conflicts between providing care and ensuring safety. Federal safety and health standards require that all employers develop injury and illness prevention programs for hazards unique to their facility or program.

WORKPLACE VIOLENCE

Workplace violence is a serious problem in the United States, and nurses are particularly vulnerable. On average, 30% of nurses report experiencing assault, abusive language, emotional or mental abuse, or sexual harassment. Patients and physicians are the most common perpetrators of physical violence against nurses; physicians, nurse managers, or other supervisors are the most common perpetrators of verbal and emotional abuse.

Studies indicate that drugs, poor staffing, hospital type and location, gangs, easy access to a hospital emergency area, long work hours, inadequate training, power and control issues, and stress contribute to violence in health care settings. (See *Creating a safe work environment.*)

Creating a safe work environment

Health care officials and nursing leaders have an ethical and legal responsibility to create and maintain a safe, healthy work environment. To do this, they need to develop policies and procedures detailing behavioral expectations, reporting mechanisms that don't discriminate against victims of workplace violence, and effective security policies and systems. Some of the initiatives that they can take include:

• documenting required employee safety and self-protection training provided for all employees by the organization
• teaching proven strategies of intervention for situations of escalating violence
• teaching caregivers to work as a team when responding to violence
• clearly stating behavioral expectations for employees, medical staff, patients, and visitors
• stating the organization's expectations for reporting instances of violence or abuse and describing appropriate documentation
• establishing a mechanism (such as the organizational ethics committee) for investigating, negotiating, and resolving conflicts and disputes.

Employee rights

When violence occurs in the workplace, employees may have claims against their employer under federal or state law. Employees may have additional legal remedies against their abusers and their employer under legal principles involving tort or contract issues. Tort cases may occur if an employer or manager intentionally or negligently violates an employee right. Cases involving contract issues may occur if the employer was negligent in providing contracted security safeguards.

Legal issues of sexual harrassment

Sexual harassment is a violation of Title VII of the 1964 Federal Civil Rights Act, which was amended by the Civil Rights Act of 1991. It's now easier for employees to prove discrimination and receive higher awards in damages.

Hospitals and other health care organizations should establish fair policies and procedures that clearly define sexual harassment. Nurses should receive consistent education about sexual harassment in the workplace, including how to recognize it and how to avoid causing it.

Some of the ways to protect yourself from becoming a victim of sexual harassment include:

• refraining from talking or joking with employees about sex, including making remarks you feel are innocent

• stopping sexually oriented conduct among employees, such as joke telling and gestures

• keeping sexually oriented materials (such as posters, cartoons, or E-mails) from being posted in the workplace

• calling employees by their name or title

• refraining from expressing sexual interest or feelings for another employee.

SEXUAL HARASSMENT

Sexual harassment in the workplace isn't unique to health care facilities. Anecdotal evidence suggests that the problem is related in part to nurses' traditionally subservient role to that of the physician in health care and the sexism underlying this problem. However, sexism and sexual harassment can and do involve same-sex advances as well as female-male situations.

From coworkers, sexual harassment is best understood as a form of violence in the workplace. It's much less about sex than it is about abuse and control issues. For this reason, sexual harassment is experienced in two forms: *quid pro quo* and *hostile workplace*.

The Latin term *quid pro quo* means "this for that." Quid pro quo sexism occurs when a manager, supervisor, or individual in a "dominant" role (such as a physician) indicates or hints to an employee or person in a "nondominant" position that he'll trade job advancement, job benefits, or other special considerations for sexual favors.

Sexual harassment may also be defined as any form of sexual hostility in the workplace. Sexual hostility can include sexually offensive jokes, pictures, innuendoes, or behaviors. Although this type of sexual harassment is commonly repeated in the work environment, with the intent to shock, annoy, and degrade the recipient, it may sometimes take only one incident to provoke a charge of sexual harassment. For example, one vice president of nursing who was her hospital's only female senior manager brought suit against the hospital when the other senior manager hired a male stripper to "perform" at a management birthday party for her. (See *Legal issues of sexual harassment*.)

From patients and visitors

Harassment may also include unwelcome or offensive verbal or physical conduct from a patient or visitor. Such acts may intimidate or threaten the nurse, be offensive, or undermine the therapeutic relationship. Such acts may be gestures or physical acts, slurs, taunting, verbal abuse or epithets, comments or jokes, or the displaying of derogatory objects, cartoons, posters, drawings, or pictures.

WHISTLE-BLOWING

Whistle-blowing refers to an employee's disclosure of illegal, immoral, or illegitimate practices under an employer's control. The American Nurses Association (ANA) Code for Nurses outlines the nurse's obligation to report acts of negligence and incompetence by other health care providers. It states that "the nurse acts to safeguard the patient and public when health care and safety are affected by incompetent, unethical, or illegal practice by any person."

The ANA guidelines on reporting incompetent, unethical, or illegal practices identify helpful parameters for judging problematic conduct. Incompetent nursing practice is measured by nursing standards, unethical practice is evaluated in light of the Code for Nurses, and illegal practice is identified in terms of violations of the law. As a patient advocate, you must be willing to take appropriate action—in short, to blow the whistle.

When to blow the whistle

Nurses are, by their professional code of ethics and licensure standards, required to act as patient advocates. Whenever nurses see other health care providers acting in a way that could endanger the health or safety of a patient, they should make a report of what they witnessed. (In many states, state law *requires* nurses to report patient endangerment.)

The concept of moral agency should guide nurses not only in situations of whistle-blowing, but also in reporting witnessed or suspected malpractice. Some states have regulations and case laws that protect nurses who speak up in cases of suspected or confirmed medical malpractice.

A health care professional who makes a mistake usually wants to ensure that it won't happen again. Correcting an error usually involves admitting the mistake, expressing honest regret, and completing an incident report. At times, though, you may encounter a health care professional who makes repeated mistakes, attempts to cover them up or minimize them, and engages in suspect or misleading behavior. To uphold the ethical standards of your profession, you need to blow the whistle.

Implications of whistle-blowing

Many nurses equate whistle-blowing with heroic self-sacrifice: a moral victory in the midst of a professional defeat. In fact, some nurses have had their reputations tarnished, lost their jobs, or been named in libel suits after reporting professional misconduct. Fortunately, such bitter retaliation isn't the norm. Keep in mind, however, that the higher the professional standing of the health care professional who commits misconduct, the greater risk you face when blowing the whistle. (See *Whistle-blowing: A systematic approach,* page 606.)

Reporting nurse misconduct

Usually, institutional channels exist through which you can report the misconduct of another nurse or nursing assistant without fear of reprisal. Typically, a nurse-manager and the personnel office assume joint responsibility for investigating allegations of misconduct. For you, the only drawback is animosity from the affected staff member— and possibly from her acquaintances or sympathizers. The benefits, though, include correcting an injustice, preventing future harm, and

Whistle-blowing: A systematic approach

As with other nursing actions, whistle-blowing can be carried out successfully if it's planned, systematic, and purposeful.

Gathering facts

Begin by gathering all the facts. Then put in writing the misconduct you want to report. Be sure to include the date and time of the incident, the person or people involved, and the source of your information. Above all, avoid accusations and personal opinions.

Stating the problem

Clearly state the problem and identify causative factors:

• Was incompetence or negligence involved?
• Were supplies adequate?
• Did equipment malfunction?
• Was facility policy at fault?

When answering these questions, try to eliminate your personal biases. If possible, review the problem with a trusted colleague.

Determining your objective

State your objective in confronting the problem. For example, you may want to eliminate threats to patient safety; eliminate illegal, immoral, or illegitimate practices; uphold professional ethical standards; or put into effect changes in facility policy.

Confronting the problem

Confront the person who committed the misconduct in a constructive, nonthreatening way. Express your concerns, and ask for an explanation of the incident. Seek reassurance that the problem will be addressed.

Making your decision

After a reasonable duration, determine if the problem has been corrected. If it hasn't, identify the pros and cons of whistle-blowing. The pros include correction of a harmful or potentially harmful situation, retained moral integrity, and an enhanced sense of moral accountability. The cons include alienation, stress and, possibly, loss of reputation, professional standing, and job. After you weigh the pros and cons, talk over the issue of whistle-blowing with your lawyer or another knowledgeable person.

Next, realistically appraise your situation. Will you be able to cope if you blow the whistle? Are you secure professionally and financially? Do you have the support of your family, colleagues, or administration?

Make your decision based on your analysis of the severity of the incident, the consequences of whistle-blowing, and your resources. If you elect to blow the whistle, carefully devise a strategy that follows facility channels.

If you're fearful of losing your job as a result of your actions, consider taking a position in another facility before you blow the whistle. If you fail to get satisfaction through facility channels, consider consulting professional organizations, regulatory agencies and, as a last resort, the press. Be sure to document each step you take.

---

strengthening your sense of moral integrity.

Reporting medical or management misconduct

If you report the misconduct of a physician, a nursing supervisor, a nurse-manager, or a member of the institution's administration, expect stiffer resistance and, possibly, more severe retaliation, especially if management has cooperated in concealing the misconduct. Be prepared for a lengthy and hard-fought battle. The accused professional may attempt to discredit you—or have you fired—rather than face the allegations honestly.

Substance abuse among nurses

The ANA estimates that 6% to 8% of nurses in the United States are addicted to alcohol or drugs. In one state study, researchers found that more than 90% of disciplinary hearings for nurses in the state were related to alcohol and drug abuse. These statistics aren't surprising in light of the high stress levels in nursing today. Nurses can experience frustration and feelings of powerlessness when trying to act as patient advocates. Frequent floating to unfamiliar units, unrealistic workloads, and long work hours may bring on fatigue and loneliness. Many nurses must shoulder tremendous family and financial obligations while trying to meet professional demands. And, of course, nurses aren't immune to the harsh social realities of modern life. Combined with the availability of controlled substances, such stressors can lead a nurse to substance abuse.

PAST ATTITUDES TOWARD SUBSTANCE ABUSE

In the past, nurses who were discovered abusing drugs or alcohol were punished. The prevailing ethic held that a nurse who abused drugs or alcohol violated the public trust and the standards of her profession and deserved to be subject to strong disciplinary action.

Nursing administrators were expected to report suspected substance abusers to their state nursing board. The board would then investigate the allegation, and if it found the nurse guilty, it would impose punishment such as revocation of her license.

In practice, though, many administrators didn't report substance abuse but chose instead to fire the offending nurse. Furthermore, colleagues of suspected substance abusers commonly didn't report their suspicions because they knew the nurses' job would be in jeopardy. Aware of the harsh treatment that awaited them, nurses who abused drugs or alcohol changed jobs frequently rather than endure the repercussions that would follow an admission of substance abuse.

Ethical perspectives

From an ethical viewpoint, this punitive approach to substance abuse left much to be desired. Administrators who simply fired a substance abuser relinquished their ethical responsibility to help nurses in need and prevent qualified nurses from dropping out of their profession. Colleagues who didn't report substance abuse abandoned the best interests of both the addicted nurse and her patients. The substance abuser usually changed jobs rather than seek help. She had little motivation to change, knowing that she was unlikely to receive understanding or rehabilitation. (See *Recognizing substance abuse*, page 608.)

Though the decision to report an impaired coworker is never an easy one, you have an ethical obligation to intervene if you suspect that a colleague is abusing drugs or alcohol. Intervening enables you to fulfill your moral obligation to your colleague: By reporting abuse, you compel her to take the first step toward regaining control over her life and undergoing rehabilitation. You also fulfill your obligation to patients by protecting them from a nurse whose judgment and care may fail to meet professional standards.

Recognizing substance abuse

Be aware that allegations of substance abuse are serious and potentially damaging. To make an accurate assessment, you need to be familiar with the signs of substance abuse, which may include:

• rapid mood swings, usually from irritability or depression to elation
• frequent absences, lateness, and use of private quarters such as bathrooms
• frequent volunteering to administer medications
• excessive errors or problems with controlled substances, such as reports of broken vials or spilled drugs
• illogical or sloppy charting
• inability to meet deadlines or minimum job requirements
• avoidance of new and challenging assignments
• increased errors in treatment, particularly in dosage computation

• poor personal hygiene and appearance
• inability to concentrate or remember details
• alcohol on the breath
• slurred speech, unsteady gait, flushed face, or red eyes
• discrepancies in narcotics supplies detected at the end of the nurse's shift
• controlled substances signed out to patients only on the nurse's shift
• patient complaints of no relief from opioids supposedly administered when the nurse is on duty
• preference for working alone or on the night shift, when supervision is minimal
• social withdrawal
• memory loss
• alcohol-induced complications, including jaundice, bruises (from falls), and delirium.

Reporting substance abuse

If you detect signs of substance abuse, your first step is to document them. Include the time, date, and place of the incident; a description of what happened, and the names of any witnesses. Be sure to leave out personal opinions and judgments.

Never personally confront or accuse the suspected nurse. After you've documented the incident, report it to, and discuss it with your nurse-manager. She'll need to gather additional information by examining patient charts, medication records (especially for opioids), and reports from patients and other nurses. After the nurse-manager completes this review, she'll try to determine if the evidence corroborates your incident report.

IV Career options

14 Nursing education 610

15 Nursing specialties 623

14 Nursing education

The registered nurse (RN) may be required to earn contact hours or continuing education units (CEUs) throughout her career in order to maintain her licensure. Each state licensing board dictates how many education hours are required to renew licensure. (See *Contact hours required by state*.) Education hours are also required to renew certifications, which we'll discuss in chapter 15. See chapter 12 for contact information on specific state boards of nursing.

Continuing education

Continuing education provides learning experiences that enhance the knowledge and skills of the practicing nurse in order to improve administration of health care.

The RN may obtain continuing education via:
- classroom education
- conference
- workshop
- satellite class
- Web cast
- internet or intranet
- teleconference
- learning module.

Education must usually be state board-certified and must provide documentation of attendance in the form of a certificate, transcript, or attendance sheet. Licensees are responsible for maintaining their own continuing education records.

Each state has individual regulations concerning the amount of continuing education, usually in the form of contact hours. A *contact hour* is a unit of measurement for organized education. Each "hour" is technically 50 minutes. A CEU is a different measurement of education hours than a contact hour. Each CEU is equivalent to 10 contact hours. So, if you attended 10 hours of continuing education, it would be equal to 1.0 CEU. It's the nurse's responsibility to know how many hours are required for each state license that she holds. Education obtained in one state may be accepted by other states. Failure to meet education requirements may result in a lapse of license.

EDUCATIONAL OPTIONS

Pursuing a higher degree in nursing may be necessary in order to advance in your current position or qualify for a new position, or you may want to continue your education for personal reasons. If you decide to return to school, you can choose from several options.

A practicing registered nurse who has an associate's degree or a hospital-based school of nursing diploma can participate in programs such as:
- bachelor's degree (RN/BSN)
- master's degree (RN/MSN)
- doctor of nursing practice (RN/DNP).

If you have a BSN you have many options as well:
- Master's degree

Contact hours required by state

Most states have a 2-year license renewal period, and nurses are required to obtain contact hours between renewal periods. Audits of educational hours are often done randomly. Some states have additional requirements, such as a minimum amount of employed hours, or education requirements for specific nursing specialties. Be sure to check with your state board of nursing for specific information.

State	Contact hours
Alabama	24 hours
Alaska	30 hours
Arizona	None
Arkansas	15 hours
California	30 hours
Colorado	None
Connecticut	None
Delaware	30 hours
District of Columbia	24 hours
Florida	25 hours
Georgia	None
Hawaii	None
Idaho	None
Illinois	None
Indiana	None
Iowa	36 hours (3 years)
Kansas	30 hours
Kentucky	14 hours (1 year)
Louisiana	5 hours (1 year)
Maine	None
Maryland	None
Massachusetts	15 hours
Michigan	25 hours
Minnesota	24 hours
Mississippi	None
Missouri	None
Montana	None
Nebraska	20 hours
Nevada	30 hours
New Hampshire	30 hours
New Jersey	30 hours
New Mexico	30 hours
New York	3 hours infection control every 4 years; 2 hours child abuse (1x for initial licensure)
North Carolina	Learning activity (Check with the National Council of State Boards of Nursing.)
North Dakota	12 hours
Ohio	24 hours
Oklahoma	None
Oregon	7 hours on pain management (1x)
Pennsylvania	30 hours
Rhode Island	10 hours
South Carolina	30 hours

(continued)

■

Contact hours required by state *(continued)*

State	Contact hour
South Dakota	None
Tennessee	None
Texas	20 hours
Utah	30 hours
Vermont	None
Virginia	None
Washington	None
West Virginia	30 hours
Wisconsin	None
Wyoming	20 hours

- Master's degree to become an advanced practice nurse
  - Clinical nurse specialist
  - Nurse practitioner
  - Nurse anesthetist
  - Nurse midwife
- Master's degree with a specialty
  - Nursing education
  - Public health
  - Nursing administration

There are also schools and universities offering post-master's certificates to RNs who hold a master's degree and wish to pursue further specialization, such as:
- wound care
- nursing education
- preoperative nursing
- informatics.

Some certificate program options may be available for the BSN as well.

TIPS FOR RETURNING TO SCHOOL

Returning to school while working full- or part-time can prove challenging. There are a few things to consider as you plan your educational pursuits.

Shop around

Once you decide on the specialty you wish to pursue, talk to professionals who hold a degree in this field, and ask some questions. Where did they go to school? Did they like the program? What were the strengths and weaknesses of the program? These questions can help you narrow down your choices.

Admission process

Once you decide on your specialty and have selected a school, you will need to begin the admission process. Read the information from the school carefully so you are fully prepared. (See *Admission requirements for college.*)

Transfer credits

When pursuing further education, you may be able to transfer some or all of your previously earned credits. Check with the admissions office, and keep this possibility in mind if you're thinking about transferring out of your current program. Lost credits may feel like wasted time and money. If the previous program wasn't accredited, credits earned with that program may not be accepted at the new institution.

Commitment

Know what's involved in earning a new degree or certificate, including time commitment, cost, and travel. Research the types of programs in

Admission requirements for college

Being knowledgeable about these admission requirements may cut down on delays for admission.

Application deadline

An application deadline is a specific date by which all application information must be received. Some schools may have a rolling application deadline, which means that applications are accepted at any time. Be aware of the date, and allow yourself plenty of time to submit all the information to the admissions committee by the deadline.

Grade point average

Some schools require a specific undergraduate grade point average (GPA). If your GPA from your original educational program was low, don't worry; the admission committee reviews the entire picture of each applicant. You will need to contact all previous schools that you attended, including your original nursing program, and have your transcripts sent directly to the school to which you are applying.

Writing sample

For some programs you may be required to submit a writing sample; this may be a paper or case study. The school will provide the guidelines for their specific requirements.

Recommendations

You will need letters of recommendation from colleagues, former faculty members, or clinical supervisors. When asking for a recommendation, provide the form (if required), a postage paid envelope, and the timeline for submission. Be sure to check back to be sure the recommendation was sent to the school and to offer a word of thanks.

Standardized tests

Based on the specific institution, you may be required to complete a standardized test before admission to a master's program, such as the Graduate Record Examination (GRE) or the Miller Analogy Test (MAT). Check with the school to determine its admission requirements. It's recommended that you use a study guide or attend a review program to help prepare for the specific test. If your undergraduate GPA is high enough, however, the GRE or MAT requirement may be waived.

your area, the estimated length of study required, and the availability of satellite schools or programs close to your home. Be aware of the requirements for the program, including clinical rotations or labs, and if there are online components for course work. (See *Time management,* page 614.) Look into the estimated cost of the program, including laboratory fees and books. Don't hesitate to contact schools and ask for detailed information. Obtain a school catalogue, schedule a visit to tour the facility and campus, and meet with current students and faculty before making a final decision.

Academic advisor

Make sure you know your academic advisor. Make a point to introduce yourself, and schedule time to discuss your educational plan. Your advisor can offer guidance on when to take specific courses, answer questions you have regarding the program, and serve as a resource on many other topics.

Funding

Check with the human resources department of your workplace to see if there's a tuition reimbursement program. If this benefit is available, gather all of the information to help with financial planning. Some reimbursement programs have

Time management

Returning to school takes energy as well as time. You may not be able to do extra shifts or work overtime while in school. Class time is only one component of going to school. Remember to schedule time for reading, going to the library, and writing papers. When asked to volunteer for just one more thing, think twice before making commitments. Keep a calendar of class dates and when papers and presentations are due, and refer to it before saying yes.

Everything you do requires time, so make the most of extra time. Plan for travel time to and from school because this can add as much as 1 hour (or more) to your class time each week. If possible, record lectures and take advantage of travel time to listen to them. Always carry required reading material with you in case some extra time pops up. In 20 to 30 minutes, you may be able to read one more chapter!

Prepare your friends, family, and employer for your return to school. It may seem that everyone will want just a little more time from you when you actually have less time to give. Make sure the people who are important to you are aware of your time commitment for school, but be sure to schedule time for them as well. Let your immediate supervisor at work know of your plans to return to school. Submit, in writing, your course or clinical schedule so that your work schedule can be adjusted accordingly.

an application deadline or operate on a "per semester" schedule and have specific dates and deadlines to submit the required information. Be aware that some employers require an employment commitment in return for financial assistance. Leaving your place of employment before fulfilling this commitment may require you to repay all or part of the tuition.

Employers and professional organizations may provide opportunities for scholarships. Ask what's available and the specific requirements attached to the scholarship. Some may require a brief essay, a list of professional accomplishments, or a commitment following graduation. With the cost of higher education, it's well worth the time to apply. Even a $100 scholarship can help pay for books and school supplies.

Equipment

In today's technological world, a computer is a necessity. Internet access is also essential for research and communication. Even if you select a program without an online component, you're required to type your papers. As a student, you will have computer access to information on the books and articles available at your institution's library. Some programs allow you to email your papers directly to faculty, saving on paper, printer ink, and time. If you need to review or expand your computer skills, check the local library or community programs for classes on basic computer use.

EDUCATIONAL PROGRAMS

RN to BSN programs

If your initial nursing education is an associate's degree or a diploma from a hospital-based school of nursing, you may wish to further your education. Pursuing a baccalaureate degree may be the first step on your educational path.

Many schools have articulation agreements that support the educational mobility of RNs and facilitate the transfer of academic credit between associate degree nursing programs and baccalaureate nursing programs. Depending on your location, there are different articulation agreements; however, most allow the transfer of 60 credits. If you have a diploma from a hospital-based school of nursing, you may be required to take the College Level Examination Program® (CLEP) exams to receive credit for courses previously taken without college credit.

Degree completion programs provide RNs with additional education and build on previous knowledge, preparing them for a higher level of practice. Many hospitals require the baccalaureate degree for management positions.

RN to BSN programs include course work to enhance professional development and discuss the current political, cultural, and social issues that impact patient care delivery. If you wish to pursue a BSN degree there are many programs available.

According to the American Association of Colleges of Nursing (AACN) there are more than 600 RN to BSN programs available in the United States. (See *Accelerated baccalaureate and master's degree programs in nursing*, pages 616 to 619.) Program length can vary from 12 to 24 months, based upon facility requirements or previous college credits. Some RN/BSN programs offer complete online degrees, provide satellite campuses, or offer a combination of classroom and online courses.

BSN degree requirements can vary from 120 credits to 126 credits. Most require a "bridge course" as a transition course. This course serves as an introductory course and will help set the pace for your continuing education. The curriculum includes standard courses including upper division English, history, and foreign language courses and other electives. Course work specific to

nursing may include health assessment, informatics, research, cultural diversity, and community health. Clinical course work varies depending upon the institution. If you are a practicing RN, clinical course work will be different from your initial education and may be completed in the evening or weekend hours.

RN to MSN programs

Some universities offer a program that allows the RN to complete a bachelor's degree and a master's of science in nursing (MSN) degree simultaneously. According to the American Association of Colleges of Nursing, there are 137 programs available in the United States for RNs with diplomas or associate degrees who are interested in pursing a master's degree. These programs prepare RNs to assume the advanced practice nursing (APN) positions of clinical nurse specialist, certified nurse midwife, nurse practitioner, and certified registered nurse anesthetist as well as prepare them for roles in nursing education, nursing administration, or public health/community nursing.

The RN to MSN program builds the BSN level content into the beginning of the program. These programs can take about 3 years to complete, depending upon the requirements of the institution, previous academic course work, and whether the student attends classes on a part- or full-time basis. Upon completion of the BSN content of the program, the student continues to MSN-level work.

Some programs offer a component of the RN to MSN program online. Check with the specific institution to determine what's available. As for clinical requirements, a program with master's degree content that prepares you for an APN role

(Text continues on page 619.)

Accelerated baccalaureate and master's degree programs in nursing

This list is based on responses to the American Association of Colleges of Nursing (AACN) 2005-2006 survey of nursing schools and on information provided by individual programs. All schools listed offer accelerated baccalaureate programs (BSN) unless otherwise indicated. Schools with accelerated master's programs (MN, MS, or MSN) are identified after the school name.

Alabama
Auburn University
Samford University
University of South Alabama (BSN and MSN)

Arizona
Grand Canyon University
North Arizona University
University of Arizona

California
Azusa Pacific University (BSN and MSN)
California State University—Long Beach
California State University—Los Angeles (MSN)
Loma Linda University
Mount St. Mary's College
National University
Samuel Merritt College (BSN and MSN)
San Francisco State University (MSN)
San Jose State University
Sonoma State University (MSN)
University of California-San Francisco (MSN)
University of San Diego (MSN)
University of San Francisco (MSN)
Western University of Health Sciences (MSN)

Colorado
Colorado State University—Pueblo
Metropolitan State College of Denver
Regis University
University of Colorado at Colorado Springs
University of Colorado at Health Sciences Center

University of Northern Colorado

Connecticut
Fairfield University
Quinnipiac University
Saint Joseph College
University of Connecticut (MSN)
Yale University (MSN)

Delaware
University of Delaware

District of Columbia
Georgetown University (BSN and MSN)
Howard University
Catholic University of America

Florida
Barry University
Florida Atlantic University
Florida International University
Jacksonville University (BSN and MSN)
University of Central Florida
University of Florida
University of Miami (BSN and MSN)
University of North Florida
University of South Florida
University of Tampa (MSN)

Georgia
Emory University
Georgia Southwestern State University
Georgia State University
Kennesaw State University
Valdosta State University

Hawaii
University of Hawaii at Manoa

Idaho
Idaho State University
Lewis-Clark State College

Illinois
Blessing-Rieman College of Nursing
DePaul University (MSN)
Lake College of Nursing
Lewis University
Loyola University Chicago
Rush University
University of Illinois at Chicago
West Suburban College of Nursing

Accelerated baccalaureate and master's degree programs in nursing *(continued)*

Indiana
Indiana University—Purdue University
Indiana University—South Bend
Marian College
Purdue University
Purdue University—Calumet
Saint Mary's College
University of Southern Indiana
Valparaiso University

Iowa
Allen College
University of Iowa (MSN)

Kansas
MidAmerica Nazarene University

Kentucky
Bellarmine University
Eastern Kentucky University
Northern Kentucky University
Spalding University
University of Kentucky
University of Louisville

Louisiana
Louisiana State University Health
  Sciences Center
Southeastern Louisiana University
University of Louisiana at Lafayette
University of Louisiana at Monroe

Maine
University of Maine
University of Maine—Fort Kent
University of Southern Maine (BSN
  and MSN)

Maryland
Johns Hopkins University
Salisbury University
University of Maryland
Villa Julie College/Union Memorial

Massachusetts
Boston College (MSN)
Curry College
MGH Inst. of Health Professions
  (MSN)
Northeastern University (BSN and
  MSN)
Regis College (MSN)
Simmons College (BSN and MSN)

University of Massachusetts—
  Amherst
University of Massachusetts—
  Dartmouth
University of Massachusetts—
  Worcester (MSN)

Michigan
Michigan State University
Northern Michigan University
Oakland University
University of Detroit Mercy
University of Michigan
Wayne State University

Minnesota
College of St. Catherine
Concordia College
Metropolitan State University
Minnesota State University—Mankato

Missouri
Barnes-Jewish College
Lester L. Cox College of Nursing
Research College of Nursing
Saint Louis University
University of Missouri—Columbia
University of Missouri—St. Louis
William Jewell College

Nebraska
Creighton University
Nebraska Methodist College

Nevada
Nevada State College
Touro University (BSN and MSN)

New Hampshire
University of New Hampshire (MSN)

New Jersey
Fairleigh Dickinson University
Rutgers, The State University of New
  Jersey
Seton Hall University
University of Medicine & Dentistry of
  New Jersey (BSN and MSN)
William Patterson University

New Mexico
New Mexico State University
University of New Mexico

(continued)

Accelerated baccalaureate and master's degree programs in nursing *(continued)*

New York
Adelphi University
Binghamton University
College of New Rochelle
Columbia University (BSN and MSN)
Dominican College
Hartwick College
Molloy College
Mount Saint Mary College
New York University
Pace University (BSN and MS)
SUNY/Downstate Medical Center
SUNY/Stony Brook
SUNY/University at Buffalo
Syracuse University
The Sage Colleges
University of Rochester (BSN and MSN)
Wagner College

North Carolina
Barton College
Duke University
East Carolina University (MSN)
University of North Carolina—Chapel Hill
Winston-Salem State University

North Dakota
Medcenter One College of Nursing

Ohio
Case Western Reserve University (BSN and MSN)
Cleveland State University
College of Mount St. Joseph (MN)
Kent State University
MedCentral College of Nursing
Medical University of Ohio (MSN)
The Ohio State University (MS)
University of Akron
University of Cincinnati (BSN and MSN)
Ursuline College
Wright State University
Xavier University (MSN)

Oklahoma
Oklahoma Baptist University
Oklahoma City University
University of Oklahoma

Oregon
Linfield College
Oregon Health & Science University (MSN)
University of Portland (MSN)

Pennsylvania
Bloomsburg University
College Misericordia
DeSales University
Drexel University
Duquesne University
Edinboro University of Pennsylvania
La Salle University
Robert Morris University
Temple University
Thomas Jefferson University (MSN)
University of Pennsylvania (BSN and MSN)
University of Pittsburgh
Villanova University
Waynesburg College
Wilkes University (MSN)
York College of Pennsylvania

South Carolina
Lander University
Medical University of South Carolina

South Dakota
South Dakota State University

Tennessee
Belmont University
Cumberland University
East Tennessee State University
Union University
University of Memphis (BSN and MSN)
University of Tennessee—Knoxville (MSN)
Vanderbilt University (MSN)

Texas
Texas Christian University
Texas Tech University Health Sciences Center
Texas Woman's University
University of Texas—Austin (MSN)
University of Texas—El Paso
University of Texas Health Science Center—Houston
University of Texas Medical Branch

Accelerated baccalaureate and master's degree programs in nursing *(continued)*

Utah
University of Utah

Virginia
Eastern Mennonite University
George Mason University
Hampton University
Liberty University
Lynchburg College
Marymount University
Norfolk State University
Shenandoah University
University of Virginia (BSN and MSN)
Virginia Commonwealth University
(BSN and MSN)

Washington
Pacific Lutheran University (MSN)
Seattle University (MSN)
University of Washington (MSN)

West Virginia
Mountain State University
West Virginia University

Wisconsin
Bellin College of Nursing
Marquette University (MSN)
University of Wisconsin—Milwaukee
(BSN and MSN)
University of Wisconsin—Oshkosh

will have more clinical content, usually requiring a minimum of 500 hours of clinical practicum. Check with the institution for the specific clinical requirement.

MSN programs

Some programs offer an MSN education *only* to the RN who has already obtained a BSN degree. These programs build on your BSN education and provide additional course work in advanced theory and practice in a specific clinical area, such as nurse practitioner, clinical nurse specialist, nurse midwife, nurse anesthetist, nurse educator, public health/community nursing, and nurse administrator. (See *Degree specialties,* pages 620 and 621.) Currently there are more than 300 master's degree programs for nurses available in the United States. These include:

• master of nursing (MN)
• master of science (MS)
• MSN.

Combination or joint master's degrees include:

• MSN and a master of business administration (MBA), or MSN/MBA

• MSN and a master's degree in public health (MPH), or MSN/MPH
• MSN and a master's degree in health administration (MSHA), or MSNS/MSHA.

Regardless of the type of program, the curriculum requirements for the master's degree are similar. All programs have a core of graduate courses which include research, health/social policy, organizational theory, role development, theoretical foundations of nursing, ethics, diversity, and health promotion and disease prevention. If you are seeking an APN degree, the core curriculum also includes health and physical assessment, physiology, pathophysiology, and pharmacology. After completing the core courses, taking courses specific to the advanced practice specialty are necessary—for example, if you're seeking a degree as a pediatric nurse practitioner, your courses will be specific to the pediatric population. If you're seeking a degree in nursing education, administration, or public health, your specific course work begins following the general graduate core courses.

Degree specialties

Specialized areas of nursing include clinical nurse leader, clinical nurse specialist, nurse administrator, nurse anesthetist, nurse educator, nurse midwife, nurse practitioner, and public/community nurse. Each position is known as an advanced practice nurse (APN).

Clinical Nurse Leader

The clinical nurse leader is a new nursing role designated by the American Association of Colleges of Nursing (AACN). Per the AACN, this role requires a master's degree and is described as a nurse who designs, implements, and evaluates client care by coordinating, delegating, and supervising the care provided by the health care team, including licensed nurses, technicians, and other health care professionals.

Clinical Nurse Specialist

A clinical nurse specialist (CNA) is an APN who focuses on a specific patient population and divides her practice into five general areas, including:
- clinical practice
- teaching
- research
- consulting
- management.
  A CNA can focus on:
- acute care
- geriatrics
- adult health
- community health
- critical care
- gerontology
- rehabilitation
- cardiovascular
- surgery
- oncology
- maternity/newborn
- pediatric
- mental/psychiatric
- women's health.

The CNA can also provide a range of care in specialty areas, such as oncology, pediatrics, and cardiac, neonatal, obstetric/gynecological, neurological, and psychiatric nursing.

Web site of interest
The National Association of Clinical Nurse Specialists: *www.nacns.org*

Nursing Administrator

The nurse administrator works in a variety of health care settings, including:
- hospitals
- long-term care facilities
- community heath care agencies.

The nurse administrator's responsibilities can include developing a plan for nursing practice in an organization, making decisions for the organization, problem solving, managing conflict resolution, managing personnel hiring and management, acting as an advocate for patients and staff, allocating resources, and preparing budgets.

Course work specific to the nurse administrator role can include strategic management, organizational behavior, health systems management, continuous quality improvement, policy development, human resources, financial management and budget planning, and leadership.

Nurse Anesthetist

A certified nurse anesthetist (CRNA) is an APN with the ability to administer anesthesia to patients. The CRNA practices in a range of settings, including:
- hospital surgical suite
- obstetrical setting
- ambulatory care surgery setting
- physicians' office
- dentists' office
- wound care center
- pain center.

The programs specific for nurse anesthetists usually require full-time enrollment and can range from 24 to 36 months. Most programs require a minimum of 1 year of acute care nursing experience. Individual programs determine what constitutes acute care nursing—for some it's 1 year in an intensive care unit; for others it may be 1 year in an emergency department.

The classroom curriculum, after completion of the core curriculum for

Degree specialties *(continued)*

a master's degree, includes anatomy and physiology, pathophysiology, and pharmacology. The clinical component of the program provides the students with a variety of clinical rotations to experience the different types of surgical settings where anesthesia is provided. All students are required to pass a national certification examination following graduation from the program and must obtain a minimum of 40 hours of continuing education every 2 years.

Web site of interest
The American Associate of Nurse Anesthetists: *www.aana.com*

Nurse Educator

The nurse educator works in the classroom and clinical setting providing education to student nurses as well as staff nurses. Nurse educators are responsible for designing, implementing, and evaluating academic and continued education programs for registered nurses. Their practice setting can include:

- hospital-based schools of nursing
- community colleges
- college universities
- community health care agencies
- hospitals
- home care agencies
- long-term care facilities.

Specific course work designed for the nurse educator includes curriculum design and evaluation, teaching strategies, clinical evaluation, and test construction and also involves a teaching practicum where the student can teach in a nursing program.

Nurse Midwife

The nurse midwife provides a range of women's health care. She provides routine prenatal and gynecological care, delivers babies in private settings and in hospitals, and follows patients postpartum.

Web site of interest
American College of Nurse Midwives: *www.midwife.org*

Nurse Practitioner

Depending upon her practice setting, the nurse practitioner (NP) carries out a number of functions in her role. The NP is authorized to practice across the nation and has prescriptive privileges of varying degrees in 49 states. There are numerous programs for nurse practitioners with a variety of practice settings available. Not all schools offer all programs.

The NP conducts physical exams; diagnoses and treats common acute illnesses and injuries; administers immunizations; manages chronic problems, such as high blood pressure and diabetes; and orders laboratory services, X-rays, and medications.

Specific NP programs include:
- Family NP
- Pediatric NP
- Adult NP
- Geriatric NP
- Women's Health Care NP
- Neonatal NP
- Acute Care NP.

Web sites of interest
American Academy of Nurse Practitioners: *www.aanp.org*
American College of Nurse Practitioners: *www.acnpweb.org*

Public Health/Community Nurse

The public health/community nurse works with the broad health care needs of a population, with a focus on the community rather than the individual patient. Nursing interventions are based on the needs of the community with a strong emphasis on disease prevention and health promotion.

Web site of interest
Association of Community Health Nursing Educators: *www.ACHNE.org*

Doctoral degree
For the nurse who possesses a master's degree and wishes to further

her education, the doctoral degree is available. Nurses with doctoral degrees teach, conduct research, and can be employed in academic settings, private business, health care arenas, and government. For academic settings, colleges and universities, the doctoral degree is preferred. There are different doctoral degrees in nursing—the doctor of philosophy (PhD) and the doctorate of nursing science (DNSc). The PhD prepares nurse scholars and researchers, and the DNSc prepares nurse scientists. Both degrees focus on research, and both are appropriate for the academic setting.

Each university determines its admission criteria. Generally, applicants are required to take the Graduate Record Examination (GRE), have a specified grade point average, submit letters of reference and a writing sample, and may be required to interview at the school. Doctoral study can be conducted on a part-time basis, although there are full-time programs available. The average time for completion of the program is 5 years, but students are usually allowed a maximum of 7 to 8 years to complete the doctoral program.

In most programs doctoral students complete specified course work and then take an examination to demonstrate mastery of the subject matter. Once successful, they become doctoral candidates and can proceed to dissertation.

The core courses in a nursing doctoral program include theory, theory development, research methodology, research analysis, philosophy, and ethics. The curriculum also includes courses that will help dissertation research.

There are programs offering a MSN/PhD degree to qualified nurses who possess a bachelor's degree. This program offers master's course work and doctoral course work simultaneously, allowing you to complete your MSN and PhD at the same time. The program can be completed in 5 years.

DNP programs
The doctor of nursing practice (DNP) is a relatively new, clinical-based degree and is similar to degrees in other practice disciplines including pharmacy (PharmD), occupational therapy, and physical therapy. The program is clinically focused, not research focused, and a dissertation isn't required. Nurses who wish to pursue an academic focus may opt for the PhD and the DNS/DNSc programs because these programs are more research oriented and require a dissertation.

15   Nursing specialties

Besides being a noble occupation dedicated to providing care and comfort to others, the nursing profession offers numerous career paths to its members. Presently, the nursing field has more than 60 specialty options. (See *Nursing specialties*.) Some specialties require formal advanced education (see chapter 14, Nursing education) while others provide on-the-job training in the form of classes, self-study, and clinical orientation.

Multiple professional organizations have formed to support their specialties and offer certification in their fields. (See *Nurse certification organizations*, pages 624 and 625.) Certification is a testimonial to the expertise of the nurses in that specialty. This chapter provides information on nursing specialties and certification and offers resources for additional information.

Nursing specialties

Here are some of the many career paths that a nurse may choose.

- Ambulatory care*
- Cardiac care*
  - cardiothoracic surgery*
  - cardiac rehabilitation
  - cardiac catheterization laboratory
- Case management*
- Community (public health)*
  - college health*
  - home health*
  - school*
  - parish
- Critical care*
  - burns
  - cardiac
  - medical
  - neonatal
  - neurological
  - pediatric
  - pulmonary
  - surgical
  - trauma
- Education
  - academic teaching
  - childbirth*
  - clinical nurse specialist*

  - diabetic teaching*
  - staff development
- Emergency*
  - acute care
  - flight*
  - transport*
- Forensics*
  - correctional nurse
  - death investigators
  - domestic violence specialists
  - legal nurse consultant*
  - nurse attorney
  - sexual assault nurse examiners*
- Gastroenterology*
- Genetics*
- Gerontology*
- Health care quality*
- HIV/AIDS*
- Holistic*
- Hospice and palliative care*
- Hyperbarics
- Infection control*
- Informatics*
- Infusion*
- Managed care*
- Medical-surgical*
- Nephrology*
  - dialysis

(continued)

Nursing specialties *(continued)*

– transplant
· Neuroscience*
· Nurse anesthetist*
· Nurse midwife*
· Nurse practitioner*
· Nursing administration*
· Obstetrical and gynecological
  – labor and delivery
  – lactation consultant*
  – perinatal*
  – postpartum
  – neonatal*
  – women's health*
  – nurse midwife*
· Nutrition support*
· Occupational health*
· Oncology*
· Operating room (OR)
  – perianesthesia*
  – perioperative*
  – postanesthesia*
· Ophthalmic*

· Orthopedic*
· Otorhinolaryngology and head-neck*
· Pain management*
· Pediatric*
· Plastic and reconstructive surgery*
· Progressive care*
· Psychiatric and mental health (behavioral health)*
  – addictions nursing*
· Publishing
· Radiology
· Rehabilitation*
· Research
· Risk management
· Sales (pharmaceutical or equipment)
· Telephone nursing*
· Travel
· Urology*
· Wound and ostomy care*

*Certification available

Nurse certification organizations

These nursing organizations offer certifications in nursing specialties.

American Association of Critical-Care Nurses
www.certcorp.org
American Academy of Nurse Practitioners
www.aanp.org
American Association of Neuroscience Nurses
www.aann.org
American Board for Occupational Health Nurses
www.abohn.org
American Board of Perianesthesia Nursing Certification
www.cpancapa.org
American Nurses Credentialing Center
www.nursecredentialing.org
Board of Certification for Emergency Nursing
www.ena.org/bcen
Canadian Nurses Association Certification Program
www.cna-nurses.ca

Certification Board Perioperative Nurses
www.certboard.org
Council on Certification of Nurse Anesthetists
www.aana.com
Infusion Nurses Certification Corporation
www.ins1.org
National Board for Certification of Hospice and Palliative Nurses
www.hpna.org
National Certification Board for Diabetes Educators
www.ncbde.org
National Certification Board of Pediatric Nurse Practitioners and Nurses
www.napnap.org
National Certification Corporation for the Obstetric, Gynecologic, and Neonatal Specialties
www.nccnet.org
Nephrology Nursing Certificate Commission
www.nncc-exam.org

Nurse certification organizations *(continued)*

Oncology Nursing Certification
   Corporation
   www.oncc.org
Orthopaedic Nurses Certification
   Board
   www.orthonurse.org/certification

Rehabilitation Nursing Certification
   Board
   www.rehabnurse.org

Ambulatory care nursing

Ambulatory care nurses treat patients on an outpatient basis. They deal with acute and chronic illness on an episodic basis, act to promote wellness and prevent illness, and help the patient maintain optimal health. They work in such settings as health care facilities, community clinics, dialysis centers, schools, workplaces, urgent care centers, and pain management centers.

Education requirements
Current RN license, on-the-job training, or orientation

Certification
Registered nurse, certified (RN, C) recognizes nurses who provide direct and indirect care to patients of all ages on an outpatient basis.

Certifying body
American Nurses Credentialing Center (ANCC)

Examination
This is a 3½-hour pen and pencil examination consisting of 125 multiple-choice questions (100 scored and 25 nonscored pretest questions). Questions focus on triage assessment, technical skills, care management, patient advocacy, interpersonal skills, cultural competency, telepractice and multimedia use, documentation, professional role, legal issues, standards of care, systems operations, performance improvement, and patient education.

Eligibility
Candidates must have:

• a diploma, associate, baccalaureate, or higher nursing degree
• unrestricted RN or APRN licensure in the United States or its territories
• practiced for the equivalent of 2 years full-time
• practiced 2,000 clinical hours caring for patients in a defined ambulatory care setting within the past 3 years
• completed 30 contact hours within the past 3 years.

Renewal
• Every 5 years
• Professional development requirements: complete minimum of two of five categories or double any single category
   – continuing education requirements: 75 contact hours (with 51% of education hours in your specialty)
   – academic courses: 5 semester hour credits (course content applicable to your area of certification)
   – presentations and lectures: 5 different presentations on your specialty
   – publications and research: one published book article or chapter, one research project, development of one educational topic in media form (such as a CD, or completion of a master's thesis or doctoral dissertation)
   – preceptorships: 120 hours
• 1,000 practice hours or option to retest

Web site
www.nursecredentialing.org

Cardiac nursing

Cardiac nurses help patients with cardiovascular disease achieve and maintain optimal cardiac health. They work in such settings as cardiac intensive care unit or critical care unit, interventional cardiology unit, cardiac catheterization and electrophysiology labs, cardiothoracic intensive care units, telemetry units, heart failure clinics, and cardiac rehabilitation units. Education requirements for all of these certifications are a current registered nurse (RN) license or on-the-job training or orientation. A critical care course may be required in some institutions.

Certification
Cardiac/vascular nurse certification (Registered Nurse, Board-Certified [RN, BC]) recognizes nurses who care for patients diagnosed with, or at risk for, cardiovascular disease.

Certifying body
American Nurses Credentialing Center

Examination
This is a 3½-hour examination consisting of 175 multiple-choice questions focusing on the care of the cardiac or vascular patient in acute and ambulatory care settings. Computer-based testing is offered year-round at more than 300 testing centers throughout the United States. Paper and pencil examinations are available in May and October.

Eligibility
Candidates must have:
• a diploma, associate, baccalaureate or higher nursing degree
• unrestricted RN or advanced practice registered nurse (APRN) licensure in the United States or its territories
• been in practice for the equivalent of 2 years full-time
• practiced 2,000 clinical hours caring for cardiac patients in the past 3 years
• completed 30 contact hours within the past 3 years.

Renewal
• Every 5 years
• Professional development requirements: complete minimum of two of five categories or double any single category
  – continuing education requirements: 75 contact hours (with 51% of education hours in your specialty)
  – academic courses: 5 semester hour credits (course content applicable to your area of certification)
  – presentations and lectures: 5 different presentations on your specialty
  – publications and research: one published book article or chapter, one research project, development of one educational topic in media form (such as a CD, or completion of a master's thesis or doctoral dissertation)
  – preceptorships: 120 hours
• 1,000 practice hours or option to retest

Web site
www.nursecredentialing.org

Certification
Critical care registered nurse (CCRN) is a certification that recognizes nurses who provide care for critically ill patients.

Certifying body
American Association of Critical Care Nurses (AACN)

Examination
This is a 3-hour examination consisting of 150 multiple-choice questions focusing on clinical judgment related to patient problems and nursing interventions. Computer-based testing is offered year-round at more than 100 testing centers throughout the United States. Paper and pencil examinations are available at the National Testing Institute.

Cardiac nursing *(continued)*

Eligibility
Candidates must have:
· an unrestricted RN or APRN license in the United States or its territories
· 1,750 hours in direct bedside care during the previous 2 years, with 875 of those hours accrued in the year preceding application caring for the acutely or critically ill patient.

Renewal
· Every 3 years
· 100 continuing education recognition points (CERPs) or reexamination
· 432 practice hours within the 3 years, with 144 of those hours in the year preceding renewal
· Education and patient care: must focus on the care or supervision of care of the acutely or critically ill patient.

Web site
www.certcorp.org

Certification
Cardiac medicine certification (CMC) is a subspecialty certification that recognizes nurses who provide care for acutely ill cardiac patients. *Cardiac surgery certification* (CSC) is a subspecialty certification that recognizes nurses who provide care for acutely ill cardiac patients during the first 48 hours after surgery.

Certifying body
AACN

Examination
This is a 2-hour examination consisting of 90 multiple-choice questions focusing on clinical judgment related to patient problems and nursing interventions. Computer-based testing is offered year-round at more than 100 testing centers throughout the United States. Paper and pencil examinations are available at the National Testing Institute.

Eligibility
Candidates must have:
· unrestricted RN or APRN licensure in the United States or its territories
· 1,750 hours in direct bedside care during the previous 2 years, with 875 of those hours accrued in the year preceding application caring for the acutely ill cardiac patient (CMC), or cardiac surgery patients during first 48 hours after surgery (CSC)
· current nationally accredited clinical nursing specialty certification.

Renewal
· Every 3 years
· 25 category "A" CERPs
· 432 practice hours within the 3 years, with 144 of those hours in the year preceding renewal
· education and patient care must focus on the care of critically ill cardiac patients (CMC) or cardiac surgery patients in the first 48 hours after surgery (CSC).

Web site
www.certcorp.org

Case management nursing

Case management nurses help coordinate health care services to patients, families, and communities with identified needs. The case manager extends her professional role to include: patient advocate, facilitator, provider, liaison, coordinator, collaborator, negotiator, educator, risk manager, and consultant. They're required to manage the assessment, planning, implementation, evaluation, and interaction of individualized health plans, as each patient may have a unique set of circumstances that challenge achieving optimal health. They work in acute care facilities, long-term care facilities, Health Maintenance Organizations, case management companies, community health centers, behavioral health centers, and rehabilitation centers.

Education requirements
A current registered nurse (RN) license, on-the-job training, or orientation; certification required in some facilities

Certification
Certified case manager (CCM) distinction recognizes nurses who provide coordination of an individualized health plan to patients, families, and communities with identified needs.

Certifying body
Commission for Case Management Certification (CCMC)

Examination
The examination is administered in April and October at specified sites. Exam content focuses on essential processes and relationships, health care management, communications and support, service delivery, psychological intervention, and rehabilitation case management.

Eligibility
Candidates must:
- have good moral character
- meet acceptable standards of quality in their practice
- possess a diploma, associate, baccalaureate, or higher nursing degree
- have unrestricted RN or advanced practice registered nurse (APRN) licensure in the United States or its territories
- obtain certification by having met predetermined qualifications by a credentialing body and having passed an examination; must be current and active and in good standing.
- qualify under one of CCMC's employment experience categories
  – 12 months full-time case management employment supervised by a CCM
  – 24 months full-time case management employment
  – 12 months full-time case management employment as a supervisor of those who provide direct case management services
- provide a complete job description
- demonstrate that they apply essential activities (assessment, planning, implementation, coordination, monitoring, evaluation, and general outcomes) within a minimum of five of the six core components
  – case management concepts
  – case management principles and strategies
  – psychosocial and support systems
  – healthcare management and delivery
  – healthcare reimbursement
  – vocational concepts and strategies.

Renewal
- Every 5 years
- 80 education hours or retest
- Verify an active license or certification

Web site
www.ccmcertification.org

Certification
Registered nurse, certified (RN, C) recognizes nurses who provide coordination of an individualized health plan to patients, families, and communities with identified needs.

Case management nursing *(continued)*

Certifying body
American Nurses Credentialing Center

Examination
This is a 3½-hour pen and pencil examination consisting of 125 multiple-choice questions (100 scored and 25 nonscored pretest questions). Questions focus on triage assessment, technical skills, care management, patient advocacy, interpersonal skills, cultural competency, telepractice and multimedia use, documentation, professional role, legal issues, standards of care, systems operations, performance improvement, and patient education.

Eligibility
Candidates must have:
• a diploma or associate, baccalaureate, or higher nursing degree
• an unrestricted RN or APRN license in the United States or its territories
• practiced for the equivalent of 2 years full-time
• practiced 2,000 clinical hours providing case management in the past 3 years
• completed 30 contact hours within past 3 years.

Renewal
• Every 5 years
• Professional development requirements: complete minimum of two of 5 categories or double any single category
 – continuing education requirements: 75 contact hours (with 51% if education hours in your specialty)
 – academic courses: 5 semester hour credits (course content applicable to your area of certification)
 – presentations and lectures; 5 different presentations on your specialty
 – publications and research: one published book article or chapter, one research project, or development of one educational topic in media form (such as a CD, or completion of a master's thesis or doctoral dissertation)
 – preceptorships: 120 hours
• 1,000 practice hours or option to retest

Web site
www.nursecredentialing.org

Critical care nursing

Critical care nurses help critically ill patients achieve and maintain optimal health. They work in such settings as general intensive care units, specialty critical care units (burns, neurological, cardiac, cardiothoracic, medical, surgical, trauma, pulmonary), and neonatal or pediatric intensive care units.

Education requirements

A current registered nurse (RN) license, on-the-job training, or orientation; critical care course may be required in some institutions

Certification

Critical care registered nurse certification (CCRN) recognizes nurses who provide care for the critically ill patient.

Certifying body

American Association of Critical Care Nurses

Examination

This is a 3-hour examination consisting of 150 multiple-choice questions focusing on clinical judgment related to patient problems and nursing interventions. Computer-based testing is offered year-round at more than 100 testing centers throughout the United States. Paper and pencil examinations are available at the National Testing Institute.

Eligibility

Candidates must have:
· unrestricted RN or advanced practice registered nurse licensure in the United States or its territories
· 1,750 hours in direct bedside care during the previous 2 years, with 875 of those hours accrued in the year preceding application caring for the acutely or critically ill patients.

Renewal

· Every 3 years
· 100 continuing education recognition points or reexamination
· 432 practice hours within the 3 years, with 144 of those hours in the year preceding renewal
· Education and patient care: must focus on the care or supervision of care of the acutely or critically ill patient

Web site

www.certcorp.org

Emergency care nursing

Emergency nurses provide emergency service for patients of all ages to help restore optimal health in acute situations. They work in acute care facilities, emergency medical services, ambulance transport services, flight rescue, or transport.

Education requirements
A current RN license, on-the-job training, or orientation; critical care course or trauma course may be required in some institutions

Certifications
Certified emergency nurse (CEN) recognizes nurses who provide emergency care for acutely ill patients.

Certifying body
Board of Certification for Emergency Nursing (BCEN)

Examination
This is a 3-hour examination consisting of 175 multiple-choice questions (150 scored and 25 nonscored pretest questions) focusing on:
- cardiovascular emergencies
- gastrointestinal emergencies
- obstetrical, gynecological, and genitourological emergencies
- maxillofacial and ocular emergencies
- neurological emergencies
- orthopedic emergencies and wound management
- psychological and social issues
- toxicological and environmental emergencies
- shock
- multisystem trauma
- communicable diseases
- professional issues.

The test is offered year-round at specified sites via computer.

Eligibility
Candidates must have:
- unrestricted RN or advanced practice registered nurse (APRN) licensure in the United States or its territories
- 2 years of experience in emergency nursing practice (recommended; not required).

Renewal
- Every 4 years
- 100 education hours, reexamination, or Internet based testing

Web site
www.ena.org

Certification
Certified flight registered nurse (CFRN) recognizes nurses who provide emergency care and air transport for the acutely ill patient.

Certifying body
BCEN

Examination
This is a 3-hour examination consisting of 175 multiple-choice questions (150 scored and 25 nonscored pretest questions) focusing on the same issues listed for the CEN examination, as well as knowledge of advanced airway care, transport considerations, safety issues, disaster management, and survival. This computer-based test is offered year-round at specified testing sites.

Eligibility
Candidates must have:
- unrestricted RN or APRN licensure in the United States or its territories
- 2 years experience in flight nursing practice (recommended; not required).

Renewal
- Every 4 years
- 100 education hours or reexamination

Web site
www.ena.org

Certification
Certified transport registered nurse (CTRN) recognizes nurses who provide emergency care and ground transport for acutely ill patients.

Certifying body
BCEN

Examination
This is a 3-hour examination consisting of 155 multiple-choice questions

(continued)

Emergency care nursing *(continued)*

(130 scored and 25 nonscored pretest questions) focusing on the same issues listed for the CEN examination as well as knowledge of advanced airway care, transport considerations, safety issues, disaster management, and survival. This computer-based test is offered year-round at specified testing sites.

Eligibility
Candidates must have:
• unrestricted RN or APRN licensure in the United States or its territories
• 2 years of experience in flight nursing practice (recommended; not required).

Renewal
• Every 4 years
• 100 education hours or reexamination

Web site
www.ena.org

Forensic nursing

Forensic nurses provide care to both victims of crime and criminals themselves, assist law enforcement personnel with collection of evidence, and evaluate injuries and circumstances involved with trauma. They work in correctional facilities, community health centers, acute care facilities, law offices, government agencies, and behavioral health facilities.

Education requirements
A current registered nurse (RN) license; advanced education with focus on forensics in the form of classes or a certificate for certain areas; certificate or certification in legal nurse consulting

Certifications
Certified forensic nurse (CFN) recognizes nurses who utilize knowledge and training in any designated field of forensic nursing.

Certifying body
American College of Forensic Examiners Institute (ACFEI)

Examination
This is a 4-hour examination consisting of 100 multiple-choice questions focusing on:
• the history of forensic nursing
• the forensic nursing process
• violence and victimology
• injury evaluation and documentation
• forensic science
• legalities
• homicide
• sexual assault
• correctional nursing
• legal nurse consulting
• domestic violence involving adults and children.

Computer-based testing is offered year-round is at specified sites.

Eligibility
Candidates must have:
• unrestricted RN or advanced practice registered nurse (APRN) licensure in the United States or its territories
• 5 years of nursing experience
• completed a formal forensic education course with a minimum of 40 contact hours, or a 3 academic hours accredited coursework
• their competency determined and documented by supervision in forensic practice
• an ACFEI membership in good standing
• two professional references.

Renewal
• Every year
• Complete 15 education hours
• Maintain active membership in ACFEI (annual renewal)

Web site
www.acfei.com

Forensic nursing *(continued)*

Certification
Sexual assault nurse examiner—adults/adolescents (SANE—AA) certification recognizes nurses who provide care, collect evidence, document events, and provide legal testimony in cases of sexual assault of adult or adolescent patients.

Certifying body
International Association of Forensic Nurses

Examination
This is a 4-hour examination consisting of 150 to 200 multiple-choice questions focusing on:
 • the dynamics of sexual assault
 • evaluation and clinical management of the sexual assault victim
 • the judicial process
 • roles of the sexual assault response team
 • professional practice trends
 • knowledge of the issues, skills, and abilities needed to perform SANE duties.
  The test is offered twice per year at specified sites.

Eligibility
Candidates must have:
 • unrestricted RN or APRN licensure in the United States or its territories
 • 2 years of nursing experience
 • completed an adult/adolescent SANE education course with a minimum of 40 contact hours, or 3 academic hours accredited coursework
 • had their competency determined by supervision in SANE practice.

Renewal
 • Every 3 years
 • 45 education hours or reexamination
 • Current practice as a sexual assault nurse within the past 3 years

Web site
www.iafn.org

Certification
Certified legal nurse consultant (CLNC) recognizes nurses who combine professional expertise with specialized training to consult on medically related legal cases.

Certifying body
National Alliance of Certified Legal Nurse Consultants (NACLNC)

Examination
This is a 2-hour examination consisting of 150 multiple-choice questions focusing on:
 • the role of the legal nurse consultant
 • the litigation process
 • liability and defense theories
 • personal injury
 • product liability
 • toxic tort
 • workman's compensation cases
 • medical records screening
 • case evaluation
 • record tampering
 • standards of care
 • testifying
 • legal and ethical issues.
  The test is offered year-round via computer-based testing at specified sites or after completion of a certification seminar.

Eligibility
Candidates must have:
 • unrestricted RN or APRN licensure in the United States or its territories
 • completed a CLNC home-study certification program or a certification seminar; nurses with 3 years of full time legal nurse consulting may challenge the examination.

Renewal
 • Every 2 years
 • 15 education hours specific to legal consulting; retest; attend the NACLNC conference or listen to audio of conference and complete test (extends certification 1 year); attend a 2-day NACLNC apprenticeship program or private NACLNC apprenticeship program (extends certification one year)

Web site
www.legalnurse.com

Gerontological nursing

Gerontological nurses care for older adult patients. They work to identify the strengths and weaknesses of the older adult to provide appropriate care that maximizes health and improves quality of life. They work in acute care facilities, long-term care facilities, community health centers, homes, and senior centers.

Education requirements

Current registered nurse (RN) license, on-the-job training, or orientation

Certification

Registered nurse, board certified (RN, BC) recognizes nurses who provide direct and indirect care to elderly patients.

Certifying body

American Nurses Credentialing Center

Examination

This is a 3½-hour, computer-based examination consisting of 175 multiple-choice questions (150 scored and 25 nonscored pretest questions). Questions focus on:
• primary care considerations of the aging population
• theory
• communication
• death and dying
• problems of the major body systems
• medications
• pain
• health-care delivery systems
• federal regulations and reimbursement issues
• professional issues
• gerontological trends and issues.

Eligibility

Candidates must have:
• a diploma, associate, baccalaureate, or higher nursing degree
• unrestricted RN or advanced practice registered nurse licensure in the United States or its territories
• practiced for the equivalent of 2 years full-time
• practiced 2,000 clinical hours caring for older patients within the past 3 years
• completed 30 contact hours within past 3 years.

Renewal

• Every 5 years
• Complete professional development requirements: complete minimum of two of five categories or double any single category
  – continuing education requirements: 75 contact hours (with 51% if education hours in your specialty)
  – academic courses: 5 semester hour credits (course content applicable to your area of certification)
  – presentations and lectures: 5 different presentations on your specialty
  – publications and research: one published book article or chapter, one research project, or development of one educational topic in media form (such as a CD or completion of a master's thesis or doctoral dissertation)
  – preceptorships: 120 hours
• 1,000 practice hours or option to retest

Web site

www.nursecredentialing.org

Informatics nursing

Informatics nurses focus on the management of medical data. They develop, implement, support, and evaluate information systems to assist nurses with direct patient care. They work in acute care facilities, computer companies, consulting firms, insurance companies, and academic settings.

Education requirements

Current registered nurse (RN) licensure; advanced education with a focus on informatics

Certification

Registered nurse, board certified (RN, BC) recognizes nurses who are involved with information management that directly or indirectly affects patient care.

Certifying body

American Nurses Credentialing Center

Examination

This is a 3½-hour, computer-based examination consisting of 175 multiple-choice questions (150 scored and 25 nonscored pretest questions). Questions focus on models and theories of informatics, system planning, analysis, design, implementation, testing, evaluation, maintenance, and support. The test also deals with information technology, management, security, and professional trends and issues.

Eligibility

Candidates must have:
• a baccalaureate or higher nursing degree or a degree in a relevant field
• unrestricted RN or advanced practice registered nurse licensure in the United States or its territories

• practiced for the equivalent of 2 years full-time
• practiced 2,000 clinical hours involved in information management, or completed 12 semester hours in informatics and completed 1,000 clinical hours in informatics within the last 3 years, or completed a graduate nursing program that included 200 practicum hours
• completed 30 contact hours specific to informatics within the past 3 years (unless they just completed a graduate program).

Renewal

• Every 5 years
• Complete professional development requirements: complete minimum of two of five categories or double any single category
  – continuing education requirements: 75 contact hours (with 51% if education hours in your specialty)
  – academic courses: 5 semester hour credits (course content applicable to your area of certification)
  – presentations and lectures: 5 different presentations on your specialty
  – publications and research: one published book article or chapter, one research project, or development of one educational topic in media form (such as a CD or completion of a master's thesis or doctoral dissertation)
  – preceptorships: 120 hours
• 1,000 practice hours or option to retest

Web site

www.nursecredentialing.org

Infusion nursing

Infusion nurses provide infusion therapy to patients through the insertion of infusion devices and administration of fluids, blood products, medications, and nutritional therapy. They also focus on infection control, technology and clinical applications, and performance improvements. They work in acute care facilities, cancer centers, long-term care facilities, homes, and ambulatory care centers.

Education requirements
Current registered nurse (RN) license; advanced education with a focus on informatics

Certification
Certified registered nurse infusion (CRNI) recognizes nurses who administer parenteral therapy to patients.

Certifying body
Infusion Nurses Certification Corporation

Examination
This is a 3½-hour, computer-based examination consisting of 150 multiple-choice questions that focus on technology and clinical applications, fluid and electrolyte therapy, pharmacology, infection control, transfusions, antineoplastic therapy, parenteral nutrition, performance improvement, and pediatrics.

Eligibility
Candidates must have:
· a diploma, associate, baccalaureate, or higher nursing degree
· unrestricted RN or advanced practice registered nurse licensure in the United States or its territories
· the equivalent of 2 years of full-time practice
· the equivalent of 1,600 clinical practice hours involved in infusion therapy within the past two years.

Renewal
· Every 3 years
· 1,000 practice hours
· 40 education hours or retest

Web site
www.ins1.org

Medical-surgical nursing

Medical-surgical nurses provide care to acute care patients. Besides physical care, they provide patient education, case management, and discharge planning as well as psychological or psychosocial support and guidance. They work in acute care facilities, outpatient centers, and long-term care facilities.

Education requirements
Current registered nurse (RN) license, on-the-job training, and orientation

Certification
Registered nurse, board certified (RN, BC) recognizes nurses who provide care to patients during acute or chronic illness, or after surgery or injury.

Certifying body
American Nurses Credentialing Center

Examination
This is a 3½-hour, paper and pencil examination consisting of 175 multiple-choice questions (150 scored and 25 nonscored pretest questions). Questions focus on biophysical and psychosocial concepts, pathophysiology, patient care issues, and current issues and trends.

Eligibility
Candidates must have:
• a diploma, associate, baccalaureate, or higher nursing degree
• unrestricted RN or advanced practice registered nurse licensure in the United States or its territories
• practiced for the equivalent of 2 years full-time
• practiced 2,000 clinical hours involved in direct patient care
• completed 30 contact hours within past 3 years.

Renewal
• Every 5 years
• Professional development requirements: complete minimum of two of five categories or double any single category
  – continuing education requirements: 75 contact hours (with 51% if education hours in your specialty)
  – academic courses: 5 semester hour credits (course content applicable to your area of certification)
  – presentations and lectures: 5 different presentations on your specialty
  – publications and research: one published book article or chapter, one research project, or development of one educational topic in media form (such as a CD or completion of a master's thesis or doctoral dissertation)
  – preceptorships: 120 hours
• 1,000 practice hours or option to retest

Web site
www.nursecredentialing.org

Nursing administration

Nurse administrators are involved in the organizational aspects of nursing. They work on a management or executive level and are involved in providing appropriate policies, procedures, and resources to deliver optimal nursing care. This is a leadership role that involves quality outcomes, staff development, standards of care, and institutional growth. Nurse administrators work in all types of health care settings.

Education requirements
Current registered nurse (RN) license; usually requires advanced education in leadership and management.

Certification
Registered nurse, certified nurse administrator, board certified (RN, CNA, BC) recognizes nurses who are involved in managing a health care facility or service. Certification may also be granted to educators of graduate level students enrolled in an administrative track or program. *Registered nurse, certified nurse administrator, advanced, board certified* (RN, CNAA, BC) has the same requirements as the RN, CAN, BC except that eligibility requires a master's degree or higher and the nurse must hold an executive position.

Certifying body
American Nurses Credentialing Center

Examination
This is a 3½-hour, paper and pencil examination consisting of 175 multiple-choice questions (150 scored and 25 nonscored pretest questions). Questions focus on facility organization, structure and environment, budget economics, reimbursement and cost containment, staffing issues, professional ethics, and legal and regulatory issues.

Eligibility
Candidates must have:
• a baccalaureate or higher nursing degree
• unrestricted RN or advanced practice registered nurse licensure in the United States or its territories
• practiced for the equivalent of 2 years full-time and in an administrative position within the past 5 years
• participated in at least seven of the following activities:
  – administration of a health care organization
  – strategic and long-range planning of a health care organization
  – development of clinical and administrative nursing goals and directions
  – development of strategic plan to achieve clinical and administrative nursing goals and directions
  – assumption of responsibility of human, material, and financial resources for specific functions and activities
  – evaluation and revision of goals, structure, activities, and resources of organized nursing services
  – problem-solving leadership
  – human resource development and management leadership
  – ongoing evaluation of organization services
  – facilitation of research
  – performed as a role model to future administrators
• have a master's degree in nursing administration or have 30 contact hours within the past 2 years (with 20 hours involved with nursing administration).

Renewal
• Every 5 years
• Practiced 1,500 hours in a middle management or higher position or provided consultation services, or provided education and supervision to nursing students for the equivalent of 12 months in the past 5 years.
• Professional development requirements: complete minimum of two of 5 categories or double any single category

Nursing administration *(continued)*

– continuing education requirements: 75 contact hours (with 51% if education hours in your specialty)
– academic courses: 5 semester hour credits (course content applicable to your area of certification)
– presentations and lectures: 5 different presentations on your specialty

– publications and research: one published book article or chapter, one research project, or development of one educational topic in media form (such as a CD or completion of a master's thesis or doctoral dissertation)
– preceptorships: 120 hours

Web site
www.nursecredentialing.org

Obstetrical and gynecological nursing

Obstetrical and gynecological nurses care for female patients with a focus on pregnancy (before, during, and after), gynecological disorders, women's health, and neonates. They also focus on education concerning childbirth, breast-feeding, infant care and well-care (such as breast self-examination). They may be involved in case management by addressing the health care needs of women, their partners, and families as well as the psychological aspects of care. They work in acute care facilities, birthing centers, community health centers, adult education centers, and doctor's offices.

Education requirements
Current registered nurse (RN) license; some subspecialties require advanced education with a focus on education or obstetrics

Certification
Registered nurse, board certified (RN, BC) recognizes nurses who provide care to the patient during childbearing years.

Certifying body
American Nurses Credentialing Center

Examination
This is a 3½-hour, paper and pencil examination consisting of 175 multiple-choice questions (150 scored and 25 non-scored pre-test ques-

tions). Questions focus on issues and trends, antepartum, intrapartum and postpartum periods, neonatal knowledge, and care of the high-risk patient.

Eligibility
Candidates must have:
· a diploma, associate, baccalaureate, or higher nursing degree
· unrestricted RN or advanced practice registered nurse (APRN) licensure in the United States or its territories
· practiced for the equivalent of 2 years full-time
· completed 2,000 clinical hours involved in direct care of the obstetric or gynecologic patient
· completed 30 contact hours within the past 3 years.

Renewal
· Every 5 years
· Professional development requirements: complete minimum of two of five categories or double any single category
– continuing education requirements: 75 contact hours (with 51% if education hours in your specialty)
– academic courses: 5 semester hour credits (course content applicable to your area of certification)
– presentations and lectures: five different presentations on your specialty
– publications and research: one published book article or chapter,

(continued)

Obstetrical and gynecological nursing *(continued)*

one research project, or development of one educational topic in media form (such as a CD or completion of a master's thesis or doctoral dissertation)
– preceptorships: 120 hours
• 1,000 practice hours or option to retest

Web site
www.nursecredentialing.org

Certification
Registered nurse, certified (RN, C) in: *Inpatient obstetric nursing* (INPT), *Maternal newborn nursing* (MN), *Low risk neonatal* (LRN), and *Neonatal intensive care* (NIC) recognizes nurses who practice in the specific fields of inpatient obstetric nursing, maternal newborn nursing, and low-risk neonatal nursing.

Certifying body
National Certification Corporation

Examination
This is a 3-hour, paper and pencil or computer examination consisting of 160 multiple-choice questions (150 scored questions and 10 nonscored pretest questions). Questions are based on which area the nurse is being certified.
– INPT: 20-week pregnancy to discharge
– MN: care of the mother and neonate in various settings (hospital, home, and community)
– LRN: care of the neonate from birth to one month and family components
– NIC: care of the critically ill neonate

Eligibility
Candidates must have:
• a diploma, associate, baccalaureate, or higher nursing degree
• unrestricted RN or APRN licensure in the United States or its territories
• practiced for 2 years with 2,000 hours of practice
• been employed in the area of testing within the past two years.

Renewal
• Every 3 years
• 45 education hours or retest

Web site
www.nccnet.org

Pediatric nursing

Pediatric nurses provide care to child patients from infancy to adolescence. They provide patient education, case management, and discharge planning as well as psychological or psychosocial support and guidance. They work in acute care facilities, outpatient centers, community centers, home care agencies, and doctor offices.

Education requirements
Current registered nurse (RN) license, on-the-job training, and orientation

Certification
Certified pediatric nurse (CPN) recognizes nurses who provide care for child patients from infancy to adolescence.

Certifying body
Pediatric Nursing Certification Board

Examination
This is a 3½-hour, paper and pencil examination consisting of 175 multiple-choice questions (150 scored and 25 nonscored pretest questions). Questions focus on concepts of child health care, acute and chronic conditions, and professional issues and trends.

Eligibility
Candidates must have:
• a diploma, associate, baccalaureate, or higher nursing degree

Pediatric nursing *(continued)*

• unrestricted RN or advanced practice registered nurse (APRN) licensure in the United States or its territories
• practiced for the equivalent of 2 years full-time
• practiced 1,800 clinical hours in pediatric nursing.

Renewal
• Every year
• Four options
  – pediatric self-assessment examination (required one time in a 7-year cycle)
  – 10 education hours or 1 semester hour
  – 5 education hours and 200 clinical practice hours
  – inactive

Web site
www.pncb.org

Certification
Registered nurse, board certified (RN, BC) distinction recognizes nurses who provide care for the pediatric patient from infancy to adolescence.

Certifying body
American Nurses Credentialing Center

Examination
This is a 3½-hour, paper and pencil examination consisting of 175 multiple-choice questions (150 scored and 25 nonscored pretest questions). Questions focus on concepts of child health care, acute and chronic conditions, and professional issues and trends.

Eligibility
Candidates must have:
• a diploma, associate, baccalaureate, or higher nursing degree
• unrestricted RN or APRN licensure in the United States or its territories
• practiced for the equivalent of 2 years full-time
• practiced 2,000 clinical hours involved in direct patient care
• completed 30 contact hours within past 3 years.

Renewal
• Every 5 years
• Professional development requirements: complete minimum of two of 5 categories or double any single category
  – continuing education requirements: 75 contact hours (with 51% if education hours in your specialty)
  – academic courses: 5 semester hour credits (course content applicable to your area of certification)
  – presentations and lectures: 5 different presentations on your specialty
  – publications and research: one published book article or chapter, one research project, or development of one educational topic in media form (such as a CD) or completion of a master's thesis or doctoral dissertation
  – preceptorships: 120 hours
• 1,000 practice hours or option to retest

Web site
www.nursecredentialing.org

Selected references 645

Index 647

Selected references

Ancheta, I. "B-type Natriuretic Peptide Rapid Assay: A Diagnostic Test for Heart Failure," *Dimensions in Critical Care Nursing* 25(4):149-54, July-August 2006.

Best Practices: Evidence-Based Nursing Procedures, 2nd ed. Philadelphia: Lippincott Williams & Wilkins, 2006.

Costello, K., and Harris, C. "An Overview of Multiple Sclerosis: Diagnosis and Management Strategies," *Topics in Advanced Practice Nursing ejournal* 6(1), 2006. Available at *www.medscape.com/viewarticle/527706.*

Czarnecki, R. "Biventricular Pacing: When One or Two Leads Aren't Enough," *Nursing 2006 Critical Care* 1(4):30-37, July 2006.

Frizzell, J.P., et al. "Acute Stroke: Pathophysiology, Diagnosis, and Treatment," *AACN Clin Issues* 16(4):421-40, October-December 2005.

Hockenberry, M.J. *Wong's Essentials of Pediatric Nursing,* 7th ed. St. Louis: Mosby–Year Book, Inc., 2004.

Huszar, R. *Basic Dysrhythmias: Interpretation & Management,* 3rd ed. St. Louis: Mosby–Year Book, Inc., 2006.

Johnston, M., et al. "Models of Cerebral Palsy: Which Ones Are Best?" *Journal of Child Neurology* 21(5):984-87, 2005.

Luerssen, M.A., and Winsch, A.L. "Identifying and Treating Gestational Diabetes Mellitus: Advances in Screening and Current Intervention," *AJN* 105(4):65-71, April 2005.

Malarkey, L., and McMorrrow, M. *Saunders Nursing Guide to Laboratory and Diagnostic Tests,* 3rd ed. Philadelphia: W.B. Saunders Co., 2005.

Murray, S., and McKinney, E. *Foundations of Maternal-Newborn Nursing,* 4th ed. Philadelphia: W.B. Saunders Co., 2005.

Nursing Journal Series: Deciphering Diagnostic Tests. Philadelphia: Lippincott Williams & Wilkins, 2007.

Orshan, S. *Maternal, Newborn & Women's Health Nursing: Comprehensive Care Across the Lifespan.* Philadelphia: Lippincott Williams & Wilkins, 2007.

Potter, P., and Perry, P. *Fundamentals of Nursing,* 6th ed. St. Louis: Mosby–Year Book, Inc., 2004.

Professional Guide to Diseases, 8th ed. Philadelphia: Lippincott Williams & Wilkins, 2005.

Seidel, H.M., et al. *Mosby's Guide to Physical Examination,* 6th ed. St. Louis: Mosby–Year Book, Inc., 2006.

Taylor, C., et al. *Fundamentals of Nursing: The Art and Science of Nursing,* 6th ed. Philadelphia: Lippincott Williams & Wilkins, 2007.

Weber, J. *Nurses' Handbook of Health Assessment,* 6th ed. Philadelphia: Lippincott Williams & Wilkins, 2007.

Xiong, L., et al. "Genetics of Alzheimer's Disease and Research Frontiers in Dementia," *Geriatrics & Aging* 8(4):31-35, April 2005.

Index

A

Abdominal quadrants, 41i
Abrasion, caring for, 311
Accelerated baccalaureate and master's degree programs, 616-619t
Achilles reflex, assessing, 35i
Acquired immunodeficiency syndrome. *See* Human immunodeficiency virus.
Admission requirements for college, 613
Adolescent
  cognitive development of, 428
  growth rates for, 413t
  moral and spiritual development of, 428
  nutritional guidelines for, 468
  psychosocial development of, 428
  sleep guidelines for, 470t
  vital sign ranges in, 6-7t
Adult, vital sign ranges in, 6-7t
Advance directives, 597-598
Advanced practice nurse, 620
Adverse drug reactions
  misinterpretation of, as age-related changes, 182t
  preventing, in older patients, 183-190t
Advocate, nurse as, 592
Agency for Healthcare Research and Quality, 573
  guidelines from, 572
Age-related changes, 64, 64t, 65i
  adverse reactions misinterpreted as, 182t
Airborne precautions, 285
  indications for, 287t
Air splint, how to use, 269i
Alginate dressings, 317
Allen's test, performing, 214i
Alloimmunization. *See* Hemolytic disease of the newborn.

Alzheimer's disease, 472-474
  managing, 473
Ambulatory care nursing, 625
American Nurses Association Standard of Clinical Nursing Practice, 572-573, 574
Amniotic fluid analysis findings, 361t
Angina, electrocardiogram changes in, 81i
Ankle strength, testing, 53i
Anthropometric arm measurements, how to take, 328i
Antibiotic peaks and troughs, 135t
Antidotes, 195t
Antiembolism stockings
  applying, 271i
  measuring for, 270i
Antimicrobial dressings, 317
Antitachycardia pacing, 115t
Anxiety disorder, 61
Apgar scoring, 397t
Apnea, characteristics of, 24i
Arousal, altered, stages of, 31t
Arterial blood gas results, 130t
Arterial oxygen saturation, monitoring, 8
Arterial pulses, palpating, 17i
Arterial puncture, technique for, 215i
Arterial ulcers, treatment algorithm for, 314i
Ascorbic acid, daily requirements of, 332t
Assessment
  in children, 446i, 447i, 450, 451
  in neonate, 396, 399
  of pain, 62-63i, 296, 297i, 453, 454t, 455
  in pregnancy by weeks, 356-357
  10-minute, 2
Asthma, 474-476
Asystole, 100-101t
Atrial fibrillation, 96-97t
Atrial flutter, 96-97t

---

i refers to an illustration; t refers to a table.

Atrial gallop, 15t
Attention deficit hyperactivity disorder, 550-551
  diagnostic criteria for, 550-551
Auscultation
  of body sounds, 7i
  cardiac, positioning patient for, 13i
  sequence for, of chest, 26i
  sites of, for tympany and dullness, 42i
  for vascular sounds, 42i
Autistic disorder, 551-553
  diagnostic criteria for, 552
Automated external defibrillator, 103

B

Babinski's reflex, eliciting, 38i
Bag-mask device, how to use, 215i
Ballottement, 4i
Bandaging techniques, 216i
Bandi's ring, 377i
Barrel chest, 23i
Basophils, effect of disease on, 124t
Biceps reflex, assessing, 35i
Biceps strength, testing, 53i
Biological dressings, 318
Biotin, daily requirements of, 332t
Biot's respirations, characteristics of, 24i
Bite, caring for, 311
Biventricular pacemaker, 109i
Bladder
  continuous irrigation of, setup for, 245i
  palpating, 49i
  percussing, 47i
Blood coagulation factors, 126-127t
Blood glucose monitoring, 217i
Blood pressure readings, classifying, 8t
Blood transfusion
  do's and don'ts of, 218
  monitoring, 219
Blunt percussion, 5i
Body mass index, calculating, 509
Body surface area, estimating, in children, 458t
Body surface nomogram, 158t
Brachial pulse, palpating, 17i

Brachioradialis reflex, assessing, 35i
Bradycardia pacing, 115t
Bradypnea, characteristics of, 24i
Brain attack. *See* Stroke.
Brain death, 595, 600
Breast cancer, 476-479
  detecting, 477
  tumor sources and sites in, 478t
Breast-feeding, positions for, 387i
Breasts, health history review of, 11
Breath sounds
  abnormal, 28t
  normal, 27t, 448t
Bronchial breath sound, 27t
Bronchovesicular breath sound, 27t
Brudzinski's sign, 38i
B-type natriuretic peptide levels, linking, to heart failure symptom severity, 131i
Buccal medications, 141
Bulge sign, 54i
Burns
  causes of, 459t
  classifying, 459
  estimating extent of, 460i

C

Cadaveric organ donors, 600
Calciferol, daily requirements of, 333t
Calcium, daily requirements of, 330t
Capillary refill, assessing, 20
Cardiac arrhythmias, types of, 94-101t
Cardiac asthma, 475
Cardiac auscultation, positioning patient for, 13i
Cardiac biomarkers, 126-127t
Cardiac conduction, 66-67i
Cardiac cycle, extra heart sounds in, 14i
Cardiac enzymes and proteins, release of, 128i
Cardiac monitoring, positioning leads for, 70i
Cardiac nursing, 626-627
Cardiac resynchronization therapy, 109i
Cardiovascular landmarks, identifying, 12i

Cardiovascular system
  in active phase of labor, 373t
  age-related changes in, 64
  health history review of, 11
  in neonate, 395t
  normal findings in, 21
  pregnancy-related changes in, 352
Caregiver, nurse as, 592
Carotid pulse, palpating, 17i
Case management nursing, 628-629
Cast
  hip-spica, 220i
  petaling, 221i
  removing, 221i
Centers for Disease Control and
    Prevention isolation pre-
    cautions, 285
Central nervous system, age-related
    changes in, 64
Central venous catheter, remov-
    ing, 223i
Central venous dressing, chang-
    ing, 235i
Central venous pressure, measuring,
    with manometer, 224i
Cerebral palsy, 553-555
  types of, 554
Cerebrospinal fluid analysis, 138-139t
Cerebrovascular accident. *See* Stroke.
Cervical effacement and dilation, 371i
Cervical readiness for labor, evaluat-
    ing, 521t
Cesarean birth, primary indications
    for, 378
Change agent, nurse as, 592
Chemistry tests, 120t
Chest
  auscultation sequences for, 26i
  palpation of, 25i
  percussion of, 26i
    sequence for, 26i
Chest deformities, 23i
Chest drainage system, assessing leaks
    in, 228i
Chest drains, troubleshooting,
    229-230t
Chest tube, removing, 231
Cheyne-Stokes respirations, character-
    istics of, 24i

Child abuse and neglect, signs of,
    455, 456
Childbearing practices, cultural con-
    siderations in, 339-340
Childhood development
  patterns of, 410t
  stages of, 410
  theories of, 411t, 412
Children. *See also specific age-group.*
  abdominal assessment in, 451
  blood pressure in, 444t
  burn prevention in, 458-459
  cardiovascular assessment in, 446i
  car safety seat guidelines for, 466t
  gastrointestinal and genitourinary
      assessment in, 450
  heart rates in, 444t
  motor vehicle and bicycle safety
      for, 465
  musculoskeletal assessment in, 451
  obesity prevention in, 469
  pain assessment in, 453
  respiratory assessment in, 447i
  respiratory rates in, 445t
  temperature ranges in, 445t
  tooth eruption in, 452i
  vital sign ranges in, by age, 6-7t
Chip tool for pain assessment, 455
Chloride, daily requirements of, 330t
Choking hazards, 463
Chorionic villus sampling, 360i
Christmas disease. *See* Hemophilia.
Chromium, daily requirements
    of, 330t
Chronic obstructive pulmonary
    disease. *See* Asthma *and* Emphy-
    sema.
Circumcision, parent teaching for, 405
Clinical nurse leader, 620
Clinical nurse specialist, 620
Clubbed fingers, evaluating, 60i
Coagulation studies, 125t
Coagulation testing, collecting speci-
    mens for, 125
Cobalamin, daily requirements
    of, 332t
Cobalt, daily requirements of, 330t
Code of ethics of International Council
    of Nurses, 594

i refers to an illustration; t refers to a table.

Collagen dressings, 318

Coma, manifestations of, 31t

Communication, effective, 10

Complete blood count with differential, 121t

Complete heart block, 98-99t

Composite dressings, 319

Condom catheter, applying, 222i

Confusion, manifestations of, 31t

Conscientious objection, 597

Consumptive coagulopathy. *See* Disseminated intravascular coagulation.

Contact hours, 610
state requirements for, 611-612t

Contact layer dressings, 319

Contact lenses, removing, 232i

Contact precautions, 285
indications for, 286-287t

Continuing education, 610-622
time management and, 614

Continuous bladder irrigation, setup for, 245i

Coordinator, nurse as, 592

Copper, daily requirements of, 330t

Crackles, 28t

Cranial nerves, 29t

Critical care nursing, 630

Croup, 555-558
effect of, on upper airways, 556i

Crutch, fitting patient for, 233i

Cultural considerations in patient care, 336-338t

Cystic fibrosis, 558-560

Cytomegalovirus, 402t

D

Dangerous drugs, 194

Death
concepts of, in childhood, 434t
defining, 595, 600

Debriding agents, 323

Decerebrate posture, 37i

Decision-making ability, standards for judging, 598

Decorticate posture, 37i

Deep ballottement, 4i

Deep palpation, 4i

Deep tendon reflexes, assessing, 35i

Deep vein thrombosis, preventing, 392

Defibrillation, safety issues with, 102

Defibrillator
automated external, 103
biphasic, 104i
monophasic, 104i
paddle placement for, 105i

Defibrination syndrome. *See* Disseminated intravascular coagulation.

Degree specialties, 620-621

Delivery, determining estimated time of, 354

Deontology, 592

Diabetes mellitus, 479-483
pathophysiology of, 480i
target numbers for, 482

Diabetic ulcers, treatment algorithm for, 315i

Dialyzable drugs, 210-212t

Direct percussion, 5i

Discharge planner, nurse as, 592

Discontinuing treatment, 597

Disorientation, manifestations of, 31t

Disseminated intravascular coagulation, 483-486
pathophysiology of, 484i

DNP programs, 622

Dobutamine infusion rates, 164-165t

Doctoral degree, 621-622

Documentation, 588-590
tips for, 589
uses of, 590

Dopamine infusion rates, 166-167t

Doppler device, how to use, 234i

Dorsalis pedis pulse, palpating, 17i

Dosage calculation
conversions for, 157
formulas for, 157

Drip rates, calculating, 162t

Droplet precautions, 285
indications for, 288t

Drowning, preventing, 464

Drug administration guidelines, 140

Drug combinations, dangerous effects of, 170-173t

Drugs that shouldn't be crushed, 191-193

Dullness as percussion sound, 6t, 27t

i refers to an illustration; t refers to a table.

Durable health care power of attorney, 597-598
Dysfunctional labor, 519-522
    hypertonic contractions in, 519, 520i, 521
    hypotonic contractions in, 519, 520-521, 520i
    uncoordinated contractions in, 519-520, 520i, 521

E

Ear canal, irrigating, 246i
Eardrops, instilling, 145
Ear drug administration, 145
Ears, health history review of, 10
ECG. *See* Electrocardiography.
Eclampsia, 524
Ectopic pregnancy, 522-524
    implantation sites of, 523i
Edema
    pitting, evaluating, 20i
    scale for, 20
Educational options, 610, 612
Educator, nurse as, 592
Egoism, 592
Einthoven's triangle, 68i
Electrical axis determination
    degree method of, 80i
    quadrant method of, 79i
Electrocardiography, 66-116
    in angina, 81i, 83i
    augmented leads in, 69i
    Einthoven's triangle and, 68i
    electrical activity and, 78i
    grid for, 71i
    limb lead placement in, 77i
    normal QTc intervals in, 72t
    positioning leads for, 70i
    posterior lead electrode placement in, 76i
    precordial lead placement in, 75i
    rhythm strips
        interpreting, 72
        normal, 71i
        patterns in, 72i
    right precordial lead placement in, 76i
    in Wellens syndrome, 82i, 84i
Emergency care nursing, 631-632

Emphysema, 486-488
Endocrine system
    in active phase of labor, 373t
    health history review of, 11
    pregnancy-related changes in, 352
Endometritis, 389
Endotracheal tube, securing, 237-238i
Enteral drug administration, 141
Eosinophils, effect of disease on, 124t
Epicardial pacemaker, 106
Epinephrine infusion rates, 163t
Erikson's theory of development, 412
Erythroblastosis fetalis. *See* Hemolytic disease of the newborn.
Erythromycin treatment for neonate, 403i
Esophageal atresia, 567-570
Ethical decisions, 591, 593
    basis of, 595
Ethical theories, 592-593
Ethics committee, 596
Evidence-based Practice Centers, 572, 573
Extravasation, antidotes for, 156t
Eye
    health history review of, 10
    irrigating, 247i
Eyedrops, instilling, 145
Eye drug administration, 145i
Eye ointment, applying, 145i
Eye patch, applying, 239i

F

Facility- and unit-specific policies and procedures as sources of standards of care, 573
Falls
    medications associated with, 181t
    preventive strategies for, in childhood, 465
Fats, types of, 334
Female genitalia, external, 45i
Female pelvis, 366i
Femoral pulse, palpating, 17i
Fetal alcohol syndrome, 535-537
    facial characteristics of neonates with, 536
    terminology associated with, 535
Fetal attitude, 370

---

i refers to an illustration; t refers to a table.

Fetal engagement and station, assessing, 372i
Fetal heart rate
  baseline irregularities in, 375i
  evaluating decelerations in, 376i
  reading monitor strip of, 374i
Fetal monitoring device
  external, 250i
  internal, 251i
Fetal positions, 369-370i
  abbreviations for, 369
Fetal presentation, classifying, 368i
Fetus
  biophysical profile and, 364t
  developmental milestones in, 358-359
  head diameters of, at term, 366i
First-degree atrioventricular block, 96-97t
FLACC Scale, pain assessment in infants and, 454t
Flatness as percussion sound, 6t, 27t
Fluoride, daily requirements of, 331t
Foam dressings, 320
Folate, daily requirements of, 332t
Folic acid, daily requirements of, 332t
Forensic nursing, 632-633
Freud's theory of development, 412
Fundus, locating, 240i
Funnel chest, 23i

G
Gait abnormalities, 36i
Gastric feeding
  administering, 241
  complications of, 242t
Gastric tube, drug delivery through, 141
Gastroesophageal reflux disease, 488-489
Gastrointestinal system
  in active phase of labor, 373t
  health history review of, 11
  in neonate, 395t
  normal findings in, 44
  pregnancy-related changes in, 352
Gastrostomy feeding button, reinserting, 243i
Genital herpes, lesions of, 46i

Genital lesions, male, 46i
Genital warts, lesions of, 46i
Genitourinary system
  normal findings in, 49
  pregnancy-related changes in, 353
Gerontological nursing, 634
Gestational hypertension, 524-527
  emergency interventions for, 526
  pathophysiology of, 525i
Glasgow Coma Scale, 32t
Glucose challenge values in pregnancy, 360t
Growth rates, expected, 413t

H
Hand hygiene, 292
Hand rubs, 292
Health care workers' rights, 597
Health history review, 10-11
Health Insurance Portability and Accountability Act, 602
Heart attack, 506-508
Heartburn, 488-489
Heart failure, 490-492
  causes of, 491t
  classifying, 490
Heart murmurs
  grading, 16
  identifying, 16t
Heart rate, calculating, 74t
Heart sounds
  abnormal, 15t
  occurrence of, in cardiac cycle, 14i
  sites of, in children, 446i
Height conversion, 9t
Height measurements
  for boys ages 2 through 18, 414t
  for girls ages 2 through 18, 416t
Hematologic system, health history review of, 11
Hematopoietic system in neonate, 395t
Hemoglobin, variations of type and distribution of, 122t
Hemoglobin monitor, bedside, 252i
Hemolytic disease of the newborn, 537-539
  Rh isoimmunization and, 527-529, 537t
Hemophilia, 560-563

---

i refers to an illustration; t refers to a table.

Heparin, administration tips for, 162
Hepatitis. *See* Viral hepatitis.
Herb-drug interactions, 174-179t
Heroic measures, 595
Herpesvirus type II, 402t
High-pitched sounds, assessing, 7i
Hip abduction in neonate, assessing, 401i
Hip fracture, 492-494
Hip-spica cast care, 220i
Hospitalization of child, minimizing trauma of, 433
Human immunodeficiency virus, 494-496
  ethical issues related to, 601-602
  ethical testing guidelines for, 602
  neonatal exposure to, 404
  testing for, 132-133t
    mandatory, 601-602
Hyaline membrane disease, 547-549
Hydraulic lift, how to use, 244i
Hydrocolloid dressings, 320
Hydrogel dressings, 321
Hyperbilirubinemia, unconjugated, 539-541
  onset-related causes of, 540
Hyperpnea, characteristics of, 24i
Hyperresonance as percussion sound, 6t, 27t
Hypertension
  blood pressure readings in, 8t
  chronic, in pregnancy, 524
  gestational, 524-527
  preeclampsia and, 524
Hypovolemic shock, emergency interventions for, 534

I

Immune system in neonate, 395t
Immunization schedule
  for catch up, 438-441t
  for persons age 0 to 6 years, 436-437t
  for persons age 7 to 18 years, 436t
Implantable cardioverter-defibrillator
  managing, 116
  placement of, 114i
  therapies delivered by, 115t
Indirect percussion, 5i

Inertia. *See* Dysfunctional labor.
Infant
  cognitive development and play of, 421t
  growth rates for, 413t
  language and social development of, 420t
  locating fontanels in, 450i
  motor development of, 418-419t
  nutritional guidelines for, 466
  pain assessment in, 454
  reflexes in, 449i
  sleep guidelines for, 470t
  solid foods and, 467t
Infection, barriers to, 289-292
Informatics nursing, 635
Informed consent, 597, 600
  obtaining, 294
Infusion nursing, 636
Insulin
  administration tips for, 162
  infusion pumps for, 160
  mixing, 159
  types of, 159t
Integumentary system
  age-related changes in, 64, 64t, 65i
  in neonate, 395t, 399
  normal findings in, 60
  pregnancy-related changes in, 353
International Council of Nurses code of ethics, 594
Intestinal obstruction, 496-498
Intracranial pressure monitoring system, setting up, 253i
Intracranial pressure, increased, signs of, 39t
Intradermal drug administration, 151I
Intramuscular injections
  modifying, 148i
  sites for, 147i
  Z-track, 149i
Iodine, daily requirements of, 331t
Iron, daily requirements of, 331t
Ischemia, 85i
Isoimmunization, 527-529. *See also* Hemolytic disease of the newborn.
  pathogenesis of, 528i
  pathophysiology of, 537i

Isoproterenol infusion rates, 163t
I.V. drug administration, 152i
I.V. infusion, initiating, 153
I.V. pump alarms, troubleshoot-
  ing, 161t
I.V. therapy
  complications of, 154-155t
  sites for, 154i

J

Job descriptions as sources of standards of care, 575
Joint Commission
  National Patient Safety Goals of,
    579-580
  as source of standards of care, 575
  standards of, 576-578
Jugular vein distention, evaluating, 19i
Junctional rhythm, 96-97t

K

Kanner's autism. *See* Autistic disorder.
Kernig's sign, 38i
Kidneys
  palpating, 48i
  percussing, 47i
Kohlberg's theory of development, 412
Kussmaul's respirations, characteris-
  tics of, 24i
Kyphosis, 52i

L

Labor
  cardinal movements of, 382-383i
  cervical effacement and dilation
    in, 371i
  comfort measures in, 377
  dysfunctional, 519-522
  evaluating cervical readiness
    for, 521t
  stages of, 367
  systemic changes in active phase
    of, 373i
  true versus false, 367
Laboratory tests
  crisis values of, 117-118t
  normal neonatal values for, 407-409t
  values for

Laboratory tests *(continued)*
  in nonpregnant patient, 363t
  in pregnant patient, 363t
Labor pain, cultural considerations
  for, 341t
Laceration, caring for, 311
Lactate dehydrogenase isoenzyme
  variations in disease, 129t
Lawsuit, reducing risk of, 590
Left bundle-branch block, 89i
  characteristic electrocardiogram
    changes in, 90i
Left ventricular hypertrophy, 87i
Leopold's maneuvers, 248i
Lethargy, manifestations of, 31t
Leukemia, acute, 498-501
  pathophysiology of, 499i
Liability insurance, choosing, 587-588
Light ballottement, 4i
Light palpation, 4i
Lipid panel, 119t
Litigation, 580-582
  avoiding, 581-582
Liver
  palpating, 43i
  percussing and measuring, 43i
Living will, 597, 598
Lochia flow, assessing, 386
Lordosis, 52i
Lower esophageal sphincter pressure,
  factors that affect, 489
Low-pitched sounds, assessing, 7i
Lund-Browder chart, 460i
Lung cancer, 501-503
  development of, 502i
Lymphocytes, effect of disease
  on, 124t

M

Macule, 59i
Magnesium
  administration guidelines for, 380
  daily requirements of, 330t
Male urethral meatus, examining, 45i
Malpractice, 580-581
  criteria for, 581
Management misconduct, reporting, 606

Manganese, daily requirements
of, 331t
Mastitis, preventing, 392
Maternal disorders, 519-535
Maternal-neonatal care, 345-409
Medical misconduct, reporting, 606
Medical-surgical nursing, 637
Menadione, daily requirements
of, 333t
Mental status, assessing, 30t
Metabolic acidosis, 130t
Metabolic alkalosis, 130t
Metabolic panel, comprehensive, 119t
Metabolic system, pregnancy-related
changes in, 352-353
Metered-dose inhaler, how to use, 142i
Mineral requirements, deficiencies,
and toxicities, 330-331t
Molybdenum, daily requirements
of, 331t
Monocytes, effect of disease on, 124t
Mood disorder, 61
Mouth and throat, health history
review of, 11
MSN programs, 619
Multiple sclerosis, 503-506
demyelination in, 504i
Muscle strength, testing and
grading, 53i
Musculoskeletal injury, 5 P's of, 54
Musculoskeletal system
in active phase of labor, 373t
age-related changes in, 64
health history review of, 11
in neonate, 395t, 401i
normal findings in, 55
pregnancy-related changes in, 353
Myocardial infarction, 85i, 506-508
locating areas of damage in, 86t
Myocardial injury, 85i
Myocardial stages, 85i

N

Nägele's rule, 354
Nasal aerosol, how to use, 143
Nasal balloon catheter, how to use,
225i
Nasal drug administration, 143
Nasal spray, how to use, 143

Nasoenteric-decompression tube,
clearing obstruction in, 256
Nasogastric tube
drug delivery through, 141
inserting, 255i
Nasopharyngeal airway, inserting, 213i
Nasopharyngeal specimen,
obtaining, 268i
National Guideline Clearinghouse, 572
National Organ Transplant Act, 601
Neck, health history review of, 11
Negligence, 580
Neonatal abstinence syndrome,
541-545
signs and symptoms of nonopioid
drug withdrawal in, 543t
signs and symptoms of opioid drug
withdrawal in, 542t
types of, 541
withdrawal scoring system for,
544-545t
Neonatal disorders, 535-549
Neonatal drug withdrawal scoring system, 544-545t
Neonatal jaundice. *See* Hyperbilirubinemia, unconjugated.
Neonatal resuscitation
algorithm for, 393i
medications for, 394t
Neonate
Apgar scoring for, 397t
assessing head of, 400i
assessing hip abduction in, 401i
assessment of, 396
average size and weight of, 396
categorizing, by gestational age, 396
chest circumference measurement
in, 249i
common skin findings in, 399
counting respirations in, 397
drug withdrawal scoring system for,
544-545t
erythromycin treatment in, 403i
evaluating respiratory status of, 398i
head circumference measurement
in, 249i
head-to-heel length measurement
in, 249i

i refers to an illustration; t refers to a table.

Neonate *(continued)*
  human immunodeficiency virus
      exposure and, 404
  neurologic assessment of, 399
  nonopioid drug withdrawal in, 543t
  normal laboratory values for,
      407-409t
  normal vital signs in, 397
  opioid drug withdrawal in, 542t
  with phenylketonuria, parent teach-
      ing for, 405
  physiology of, 395t
  premature, parent teaching for, 404
  preterm, 544-547
  preventing heat loss in, 397
  sutures and fontanels in, 400i
  TORCH infections and, 402t
  vital sign ranges in, 6-7t
  vitamin K administration in, 403i
Nephrostomy tube, taping, 257i
Neurologic system
  in active phase of labor, 373t
  health history review of, 11
  in neonate, 395t, 399
  normal findings in, 40
Neuropathic pain, 298
Neutrophils, effect of disease on, 123t
Niacin, daily requirements of, 332t
Nitroglycerin infusion rates, 163t
Nitroprusside infusion rates, 168-169t
Nociceptive pain, 298
Noncontact normothermic wound
    therapy, 325
Nonmaleficence, organ donation
    and, 599
Nonopioid drug withdrawal, signs and
    symptoms of, in neonate, 543t
Nonstress test, interpreting results
    of, 362t
Nose, health history review of, 11
Nose drops, instilling, 143
Numerical pain rating scale, 62
Nurse anesthetist, 620-621
Nurse certification organizations,
    624-625
Nurse educator, 621
Nurse midwife, 621
Nurse misconduct, reporting, 605-606
Nurse practice acts, 582

Nurse practitioner, 621
Nursing administration, 638-639
Nursing administrator, 620
Nursing education, 610-622
Nursing specialties, 623-641
Nutritional disorders, evaluating,
    326-327t
Nutritional problems, detecting, 329

O
Obesity, 508-509
Objective data, 10
Obligationism, 593
Obstetrical and gynecological nursing,
    639-640
Obstetric history
  formidable findings in, 347-348
  taking, 346
Obtundation, manifestations of, 31t
Older adult
  pharmacokinetics in, 180i
  preventing adverse drug reactions
      in, 183-190t
  vital sign ranges in, 6-7t
Opioid drug withdrawal, signs and
    symptoms of, in neonate, 542t
Oral airway, inserting, 213i
Oral drug administration, 141
Ordinary versus extraordinary meas-
    ures, 595, 597
Organ transplantation, 599-601
  approaching potential donor's family
      and, 600
  cadaveric donors and, 600
  National Organ Transplant Act
      and, 601
  nonmaleficence and, 599
  protecting potential donors' rights
      in, 599
  Uniform Anatomical Gift Act
      and, 600
Otitis media, 563-566
  site of, 564i
Oxytocin administration, 378
  complications of, 379
Oxytocin challenge test, interpreting
    results of, 362t

PQ

Pacemaker
assessing function of, 113
biventricular, 109i
codes for, 110
leads for, 109i
malfunction of, 111-112i
permanent, placing, 108i
spikes and, 110i
temporary, 106
pulse generator for, 107i
types of, 106, 106i
Pain
assessment of, in children, 453,
454t, 455
assessment tools for, 62-63i, 296,
297i
behavior checklist for, 298
differentiating acute and chronic,
63t, 297t
responses to, 296, 453
treating, 299
types of, 298
Palpation
of chest, 25i
of liver, 43i
techniques for, 4i
Pantothenic acid, daily requirements
of, 332t
Papule, 59i
Parametritis, 389
Parent teaching
for circumcision care, 405
for neonate exposed to human immunodeficiency virus, 404
for neonate with phenylketonuria, 405
for premature neonate, 404
Parkinson's disease, 509-512
neurotransmitter action in, 510i
Paroxysmal supraventricular tachycardia, 94-95t
Patellar reflex, assessing, 35i
Pathologic retraction ring, 377i
Patient Care Partnership, 575
as source of standards of care, 581
Patient-controlled analgesia, administration tips for, 162
Patient interview, 10

Patient's Bill of Rights. *See* Patient
Care Partnership.
Pediatric care, 410-470
Pediatric coma scale, 448t
Pediatric disorders, 550-570
Pediatric fluid needs, calculating, 461
Pediatric health history
age-specific interview and assess-
ment tips for, 442-443
obtaining, 440-443
Pediatric medication dosage, calculat-
ing, 457
Pediatric nursing, 640-641
Pelvic cellulitis, 389
Pelvis, female, 366i
Penetrating wound, caring for, 311
Penile cancer, lesions of, 46i
Percussion
of chest, 26i
sequence for, 26i
of liver, 43i
techniques for, 5i
Percussion sounds, identifying, 6t, 27t
Percussion and vibration as chest
physiotherapy techniques, 260i
Percutaneous endoscopic gastrostomy
site, caring for, 261i
Percutaneous endoscopic jejunostomy
site, caring for, 261i
Pericardial friction rub, 15t
Pericarditis, electrocardiogram
changes in, 91i
Perineal lacerations, classifying, 382
Peritonitis, 389
Personality disorder, 61
Personal safety in workplace, 603-606
Pharmacokinetics in older adult, 180i
Phenylketonuria, parent teaching
for, 405
Phosphorus, daily requirements
of, 330t
Phototherapy, performing, 406
Physiologic jaundice of the newborn.
See Hyperbilirubinemia, uncon-
jugated.
Piaget's theory of development, 412
Pigeon chest, 23i
Placenta previa, 529-532
types of, 530i

---

i refers to an illustration; t refers to a table.

Plasma and plasma fractions, transfusing, 219
Play, importance of, 433
Pleural friction rub, 28t
Pneumatic antishock garment, applying, 262i
Poison prevention, 464
Popliteal pulse, palpating, 17i
Positioning patients, 263-265t
Posterior tibial pulse, palpating, 17i
Postoperative care, 295
Postpartum hemorrhage, 532-535
Postpartum period
assessing excessive vaginal bleeding in, 388i
maternal self-care for, 391-392
phases of, 385t
psychiatric disorders in, 390t
Potassium, daily requirements of, 330t
Potassium-rich foods, 335
PQRST mnemonic device for pain assessment, 62, 296
Practice roles, 592
Preeclampsia, 524
Pregnancy. *See also* Pregnant patient.
assessment findings in, by weeks, 356-357
dealing with discomforts of, 355-356t
fundal height throughout, 354i
glucose challenge values in, 360t
physiologic adaptations to, 352-353
positive signs of, 351t
presumptive signs of, 349-350t
probably signs of, 350t
summarizing information related to, 347
types of hypertension in, 524
Pregnancy-induced hypertension. *See* Gestational hypertension.
Pregnant patient. *See also* Pregnancy.
laboratory values for, 363t
recommended daily allowances for, 365t
Prehypertension, blood pressure readings in, 8t
Premature ventricular contraction, 98-99t
Preoperative care, 294

Preschooler
cognitive development of, 425
growth rates for, 413t
language development and socialization of, 425
moral and spiritual development of, 426
motor development of, 424t
nutritional guidelines for, 468
play of, 425
psychosocial development of, 425
sleep guidelines for, 470t
Pressure ulcers, management algorithm for, 312i
Preterm neonate, 544-547
Provant Wound Closure System, 323
Psychiatric disorders, 61
Psychogenic pain, 298
Psychological status, health history review of, 11
Psychotic disorder, 61
Public health/community nurse, 621
Puerperal infection, signs and symptoms of, 389
Pulse oximeter
how to use, 258i
troubleshooting problems with, 259
Pulse oximetry, 8
Pulses
arterial, palpating, 17i
grading, 18
waveforms for, 18i
Pupil
abnormal response of, 33t
grading size of, 34i
Pyridoxine, daily requirements of, 332t

R

Radial pulse, palpating, 17i
Rapid assessment, 2
Recommended daily allowances for pregnant women, 365t
Rectal drug administration, 146
Red cell indices in anemias, 122t
Religious beliefs and practices, 342-345t
Renal failure, acute, 512-514

---

i refers to an illustration; t refers to a table.

Renal system
in active phase of labor, 373t
in neonate, 395t
Reportable diseases and infections, 293
Reproductive system
health history review of, 11
in neonate, 395t
Resonance as percussion sound, 6t, 27t
Respiratory acidosis, 130t
Respiratory alkalosis, 130t
Respiratory assessment landmarks, 22i
Respiratory distress syndrome, 547-549
Respiratory drug administration, 142
Respiratory patterns, abnormal, 24i
Respiratory syncytial virus infection, 566-567
Respiratory system
in active phase of labor, 373t
age-related changes in, 64
health history review of, 11
in neonate, 395t, 397, 398i
normal findings in, 28
pregnancy-related changes in, 352
Retinol, daily requirements of, 333t
Rh incompatibility. *See* Isoimmunization.
Rhonchi, 28t
Rhythm, methods of measuring, 73i
Riboflavin, daily requirements of, 332t
Right bundle-branch block, 87i
characteristic electrocardiogram changes in, 88i
Right to die, 593-595, 597-598
Right to refuse treatment, 597
RN to BSN programs, 614-615
RN to MSN programs, 615, 619
Rubella, 402t
Rule of Nines, 460i

S
Safe work environment, creating, 603
School-age child
cognitive development of, 427
growth rates for, 413t
language development and socialization of, 426
School-age child *(continued)*
moral and spiritual development of, 427
motor development of, 426
nutritional guidelines for, 468
psychosocial development of, 426
pubertal changes in, 427
sleep guidelines for, 470t
Scoliosis, testing for, 52i
Secondary sex characteristics, development of, 429
Second-degree atrioventricular block, 98-99t
Selenium, daily requirements of, 331t
Septic pelvic thrombophlebitis, 389
Sequential compression therapy, 266i
Sexual harassment in the workplace, 604-605
legal issues of, 604
Sexual maturity
in boys, 430i
in girls, 431-432i
Shoulder dislocation, immobilizing, 244i
Silverman-Anderson index for neonatal respiratory status, 398i
Sinus bradycardia, 94-95t
Sinus rhythm, 93i
Sinus tachycardia, 94-95t
Skeletal system, anatomy of, 50-51i
Skin
age-related changes in, 64t
anatomy of, 55i
color variations in, 57t
comprehensive assessment of, 56
effects of aging on, 65i
functions of, 56
Skin lesions
common configurations of, 58i
illuminating, 59
primary, 59i
Skin turgor, evaluating, 57i
Sling, making, 267i
Social contract theory, 593
Sodium
daily requirements of, 330t
reducing intake of, 335
Somatic pain, 298
Somatoform disorder, 61

Specialty absorptive dressings, 321
Sputum specimen, obtaining, with
    suction catheter, 268i
Standards of care, 572-590
    sources of, 572-573, 575
State boards of nursing, 583-586
State nurse practice acts and guide-
    lines as sources for standards of
    care, 575
Steeple sign, 557i
Stridor, 28t
Stroke, 514-516
    preventing, 516
Structures and systems review, 10-11
Stump, wrapping, 272i
Stupor, manifestations of, 31t
Subcutaneous drug administra-
    tion, 150i
Subjective data, 10
Sublingual medications, 141
Substance abuse among nurses,
    607-608
    past attitudes toward, 607
    recognizing, 608
    reporting, 608
Sudden infant death syndrome, pre-
    ventive strategies for, 462
Suicide
    answering threat of, 456
    warning signs of, 456
Sulfur, daily requirements of, 330t
Summation gallop, 15t
Suppository, inserting, 146i
Surgery, preparing child for, 435t
Surgical verifications, 295
Swathe, applying, 272i
Symptom, evaluating, 3i
Synchronized cardioversion, 105
Syphilis, lesions of, 46i
Systems review, 11

T

Tachypnea, characteristics of, 24i
Tactile fremitus, checking for, 25i
Teleology, 593
Temperature conversion, 10t
Temper tantrums, handling, 462
10-minute assessment, 2

Terbutaline, administration guidelines
    for, 381
Theological ethics, 593
Therapeutic drug monitoring guide-
    lines, 196-209t
Thermogenic system in neonate,
    395t, 397
Thiamine, daily requirements of, 332t
Third-degree atrioventricular block,
    98-99t
Thoracic kyphoscoliosis, 23i
Thyroid panel, 119t
Tocopherol, daily requirements
    of, 333t
Toddler
    cognitive development of, 423
    growth rates for, 413t
    language development of, 422t
    motor development of, 422t
    nutritional guidelines for, 466
    play of, 424
    psychosocial development of, 423
    sleep guidelines for, 470t
    socialization of, 423
Toilet training, 463
Tooth eruption, sequence of, 452i
Topical drug administration, 144
TORCH infections, 402t
Toxoplasmosis, 402t
Tracheal breath sound, 27t
Tracheal cuff pressure, 273i
Tracheal suctioning
    closed, 276-277i
    open, 274-275i
Tracheoesophageal anomalies, 568i
Tracheoesophageal fistula, 567-570
Tracheostomy cuff, deflating and in-
    flating, 279
Tracheotomy, bedside, assisting
    with, 278i
Transcultural communication, 336
Transcutaneous electrical nerve stimu-
    lation electrodes, position-
    ing, 280i
Transcutaneous pacemaker, 106, 106i
Transfer board, how to use, 281i
Transfusion
    of blood, 218-219
    of plasma and plasma fractions, 219

i refers to an illustration; t refers to a table.

Transparent film dressings, 322
Transparent semipermeable dressing, applying, 236i
Transvenous pacemaker, 106
Triceps reflex, assessing, 35i
Triceps strength, testing, 53i
Tuberculosis, 516-518
Tumor markers, 121t
Turbo-inhaler, how to use, 142i
2-hour postprandial plasma glucose levels by age, 131i
Tympany as percussion sound, 6t, 27t

U
Umbilical cord prolapse, 384i
Uniform Anatomical Gift Act, 600
Urinary catheter, inserting, 226-227
Urinary system, health history review of, 11
Urine hormones, 136-137t
Urine specimen, aspirating, 269i
Urine tests, 135t
Uterine contractions, types of, 520i
Uterine involution, 386i

V
Vacuum-assisted closure device, 324
Vaginal drug administration, 146
Vascular sounds, auscultating for, 42i
Venous access site, taping, 282i
Venous ulcers, treatment algorithm for, 313i
Ventricular fibrillation, 100-101t
Ventricular gallop, 15t
Ventricular tachycardia, 100-101t
Vesicle, 59i
Vesicular breath sound, 27t
Viral hepatitis
    serodiagnoses of, 134t
    test panel for, 134
Virtue ethics, 593
Visceral pain, 298
Visual analog scale for pain assessment, 62i
Visual field defects, 34i
Vital signs, ranges in, by age, 6-7t
Vital signs monitor, electronic, 254i
Vitamin A, daily requirements of, 333t

Vitamin B_1, daily requirements of, 332t
Vitamin B_2, daily requirements of, 332t
Vitamin B_3, daily requirements of, 332t
Vitamin B_6, daily requirements of, 332t
Vitamin B_{12}, daily requirements of, 332t
Vitamin C, daily requirements of, 332t
Vitamin D, daily requirements of, 333t
Vitamin E, daily requirements of, 333t
Vitamin K
    administering, to neonate, 403i
    daily requirements of, 333t
Vitamin requirements, deficiencies, and toxicities, 332-333t

WXY
Walker, how to use, 283i
Warming system, 284i
Warm-Up Therapy System, 325
Weight conversion, 9t
Weight measurements
    for boys ages 1 through 18, 415t
    for girls ages 1 through 18, 417t
Wellens syndrome, 82
    electrocardiogram changes in, 82i, 83-84i
Wheezes, 28t
Whistle-blowing, 605-606
    implications of, 605
    systematic approach to, 606
White blood cell differential values, 123
    influence of disease on, 123-124t
Wolff-Parkinson-White syndrome, electrocardiogram changes in, 92i
Wong-Baker faces pain-rating scale, 63i, 297i
Workplace violence, 603
Wound fillers, 322
Wounds
    assessing characteristics of, 301
    assessing drainage from, 302t
    classifying, by depth, 304i
    determining age of, 301t

i refers to an illustration; t refers to a table.

Wounds *(continued)*
    failure of, to heal, 307-308t
    healing complications and, 309i
    making care decisions about, 300
    managing, according to color, 310t
    measuring, 303i, 305i
    measuring tunneling of, 306i
    selecting dressing for, 316i
    traumatic, caring for, 311

Z

Zinc, daily requirements of, 331t
Z-track injection, 149I

---

i refers to an illustration; t refers to a table.

Notes

Notes